The Biological Basis of Nursing: Cancer

In line with a number of new governmental initiatives, the Department of Health has prioritised improving cancer treatment and research, and is providing greater resources for cancer care. Nurses and their colleagues are at the forefront of these changes.

The Biological Basis of Nursing: Cancer presents specialised biological information on what cancer is, how it damages the body, and how cancer treatments work. Engaging, accessible and illustrated throughout, this unique text:

- explains the basic biology of cancer
- discusses the biology of a wide range of common cancers
- identifies and explains the biological causes of cancer
- explains drug action in chemotherapy and analgesia
- explains the link between diet and cancer, and how diet is important in cancer therapy
- discusses the biological basis of a range of nursing skills linked to cancer.

This book will provide nurses with the essential knowledge required for working with cancer patients and their families, and will enable them to work with current and new forms of cancer treatment. It will also be of great use to clinical staff and nurse educators.

William T. Blows RMN, RGN, RNT, OStJ, BSc (Hons), PhD, is Lecturer in Applied Biological Sciences at St Bartholomew's School of Nursing and Midwifery, City University, London. He is the author of *The Biological Basis of Nursing: Clinical Observations* (2001) and *The Biological Basis of Nursing: Mental Health* (2003) also published by Routledge.

NURSING/CANCER CARE

The Biological Basis of Nursing: Cancer

William T. Blows

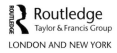 Routledge
Taylor & Francis Group

LONDON AND NEW YORK

First published in 2005 by Routledge
2 Park Square, Milton Park, Abingdon,
Oxfordshire, OX14 4RN
Tel: +44 (0)20 7017 6000
Fax: +44 (0)20 7017 6699

Simultaneously published in the USA and
Canada
by Routledge
29 West 35th Street, New York, NY 10001

*Routledge is an imprint of the Taylor & Francis
Group*

© 2005 William T. Blows

Illustrations by Oxmed

Typeset in Great Britain by
J&L Composition, Filey, North Yorkshire

Printed and bound in Great Britain by
TJ International, Padstow, Cornwall

British Library Cataloguing in Publication Data
A catalogue record for this book is available
from the British Library

*Library of Congress Cataloging in Publication
Data*
Blows, William T., 1947–
  The biological basis of nursing. Cancer/
  William T. Blows.
      p. ; cm.
  Includes bibliographical references and
  index.
  ISBN 0–415–32745–8
  (hardback : alk. paper) –
  ISBN 0–415–32746–6
  (pbk. : alk. paper)
  1. Cancer. 2. Cancer–Nursing.
  [DNLM: 1. Neoplasms–nursing.
  2. Neoplasms–pathology.
  WY 156 B657b 2005]   I. Title: Cancer.
  II. Title. RC262.B53 2005
  616.99′40231–dc22

ISBN   0 415 32745 8 (Hbk)
         0 415 32746 6 (Pbk)

Contents

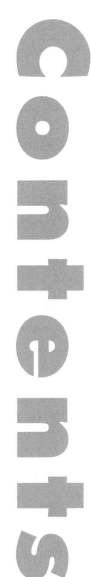

12 The treatment of cancer 319

Figures

Tables

Preface

It seems that, to most people, biology is nothing more than a subject that is taught at school and at university, but after that it has no relevance to a person's everyday life. People appear to live their lives with no regards to biology, becoming preoccupied with such matters as money, holidays, work, or looking good to their friends. Yet, whilst these things are important, life is very much the opposite of the view that biology is irrelevant. Life is all about biology. We are made from biological components; day by day, minute by minute, even second by second we must satisfy the biological needs of our cells, like oxygen and water. And we live in, and interact with, a biological environment. So, far from being just a subject at school, biology is the very *stuff of life*. Without it we simply don't exist, and our health is totally dependent on getting the biology right.

This means we need to give biology greater conscious thought every day if we are to stay healthy. Smoking is one good example of where this conscious thought is often seriously lacking. The biology related to smoking is simply swept under the carpet and forgotten by the smoker. It is well understood, and has been for some time, that smoking is *the worst health hazard* known to man, yet millions still smoke. The worst figures are for women and youngsters, whilst smoking in men is actually falling. Daily, smokers throw all caution to the wind and gamble with their health, indeed with their life. In the short term this may sound rather dramatic, but the real test comes with time, when years later the smoker is fighting cancer. Smokers cannot ignore the consequences of their actions for ever. With the development of ill health, they will have to face the stark reality of what their habit has done to them, not only cancer, but a host of other smoking-related diseases. Smoking causes a general deterioration in health over the years, opening the doors for all manner of disorders. Cancer remains one of the major problems, where prevention is most certainly better than the cure, and for many cancers there still is no cure.

But whilst a cure for cancer is difficult, prevention is perhaps simpler, a choice of a healthy lifestyle, which includes whether to smoke or not to smoke. And it is at the moment of that choice that, in an ideal world, biology should be right there, in their conscious thoughts, guiding and informing that choice. But for most people it isn't. So the choice is then based on other factors, like 'is it grown up to smoke?' or 'will I look silly to my friends because they smoke and I don't?' or simply due to curiosity. So smoking is started for all the wrong reasons, and the health services must then try to *pick up the pieces*, to correct the biological problems that this one wrong decision causes, like cancer, heart disease, vascular disease, and many others, some thirty or forty years later in life. Such choices made when we are young affect the rest of our lives. The question needs to be asked, are we doing enough to help and guide young people to make the correct health-related choices? Many young people do not understand the long-term consequences of their actions, and this should be addressed as a key component of any health strategy. Nurses should be among those offering advice to young people about health-related choices, but sadly too many nurses (and even doctors!) smoke. A notice on the wall of one ward originally stated 'Ask your nurse how to stop smoking', but was altered by hand to read 'Ask your nurse to stop smoking'. Is this a sad reflection of the reality of a health-caring profession?

The Department of Health has issued a number of publications with regards to improving the health of the nation, with a marked improvement in cancer services and a reduction in smoking as some of the targets. The NHS Plan (DOH 2000) includes a number of initiatives, and cancer is becoming a priority. The Cancer Plan is part of this strategy, where the commitment is towards ironing out inequalities of services, reducing waiting times, setting standards of care, improving cancer treatments and research, and providing greater resources for cancer care, particularly doctors and nurses. So nurses will, with their medical colleagues, be at the forefront of these changes, and they will need the specialised biological understanding of what cancer is, how it damages the body and how cancer treatments work.

This book puts this knowledge first, the knowledge that is so easily ignored as part of everyday life. It offers an explanation of the genetic mechanisms involved in malignancy, the cellular changes in metastases, how viruses, chemicals and radiation are involved in changing a normal cell to malignancy, and how chemotherapy can attack malignant cells. This is all vital for nurses in order that they can address the patients' and their relatives' concerns, and to be able to assist in the current and new waves of cancer treatment, like cancer vaccines, that will be available soon. The 'Nursing Skills' sections of this book are specifically not included in order to describe the performance of the skill (there are several good books that serve this function well), but it is intended to add to the discussion related to the biology of the skill.

The author would like to thank the following people: Maria Dingle, Alison Coutts and Barbara Novak, all lecturers in the Department of Applied Biological Sciences, St Bartholomew School of Nursing, City University, for proof reading sections of the book; David Blows for his assistance during the final preparation of this book for submission; and Lili Zhang-Lheureux for her professional comments and insight into acupuncture as a therapy.

William T. Blows
July 2004

Reference

Department of Health (DOH) 2000 *The NHS Plan*, Department of Health.

Chapter 1

Cell biology and cancer

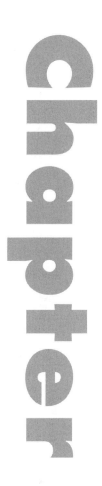

- Introduction
- The cell
- The cell cycle and growth
- Tissues of the body
- The malignant cell
- A classification of malignancy
- Key points

Introduction

We are made from cells, and cells are the functional unit of life. This means that life exists at cellular level. In single cell animals (like amoeba) the one cell does everything the animal needs to live. In the human (and other multicellular animals) however, individual cells provide only a contribution towards the life of the whole being. Cells are specialised in their function, and as such each individual cell plays just a small part in the total existence of its owner. No single cell can exist without the contribution of all the others. This is both good and bad for humans. Good because a single cell animal is unable to achieve what multicellular animals can. This is because it is not possible to pack the sophisticated biochemistry that makes up a multicellular animal's complex life into just one cell. The burden must be shared over millions of cells. By doing just that humans can build fast cars, understand the atom and walk on the moon. How many amoebae can claim those achievements? But it is also bad because failure of just a few specialised cells can jeopardise the very existence of all the others, and this is what happens in cancer.

The cell

The cell is the functional unit of the body. In humans and animals, the type of cell is known as a **eukaryotic** cell, whilst bacteria are **prokaryotic** cells (Figure 1.1). Eukaryotic cells are larger than prokaryotic cells; they have more membranes (including organelles surrounded by membranes) than prokaryotes (which do not have organelles). Bacteria have complex cell walls which eukaryotic cells do not have, and, unlike bacteria, eukaryotes have a fully formed nucleus and chromosomes.

Being multicellular, humans are made from 10^{14} cells (that is 100,000,000,000,000 cells). All these are derived from a single fertilised ovum. From this ovum the earliest cell divisions create a collection of cells that are all the same, but later growth in cell numbers allows the start of another process called **differentiation**. This means that cells begin to take on specific specialised roles, so that they will start to become tissues like blood, bone and brain. Every cell that has a nucleus also has the entire set of genes needed to make the whole body, but of course not all cells need this. The majority of genes will be switched off in most if not all cells, and only those genes needed for the cell's specialist function will remain active.

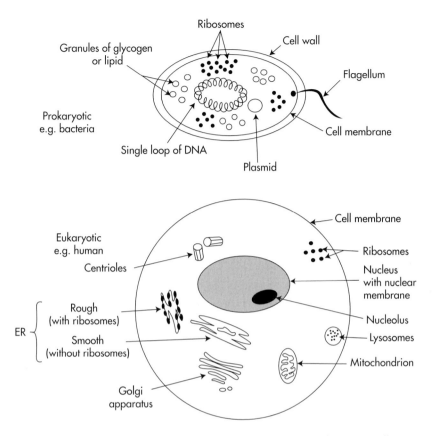

FIGURE 1.1 The prokaryote and eukaryote cells. The prokaryote cell is usually smaller with no definite nucleus, i.e. no nuclear membrane and no nucleolus. There is a cell wall in prokaryotes that eukaryotes do not have. The DNA of prokaryotes comes in a single loop, unlike the complex chromosomes found in eukaryotes. Some prokaryotes have a small additional loop of DNA called a plasmid, and some have a tail-like flagellum, both structures not found in eukaryotes. Mitochondria, endoplasmic reticulum (ER) and Golgi apparatus are features of eukaryotes.

Cells are made from **protoplasm**, which is mostly water with proteins, amino acids (broken down components of proteins), minerals (e.g. potassium) and other nutrients (e.g. glucose). Surrounding this protoplasm is a **cell membrane** (or **plasma membrane**) which is semi-permeable, i.e. it allows passage of some things through, including nutrients (entering the cell) and wastes (leaving the cell), and the gases **oxygen** (O_2)(entering the cell) and **carbon dioxide** (CO_2)(leaving the cell) (Figure 1.2). Most cells also have a nucleus surrounded by a membrane (the **nuclear membrane**) which is also

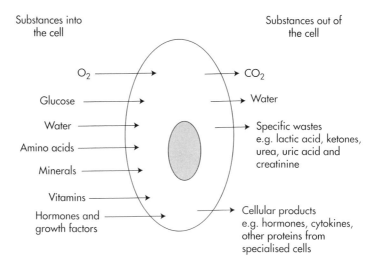

FIGURE 1.2 The input and output of the cell.

semi-permeable, with holes of a size that allows only the passage of molecules small enough to enter or leave the nucleus, e.g. **messenger ribonucleic acid (mRNA)**(see p. 13).

Cells have a series of **organelles** which carry out the various processes needed for life. In this regard, organelles are like '*mini-organs*' (hence the term *organelle*), but there the comparison ends. Organs, like the heart, are made from millions of cells, but organelles are not themselves made of cells. It is not possible to have structures made from many cells inside a single cell. That would be like saying a single house brick is made from many house bricks; it just makes no sense at all. So a definition of an organelle is 'a membrane-bound protein structure which carries out a specific function inside a cell'. Most of the organelles exist within the **cytoplasm** of the cell, i.e. that component of the protoplasm outside the nucleus, between the cell and nuclear membranes. One important organelle occurs inside the nucleus, the nucleolus. Table 1.1 is a list of the organelles found in a cell and their functions.

The nucleus, chromosomes and genes

The nucleus is that part of the cell that has a key central control over all cellular activities. This is because the nucleus houses the **genes** that code for the proteins involved is nearly all cellular functions. Genes are stretches of the molecule **deoxyribonucleic acid (DNA)**(Figure 1.3). Genes determine two things with regards to pro-

TABLE 1.1 The cellular organelles

Organelle	Description / function
Cytoplasmic	
Mitochondria	Produce energy in the form of adenosine triphosphate (ATP)
Ribosomes	Produce proteins from amino acids according to instructions from deoxyribonucleic acid (DNA)
Vacuoles	Storage spaces within the cytoplasm
Lysosomes	Specialised vacuoles containing digestive enzymes
Rough endoplasmic reticulum (ER) (ER with ribosomes)	Cytoplasmic spaces bound by a continuous membrane within which proteins are produced, modified and packaged
Smooth endoplasmic reticulum (ER) (ER without ribosomes)	Cytoplasmic spaces bound by a continuous membrane within which fat-based products are modified and packaged
Golgi apparatus	Cytoplasmic spaces bound by a separate membrane system within which products from ER are further modified, packaged and distributed or secreted from the cell
Centrioles	Structures outside the nucleus that form the nuclear spindle during cell division (called mitosis)
Nucleic	
Nucleolus	Produces the components of ribosomes

tein production: (1) they determine which amino acids will be in the finished protein, and (2) in what sequence these amino acids will occur. In the nucleus of human cells are found the 46 chromosomes which make up the **karyotype** (Figure 1.4). A chromosome is one complete molecule of DNA, and the larger chromosomes can contain many genes. The karyotype is an artificial assemblage of the chromosomes where the **homologous** chromosomes have been placed together in a numerical sequence from 1 to 22 (called **autosomes**) plus one pair of sex chromosomes. Homologous means 'the

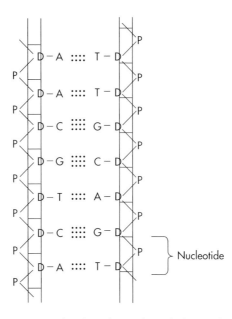

FIGURE 1.3 The DNA molecule. The sides of the molecule are made of nucleotides. Each nucleotide has a sugar (D=deoxyribose) and a phosphate (P) component with a base attached. There are four possible bases; adenine (A) links with thymine (T), and guanine (G) links with cytosine (C). Between adenine and thymine are two hydrogen bonds (two dotted lines), and between cytosine and guanine are three hydrogen bonds (three dotted lines). Many connected nucleotides create a molecule of incredible length that is coiled into a double helix.

same' because we inherit one set of 23 chromosomes from one parent, and one set of 23 chromosomes from the other parent. So number one chromosome from the father is 'the same' as number one chromosome from the mother, and so on with the other chromosomes. Both number one chromosomes carry the same genes as each other, and therefore they are homologous. This means that the cell has two versions of every gene, the version from one parent and the version from the other parent. These alternative versions of the same gene are called **alleles**. Chromosomes certainly do not exist laid out like a karyotype inside the nucleus; they occur mixed up as separate chromatin threads. The karyotype is, however, a convenient way for us to organise chromosomes for the purpose of examination. Chromatin, the substance of chromosomes, is made from DNA and its packaging proteins called **histones**. Long chromatin threads are coiled to form **chromatid** strands. Chromatid strands are copied in the cell cycle in the S stage (see p. 12), and from here to anaphase of

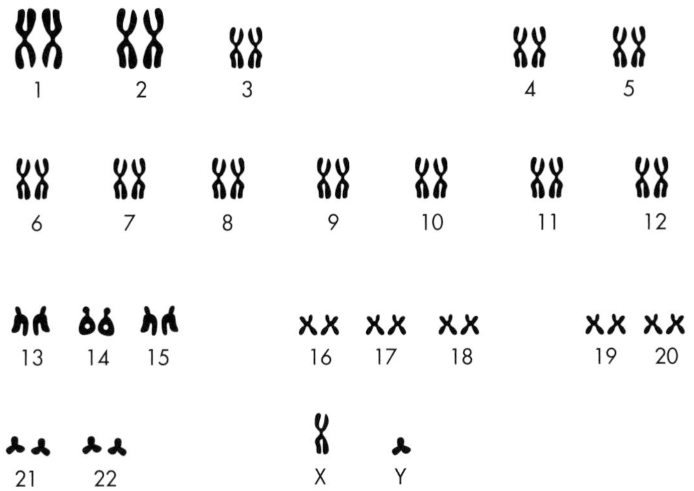

FIGURE 1.4 The human karyotype. This is an artificial presentation of the 46 chromosomes in the nucleus of the cell. Matching pairs are numbered 1 to 22 (the autosomes) and X+Y (the sex chromosomes). This is a male karyotype because it contains both X and Y. The female karyotype would contain X and X. Normally, in the nucleus, the chromosomes are jumbled and not visible, except during mitosis. (From Blows 2003, Figure 5.1.)

mitosis (see p. 10) chromosomes consist of two identical chromatid strands (called **sister chromatids**) joined at one point called a **centromere**. Deoxyribonucleic acid (DNA) has four **bases** mounted on a **sugar-phosphate** backbone (the sugar is **deoxyribose**). Two strands of DNA twist round each other in a double helix form and the bases are linked across from one strand to the other (see Figure 1.3). The four bases are **adenine, thymine, cytosine** and **guanine**, where adenine and thymine link together, and cytosine and guanine link together across the strands. The linkage is in the form of **hydrogen bonds**, two such bonds between the adenine and the thymine, three such bonds between the cytosine and the guanine. Hydrogen bonds are weak links that can be separated when the two strands come apart, and reformed when the molecule joins up again. This happens for protein synthesis and during replication of DNA (see the S phase of the cell cycle, p. 12).

The cell cycle and growth

Cells grow in two ways. They grow in size (known as **auxetic growth**) and they grow in numbers (known as **multiplicative**

growth). Size growth is limited because the volume of a cell (the cytoplasm that contains the metabolism) grows faster than the surface area (the cell membrane through which the nutrients and oxygen must pass) (see cell membrane, p. 3). Another way of putting this is to say that the volume grows by the *radius cubed* (radius³) whilst the surface area grows by only the *square of the radius* (radius²). Therefore metabolism in the volume outstrips the nutriment supply available through the surface area, and the cell must then divide into two **daughter cells** in order to reduce the volume. So the overall size of any multicellular life form on Earth is dependent on the limits of multiplicative growth rather than auxetic growth, which is already severely limited. This also explains why single cell organisms, like amoeba, are always so small.

Cells undergo a cycle of events know as the **cell cycle** (Figure 1.5). This involves both cell division (called **mitosis**) and the period between two successive divisions (a period called **interphase**). Mitosis is the division of most cells, i.e. all cells except for the **gametes**, which

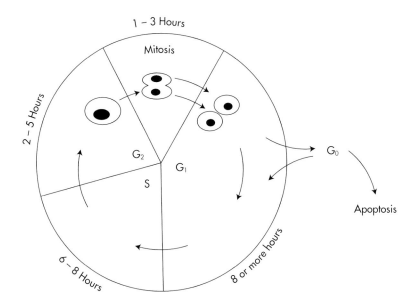

FIGURE 1.5 The cell cycle. After mitosis, the daughter cells arrive in G_1, the first and longest of two growth phases. From here, if there is any problem with the DNA the cell may go to G_0, and return to G_1 if the DNA is recoverable. If not, the cell may die (apoptosis). The S phase is a period of DNA replication, followed by a shorter growth phase, G_2, which prepares the cell for mitosis (cell division) again.

are the female **ova** ('egg' cell) and the male **sperm**. These divide by a different process, called **meiosis**.

Mitosis and cytokinesis

Mitosis, as seen in most tissue cells, is the division of the cell nucleus. It consists of a sequence of phases, namely (in order) **prophase**, **metaphase**, **anaphase** and **telophase**. **Cytokinesis** follows on from mitosis, and is the division of the cytoplasm (Figure 1.6).

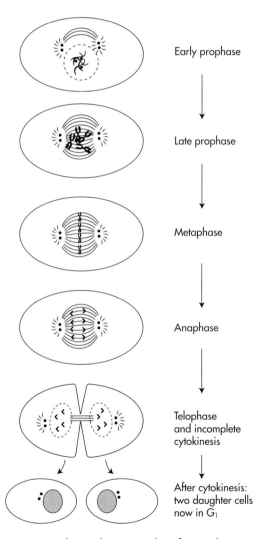

Early prophase

Late prophase

Metaphase

Anaphase

Telophase and incomplete cytokinesis

After cytokinesis: two daughter cells now in G_1

FIGURE 1.6 Mitosis and cytokinesis. The four phases of mitosis are prophase, metaphase, anaphase and telophase, followed by division of the cytoplasm, called cytokinesis. See text for details.

Prophase

This is the earliest and longest time of mitosis when preparations for division are well under way. During this phase chromatin threads (see p. 6), which were previously invisible, coil up and condense to form visible chromosomes, each chromosome consisting of a pair of sister chromatids joined at a centromere. Also in prophase the nucleolus becomes invisible and may be dispersed throughout the nucleus. Then the nuclear membrane breaks down and can no longer be seen. At this point, because the nuclear boundary has gone, the cell has no recognisable nucleus; a condition retained until the later stages of mitosis. The **centrioles** (see Table 1.1 and Figure 1.6) duplicate during prophase and these pairs migrate to positions at the apposing pole to each other. From these structures the mitotic spindle develops on both sides. The spindle is a protein framework of **microtubules**, which grows outward and crosses the space originally occupied by the nucleus. The two halves of the spindle do not quite meet but, instead, the chromosomes come between them and attach to both halves of the spindle via the chromosomal centromeres (Figure 1.6 and see p. 7).

Metaphase

This is much shorter, and consists of the chromosomes adopting a central position along the equatorial plane of the spindle. There are 46 chromosomes in the human cell and these must be divided between the two new cells, so each will receive 46 single separate chromatid strands.

Anaphase

This is the brief phase of chromosomal movement, when the spindles on both sides retract pulling the chromosomes into their separate chromatid strands. One chromatid strand will be dragged to one side of the cell, the other chromatid strand is dragged to the other side of the cell (Figure 1.6).

Telophase

This is almost the reverse of prophase. The chromatid strands disappear by uncoiling and becoming thread-like again as the two new nuclear membranes surrounding the chromatids are restored. This means that for a brief moment, before the rest of the cell divides, the cell has two nuclei. The nucleolus is also restored within each of these nuclei.

Cytokinesis

This is not part of mitosis, but is the division of the remaining cytoplasm, completing the process of producing two separate daughter cells (Figure 1.6). The plasma membrane is produced in sufficient quantities by both cells to span completely between them, cutting the cytoplasm in half. Division of the cytoplasm also involves equal distribution of the organelles between the two new cells.

Interphase

This is the period between one mitotic event and the next. Early cell scientists thought of this as the resting period for the cells, but we now know that the cell is very active during all stages of interphase. These stages of interphase are, in order of sequence from mitosis, G_0, G_1, S and G_2 (see Figure 1.5).

G_0

This is an indefinite period during which the cell is carrying out its normal metabolic functions, but it is not preparing for further division. Some cells, like most **neurons** (nerve cells), remain in G_0 and never divide. Others, like bone marrow stem cells, divide so quickly that they spend little if any time in G_0 (see p. 94).

G_1

This is the first of two growth phases (G for growth) in preparation for further cell division. Having grown in numbers from one cell to two during mitosis (multiplicative growth), the cells undergo some auxetic growth (see p. 7), with a corresponding increase in organelle numbers. Organelle numbers must meet the needs of the two further daughter cells produced at the next mitosis. All the new components must be synthesised from proteins and lipids, using glucose as an energy source, and these components must all be imported into the cells through the cell membrane (see p. 4). This is a major metabolic exercise, and the enzymes that drive this metabolism must all be produced in sufficient quantities. By the end of G_1 both cells should be ready to proceed to the next stage; the S stage.

The S (or synthesis) stage

This involves the production of DNA and the proteins (called **histones**) that are used for packaging the DNA. This provides enough DNA for the future daughter cells after the next mitosis.

G_2

This is the second of the two growth phases. At this point final preparations for mitosis take place including further essential protein synthesis and completion of centriole replication.

G_0 and cell cycle control

G_0 is the stationary phase of the cell cycle when the cell is not preparing for division. Stationary does *not* mean inactive, since the cell is carrying out its normal cellular functions during this time. Also, during the cell's stay in G_0, certain checks are made by the cell to assess the integrity of the DNA following mitosis. With chromosomes being pulled in two different directions during anaphase (see p. 10) it is possible that DNA was damaged, and this damage needs repair. Failure to do this could result in the damage being duplicated in the S stage of interphase, ready to be incorporated into each new daughter cell. In other words, the damage (i.e. gene error), not only affects the current cell but will be passed onto the future generations of daughter cells, a situation that occurs in cancer.

There are several genes (and their corresponding proteins) involved in stopping the cell in G_0 to allow for DNA assessment and possible repair. Three important genes that cause a halt to cells in G_0 are *TP53*, *CDKN2A* and *RB1* (see also p. 13). The gene *TP53* is located on chromosome 17. The location of all genes is called the gene **locus**, i.e. the address on the chromosome where the gene is found. In the case of *TP53*, the locus is 17p13.1, where 17 is the chromosome number, p means the short arm of the chromosome (i.e. above the centromere) and 13.1 is the location counted away from the centromere. *TP53* codes for a powerful protein called **p53**, which has a number of vital functions. It is a **transcription factor**, which means it binds to multiple locations on DNA and controls gene transcription, i.e. the replication of the DNA code into **messenger RNA (mRNA)**. This has a major influence over protein synthesis. But even more important is the role of p53 in stopping the cell cycle in G_1, the mechanism of which is seen in Figure 1.7. Linked to this is the role of p53 in **apoptosis** (also called **programmed cell death**). This is the ultimate control on cell replication, where cells with irreparable DNA damage are prevented from replication by dying. Although the cell is lost, it can be replaced by the replication of cells with normal DNA. This is a crucial control that prevents those cells with devastating DNA errors from surviving into the next generation. Gene mutations of *TP53* itself lead to loss of this cellular control, and result in cells with extensive DNA damage (gene mutation) being duplicated into the daughter cells. This problem is thought to be associated with about 50% or more of human cancers (see p. 40).

The *RB1* gene is located at 13q14.3 (read as shown for *TP53*; here q is the long arm of the chromosome below the centromere). This gene codes for the protein **pRB**, another powerful inhibitor of the cell cycle in G_1. The pRB protein binds and blocks the function of a transcription factor called E2F1, the function of which is essential for the cell to progress round the cycle. This loss of E2F1 function in G_1 causes blockage of further progression of the cell. The protein pRB is, itself, switched on (activated) or switched off (deactivated) by the action of other proteins called **cyclins** and **cyclin-dependent kinases (CDK)**. A particular type of cyclin (called **D-type cyclin**) forms a complex with two kinases (called **CDK4** and **CDK6**) and this complex inhibits the function of pRB. This allows E2F1 to function normally and the cell will continue around the cell cycle from G_1 into the S stage (see Figure 1.7). Mutations of gene *RB1* are associated with a tumour of the eye called a **retinoblastoma** (RB stands for retinoblastoma) (see p. 41).

One further gene involved in cell cycle control is *CDKN2A* (also called *MTS1* and *INK4A*). The locus for this gene is 9p13, and it codes for two different proteins, **p16** and **p19** (p19 is also called **ARF**, meaning Alternative Reading Frame). The p16 protein inhibits the CDKs, thus allowing the pRB to function normally. The p19 (ARF) protein is important in maintaining the normal levels of p53 in the cell (see p. 14). Loss of either protein due to gene mutations causes failure to control the cell cycle (see Figure 1.7), and is seen in

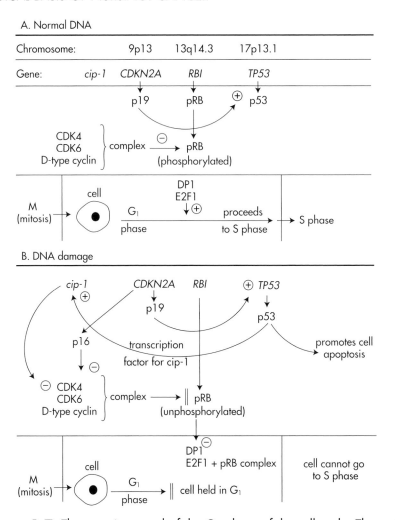

Figure 1.7 The genetic control of the G_1 phase of the cell cycle. The main genes involved are *cip-1*, *CDKN2A*, *RB1* and *TP53*. A. The cell with normal DNA. pRB (the protein product of *RB1*) is phosphorylated (a means of deactivating the protein) by a complex formed from CDK4, CDK6 and D-type cyclin. The deactivation of pRB allows the DP1+E2F1 complex to promote passage of the cell from G1 to the S phase of the cell cycle. B. The cell with DNA damage. Protein products from *cip-1* and *CDKN2A* (p16) inhibit the CDK+cyclin complex, and this in turn releases pRB (unphosphorylated) so it can bind to the DP1+E2F1 complex. This binding blocks the role of the complex so the cell cannot proceed to the S phase, and it halts in G1. The *cip-1* gene was activated by an increase in p53, the protein product from *TP53*, since p53 is a transcription factor for *cip-1*. The increase in p53 occurs as a result of the DNA damage. p19 from *CDKN2A* helps to regulate the correct amount of p53 in the cell. One function of p53 is to promote apoptosis (cell death) when DNA damage is too great for repair. Gene mutations in all four genes are seen in various cancers, where the cell cannot be stopped in G_1 and will go round the cell cycle rapidly and multiply uncontrollably.

cases of **melanoma** (see p. 247) and a range of other tumours (Strachan and Read 2001).

Tissues of the body

Cells are grouped into **tissues**, and there are two major categories of structural tissues in the body, the **epithelial** and **connective** tissues, plus tissues of specialist function such as the nervous system, blood (i.e. bone marrow), muscle and the lymphatic system.

Epithelial tissues

Epithelial tissues are the simplest tissues, and they tend to line surfaces, e.g. cavities or tubes. They are made from a single layer of cells (called **simple**) or multiple layers of cells (called **stratified**) resting on a **basement membrane**. The cells may be **squamous** (i.e. flat), **cuboid** (i.e. blocks, like dice) or **columnar** (i.e. tall)(Figure 1.8).

    Simple squamous epithelium is a single flat layer of smooth cells (i.e. pavement-like) that provides a smooth surface *inside* blood vessels (the **endothelium**) and *inside* the heart (the **endocardium**), and forms the walls of lymphatic vessels and air sacs in the lungs (called **alveoli**). It is also found in other membranes (e.g. the membrane around the heart called the **pericardium**).

    Simple cuboid epithelium lines the glands and ducts leading from the glands, and is also found in the **renal tubules** (i.e. part of the **nephron**, the functional unit of the kidney).

    Simple columnar epithelium is found lining the gall bladder, the stomach and the intestines. It is also found in digestive glands and the respiratory tract. In many of these sites it forms **mucous membrane**. In mucus membrane some cells are called **goblet cells** because of their cup-like shape, and these secrete mucus. Respiratory mucous

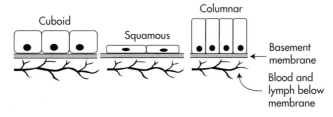

FIGURE 1.8 Cuboid, squamous and columnar epithelium on basement membrane. Beneath the basement membrane are blood and lymph vessels.

columnar cells also have **cilia**, tiny hair-like projections which can perform a sweeping action to filter the air we breathe in.

Stratified (multilayered) squamous epithelium covers the surface of the body as **epidermis**, the outer layer of the skin. The living cells of the epidermis are roughly square and occur at the base of the layers where they are constantly dividing. The new cells created migrate upward through the various layers, and during this process they produce a protein called **keratin**. As this fills the cytoplasm the cell flattens and dies. In the upper (outer) layers these dead flat cells flake off and are lost (on the scalp this is commonly known as **dandruff**). This tissue forms a tough outer layer to the body where erosion of the body surface is likely, and constant replacement from the basal layers is necessary. It is also found in the mouth, oesophagus and vagina.

Stratified cuboidal epithelium consists of multiple layers of square cells found in **sweat glands** (glands in the skin secreting sweat), **sebaceous glands** (tiny glands attached to the base of hairs in the skin, and secreting **sebum**, an oily fluid which lubricates the hair) and the **ovaries** and **testes** (i.e. the **gonads**).

Stratified columnar epithelium comprises a superficial layer of columnar cells on top of several layers of cuboidal cells. This forms moist surfaces such as inside the larynx, parts of the pharynx and the urethra, and lines the ducts of both the **salivary glands** and **mammary glands** (the breasts). This tissue allows the movement of substances over its surface, like saliva and breast milk along the ducts.

Pseudostratified columnar epithelium (pseudo means 'false') is a single layer of cells with nuclei at different heights, giving a false impression of several layers. Careful examination reveals, however, that all the cells are in contact with a basement membrane, but they do not all reach the superficial surface (Figure 1.9). This is found in large excretory ducts of the male reproductive system, the nasal cavity and other parts of the respiratory tract. Like stratified columnar epithelium this tissue allows the movement of substances over its surface and secretes fluid.

Transitional epithelium consists of cells which change shape, from cuboid to flat and back again, when stretching is required, e.g. it lines the urinary bladder and stretches during bladder filling.

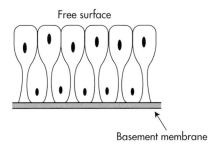

Free surface

Basement membrane

FIGURE 1.9 Pseudostratified epithelium. It appears as two layers but is in fact only one layer of cells with varying height of the nuclei.

Connective tissues

Areolar connective tissue is the most commonly found connective tissue in the body. It is made from a loose collection of two different fibres interwoven together in a mesh with scattered cells throughout. The first of these fibres is **collagen**, a very common structural protein found in many sites around the body. These fibres are tough and give strength to the tissue. The second is **elastic fibres**, and as the name suggests these are stretchy and provide some elasticity to the tissue. Among the cells are those of the immune system (i.e. **macrophages**) and those that help to produce the tissue (i.e. **fibroblasts**). Areolar tissue is ubiquitous, i.e. it is almost everywhere, and in most places areolar tissue is used as packaging around blood vessels, nerves and organs.

Dense, collagenous tissue is like areolar except it is packed with collagen but with no elastic fibres. This is a very tough tissue in either of its two forms: regular or irregular. In regular collagenous tissue the collagen fibres all lay parallel in bundles, allowing the tissue to have a great tensile strength. Such strength is needed in tendons and ligaments that pull on bones. Irregular tissue has the fibres all mixed up and laying at many different angles. The dermis of the skin is one good example of this type.

Elastic connective tissue has many yellow elastic fibres which are extensively branched, forming a network. The spaces in this net contain fibroblasts and small amounts of collagen. Elastic tissue allows stretching with recoil plus support and suspension of other structures. It is found in the stomach wall, the largest arteries and parts of the trachea, vocal cords, bronchi and the heart.

Adipose connective tissue is made from fat cells called **adipocytes**. The cytoplasm of adipocytes is packed with lipid displacing the nucleus to one side. About 10% of the average adult body weight is adipose tissue. Adipose tissue forms under the dermis of the skin where it helps to insulate against excessive heat loss. It is also found around internal organs where it helps to provide a protective cushion against potential injury. Adipose tissue is also a valuable food reserve since fat is the body's second line energy source after glucose (see p. 305).

Reticular connective tissue is a latticework of fine multibranching interwoven fibres forming a web-like structure with **reticular cells** in the spaces. This is found inside the liver, spleen, lymph nodes, tonsils, stomach and intestinal wall and it supports adipose tissue.

Cartilage

Cartilage is the toughest of the connective soft tissues and is mostly associated with the skeleton and bone function. The three cartilage types seem to be very similar to areolar, dense collagenous and elastic connective tissues, the difference being the tough, dense, gel-like matrix within which the fibres and cartilage cells (called **chondrocytes**) are set.

Hyaline cartilage is a network of collagen fibres in a gel-like matrix. The joint ends of long bones, where it is called **articular cartilage**, are a good example of hyaline cartilage. Here it needs to be tough to withstand erosion from joint movements and, in the case of the legs, weight-bearing pressures. Other sites include the tracheal and laryngeal cartilages, the bronchial cartilages, the nose (below the bridge) and the **costal cartilages** which link the ends of the ribs to the **sternum** (or breast bone). Toughness at the joint ends is tempered with flexibility in places like the nose and ribs.

Fibrocartilage consists of bundles of collagen fibres packed together in a tough gel-like matrix. The addition of collagen to the matrix gives fibrocartilage the quality of being the toughest soft tissue in the body. As such, it is found in places like the **intervertebral discs** (cartilaginous pads between the vertebrae of the spine) where weight bearing and spinal movements put great strain on soft tissues. A supportive role for fibrocartilage is found in the **meniscus** (specialised stabilising cartilages within the knee joints) and surrounding the rims of joint sockets.

Elastic cartilage is a concentration of dense elastic fibres in matrix. Flexibility coupled with the ability to retain the original shape is important for this tissue. It is found in the external ear, the nasopharynx, the larynx and the **epiglottis** (the flap in the larynx that guards the entrance to the trachea, preventing inhalation of food and drink during swallowing). For further information on the various tissue types see Martini (2004).

Bone tissue

Bone is the second hardest tissue in the body, only tooth enamel is harder than bone. Bone tissue makes up the skeleton, which provides shape and support for the body, protection for vital organs (e.g. the skull protects the brain), co-ordinated movement through a system of joints, anchorage for muscles and critical storage for calcium (Martini 2004). Bone is made from organic and inorganic components (Figure 1.10). The organic components are the cells (called **osteo-cytes**) and the cellular products, notably proteins like collagen (see p. 17). The inorganic components are the minerals, mostly calcium compounds like **calcium phosphate** and **calcium carbonate**. The

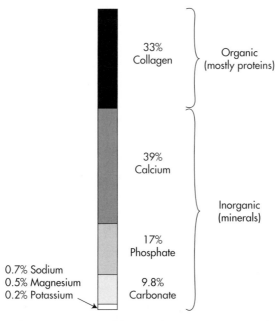

FIGURE 1.10 The composition of bone. The organic material (cells and cellular proteins like collagen) occupies about 33% of the content. The inorganic material (minerals, mostly calcium) occupies the remainder.

inorganic minerals form crystals along the protein framework, with the cells living in spaces. There are two types of bone tissue: **compact** bone and **cancellous** (or **spongy**) bone. The two hundred bones in the skeleton (plus six in the ears) have an outer casing of compact bone with the spongy bone inside. This cancellous spongy bone has many spaces in it, like honeycomb, and these spaces are filled with **bone marrow** (see p. 94). The next time you eat a honeycomb bar covered in chocolate think of it as having a similar structure to a long bone, i.e. the honeycomb is the spongy bone inside and the chocolate is the compact bone outside. Unlike the skeletons seen in museums and biology laboratories, living bone is not a dry material. In life it has a rich blood supply and contains about 20% water. It also has many living, reproducing cells, and it can grow and heal if injured. Bone has an outer membrane called the **periosteum** which houses another type of cell (called **osteogenic** cells), which are vital in the healing process and can become new osteocytes.

Muscle tissue

There are three muscle types in the body (Figure 1.11) (Martini 2004). **Skeletal muscle** is the type we are all aware of, i.e. that of the

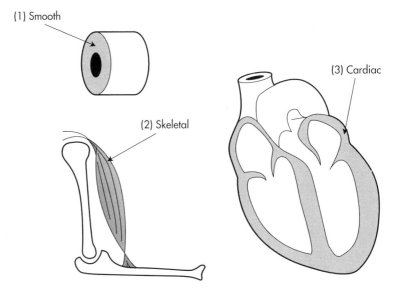

(1) Smooth

(3) Cardiac

(2) Skeletal

FIGURE 1.11 Three types of muscle. (1) Smooth muscle is found in the walls of tubes like blood vessels and the gut wall; (2) skeletal muscle is found in the muscles attached to bones; (3) cardiac muscle is only found in the myocardium of the heart.

trunk, neck and limbs. It is attached to bones and works by voluntary control. Under the microscope is appears as very long, thin, cylindrical cells called **myocytes**. These cells are striated (which means striped) or banded in appearance. Their role is voluntary movement, controlled by the brain via the **motor nervous system**. **Smooth muscle** is involuntary muscle (i.e. we have no control or awareness of it function). It is found in the walls of the digestive tract, the blood vessels and the respiratory tract. Under the microscope the cells are spindle shaped and have no stripes. It is controlled by the **sympathetic** component of the **autonomic nervous system**. **Cardiac muscle** is a specialised heart muscle, found only in the **myocardium**, the middle layer of the heart wall. As such it is involuntary in function, controlled by both the autonomic nervous system and its own internal conduction system. Under the microscope it consists of long, cylindrical, branched cells which, like skeletal muscle, have stripes (or bands).

Blood tissue

Blood is a tissue in fluid form. This is because blood must circulate around the body and supply all the other tissues with oxygen and nutrients, and remove waste. We have about five litres (5000 ml) of blood in the adult body, and of this about 55% is the fluid component called **plasma**. The other 45% is the **formed elements** (a collective term which means the various cells of the blood)(Figure 1.12). The plasma is mostly water (i.e. about 92% of plasma is water), but it also has a wide range of other substances dissolved in it. These substances include many kinds of proteins, amino acids, glucose, minerals, vitamins, hormones, the gases oxygen and carbon dioxide, and waste of various kinds, particularly **urea** (nitrogenous waste from proteins). Plasma is also the mechanism for the distribution of heat around the body, rather like a central heating system.

The cells in the plasma fall into three main categories. Almost 99.9% of the cells in the blood are the **erythrocytes** (**red blood cells**, or **RBC**), and these carry much of the blood gases; oxygen and carbon dioxide. These gases are mostly transported by the molecule **haemoglobin** (**Hb**) which fills the erythrocytes. One haemoglobin molecule has four **globin** proteins, each containing a **haeme** component, and at the core of the haeme part is an iron atom. Therefore one haemoglobin molecule can carry four oxygen molecules (4 × O_2). Each RBC contains about 250 million Hb molecules, and can

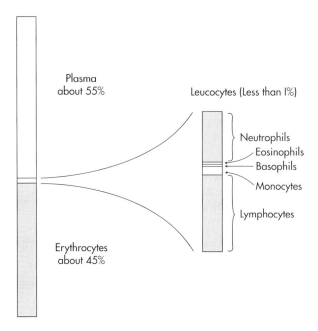

Plasma
about 55%

Leucocytes (Less than 1%)

Neutrophils
Eosinophils
Basophils
Monocytes

Lymphocytes

Erythrocytes
about 45%

FIGURE 1.12 The composition of blood. Plasma at about 55% of the volume, and red cells (erythrocytes) at about 45% of the volume leave very little (less than 1%) for the white cells (leucocytes).

therefore carry one billion oxygen molecules when fully saturated. The globin component carries around 20% of the carbon dioxide transported in the blood.

About 0.1% of the blood cells are **leucocytes** (**white blood cells**, or **WBC**) and **thrombocytes** (or **platelets**). The role of WBCs is to fight infection; they are a major component of our immune system (see p. 66). Platelets prevent blood loss in a number of ways, especially by sparking off the blood clotting process, creating a blood clot (or **thrombus**). Blood cells are derived from stem cells in bone marrow, a process which is called **haemopoiesis** (or **haematopoiesis**) which means 'blood forming'. More details about blood occur in Chapter 4 (see p. 94).

Lymph tissue

The **lymphatic system** is a key component of the immune system of the body. Lymph, like blood, is mostly water, and it is derived from, and returns to, blood plasma. Lymphatic vessels drain excess fluid from the tissues and this fluid is filtered in **lymphatic glands** (or nodes), where unwanted and potentially harmful foreign substances (called **antigens**) are removed and destroyed by **lymphocytes** (see p. 96). The lymphatic system is described in more detail in Chapter 9 (see p. 232) and in Chapter 4 (see p. 104) because the system is involved in both the fight against cancer and its spread.

Nerve tissue

Nervous tissue makes up the brain and the spinal cord (collectively called the **central nervous system**, or **CNS**) and the nerves (called the **peripheral nervous system**, or **PNS**). The functional cell of nerve impulse conduction is the **neuron** (Figure 1.13). These are highly specialised cells which have mostly lost the ability for replication (i.e. they remain in G_0 of the cell cycle, see p. 11). They create impulses (known as **action potentials**) which pass down long fibres (called **axons**) extending from the cell body (Martini 2004). These fibres link up with either other neurons, or other cells (e.g. muscular

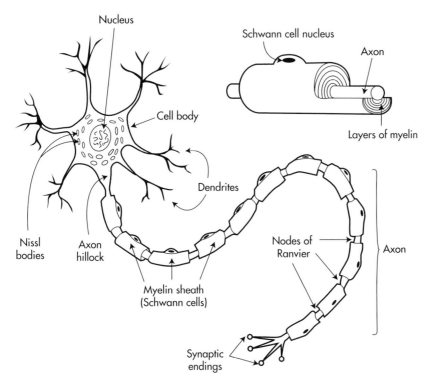

FIGURE 1.13 The neuron (or nerve cell). It consists of a cell body with dendrites and a long axon usually covered with a myelin sheath. (From Blows 2003, Figure 2.1, and Blows 2001, Figure 7.2.)

23

or glandular cells) and the impulses increase (or reduce) activity in those cells, thus having some control over the function of many cells. Supportive cells of the nervous system (called **neuroglia**, or more simply **glial cells**, or **glia**) do not produce or convey impulses, but they play a vital role in maintaining neuron function (see p. 244).

The malignant cell

Tumours are either **benign** or **malignant** (Kumar *et al.* 1997). The difference between them is of the utmost importance. Benign tumours are more common than malignant tumours, and they are potentially less dangerous (Table 1.2). Misunderstanding of the diagnosis by the patient or their relatives can be extremely distressing, for the following reason.

The word **cancer**, which is used for particular tumours, is also used in the astrological charts as the star-sign of cancer ('the crab'). The connection between these two very different concepts is said to be from the way malignant tumours form a central mass in the body with leg-like infiltrations extending out into the surrounding tissues,

TABLE 1.2 Benign versus malignant tumours

Benign tumours	*Malignant tumours (cancers)*
Common	Rarer, becoming more common in the elderly
Cells of the tumour are the same as the tissue of origin	Cells of the tumour are usually very unlike the tissue of origin (i.e. they are atypical)
Growth is slow. The tumour is encapsulated and grows by expansion, not infiltration (i.e. *not* like a crab)	Growth is usually fast. The tumour has no capsule and grows by infiltration (i.e. looks like a crab)
Does *not* produce metastases (see p. 229)	Can (and often does) produce metastases
Does cause complications by obstructing tubes, blocking blood flow, putting pressure on surrounding structures, producing excess hormones (see pp. 35–36), and other problems	Dangerous. Can spread to other parts of the body, cause tissue erosion, bleeding, obstruction, anaemia (see p. 100), necrosis (see p. 332), cachexia (see p. 305) and death

rather like the body of a crab with legs extending outwards. The use of the word 'cancer' (the star sign) to describe a tumour would seem a very trivial matter, but it does have one very serious point. The fact that a crab has legs indicates the infiltrative nature of the tumour, growing into the surrounding structures. Only tumours that are truly malignant do this. Most non-malignant (i.e. benign) tumours do not infiltrate in this manner, only doing so after they have turned malignant. Therefore, the word cancer *must only be used in the context of malignant infiltrative tumours*, but never used for tumours that are non-malignant and non-infiltrative. If a health-care professional was to use the word cancer inappropriately to a patient with a non-malignant tumour, or to their relatives, this could easily lead to mis-understanding, confusion, unnecessary fear and even anger by the patient about their treatment and prognosis.

When a **biopsy** (a small sample of tissue from a growth) is taken it will be examined in the laboratory for abnormalities, a process known as **histopathology**. This means cutting a thin section through the tissue for light microscopic examination. Close detailed examination of this kind reveals if the tissues and the cells are normal or not, and it is therefore a key step in the diagnosis of the problem. Normal epithelial cells appear regular in shape and size and they are well organised, like disciplined soldiers on parade. They also have regular-shaped nuclei and small round nucleoli. Most normal epithelial cells will be positioned along a **basement membrane** which acts as a flat surface along which the cells are anchored in place (see p. 15). Basement membranes are a vital component in the understanding of how cancers spread, as we will see. Below the basement membrane are blood and lymph vessels supplying the tissue (see Figure 1.8).

Cancer cells are somewhat different in appearance, having variable shapes for both the cell and the nucleus, large nucleoli and a loss, or disruption, of the basement membrane (King 2000). This last feature allows the malignant cells to gain access to the blood and lymph for the purposes of spread to other parts of the body. Malignant tissues also show a disturbance to the tissue **architecture**, i.e. the way the tissue is structured. Normally, there is a set ratio between the number of epithelial cells and the number of **stromal** cells in the extracellular fluid. Think of the epithelial cells as being the ones that are carrying out the tissue function, while stromal cells form the matrix, or packaging around the epithelial cells. Disruption of the architecture may well mean an increase in the ratio of epithelial to stromal cells, e.g. in a carcinoma, due to excessive epithelial growth. It may also mean disruption to the structure, as in the loss of the basement membrane, so the tissue looks abnormal.

Hyperplasia (Figure 1.14) is the term used to describe an increase in auxetic growth (see p. 7) in a tissue, i.e. the cells have grown in larger than expected numbers causing the tissue to thicken and become a mass. Hyperplasia is normal in some parts of the body, but unexpected (and therefore suspicious) in other parts of the body. For example, consider two areas of the skin, one being the sole of the foot, the other being the back of the hand. They are very different, the sole of the foot has undergone hyperplasia causing thickening of the epidermis of the skin. This is due to the stress of weight bearing, to which the back of the hand is not subjected. The hyperplasia on the foot is specifically to protect the foot against excessive erosion as it contacts the ground (or the inside of the shoe). You can imagine that erosion could be a major problem at some sites across the body, and hyperplasia is the natural body response to this problem. Hyperplasia becomes suspicious when it occurs at sites not subject to significant erosion. Here, the hyperplasia is not a response to erosion stresses but is caused by something else; and this could be the early stages of malignancy. It is important to recognise that cells in hyperplasia still look normal but they have developed a tendency to speed

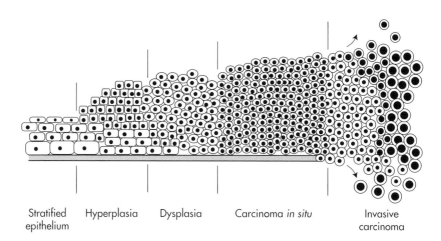

| Stratified epithelium | Hyperplasia | Dysplasia | Carcinoma *in situ* | Invasive carcinoma |

FIGURE 1.14 The stages of cancer development. Here, stratified epithelium passes through hyperplasia (overgrowth of normal cells), through dysplasia (disorganised tissue structure), through carcinoma *in situ* (changes to a malignant cell type) to invasive carcinoma (which has breached the basement membrane and released metastases).

up their cell cycle and reproduce faster. This may well be due to a genetic mutation (see p. 38).

Eventually, some cells from the hyperplasia may undergo further genetic change and this not only increases further the rate of cell division but it causes the cell appearance and its orientation within the tissue to change abnormally. This is then called a **dysplasia** (otherwise known as **atypical hyperplasia** because the cells have changed appearance)(see Figure 1.14), and it potentially marks a stage towards malignancy, called **pre-malignancy**. So far the growth has remained within the basement membrane, and there are at this stage no cells which have left the cell mass. If the pathologist finds hyperplasia during his histopathology examination, this would cause suspicion and be reviewed again at a later date. But the discovery of dysplasia would require more urgent attention, possibly excision of the affected tissues. This would be even more important if the dysplasia was classified as *high grade*, i.e. more advanced.

As the tissues become more abnormal and grow faster the mass becomes malignant. This means that growth in these cells is **autonomous**, i.e. growth is self-sustaining and has no bearing on the needs of the body. It no longer responds to the normal signals or controls of growth, the **hormones** and **cytokines** (see p. 35). If this mass has not yet broken through the basement membrane, nor has it yet shed any loose malignant cells (called **metastases**, see p. 229) the mass is called **carcinoma** *in situ* (see Figure 1.14). Once the tumour has breached the basement membrane it becomes an **invasive carcinoma** (see Figure 1.14). At this point it will be shedding metastases which now have access to the blood and lymph vessels below the basement membrane, and these can now be transported around the body. Metastatic cells in the lymph will populate the local lymph nodes (always a sign of cancer spread), and malignant cells in the blood will be delivered to other organs and could form secondary growths there.

In any malignant mass, many cells are dividing at the same time to form different **cell lines** (Figure 1.15). Cell lines are colonies of cells which have the same (or very similar) characteristics because they are all derived from the same parent cell. But the presence of many different parent cells in the original mass due to different genetic mutations results in a large number of different cell lines within the same tumour (see Figure 1.15). So it is possible that any two cells from the same tumour may be significantly different to each other. This has a bearing on the management of the cancer, as some

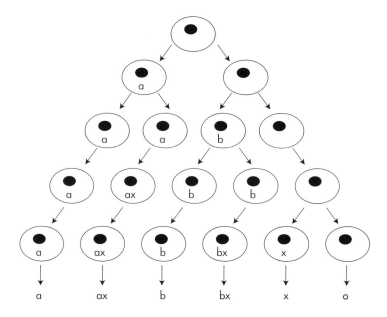

Figure 1.15 An example of cell lineage in a tumour. The original cell at the top has no mutations. Of the two daughter cells from this original, one has developed a gene mutation ('a'), the other has not. The daughter cells from the 'a' mutated cell both carry the 'a' mutation, whilst the non-mutated cell has one daughter cell that has developed another mutation (b), the other does not. And so various combinations of cell divisions and genetic mutations in this simple example result in cell lines with 'a', 'ax', 'b', 'bx', 'x' and 'o' ('o' = no mutations) all within the same tumour. It can be seen from this that some treatments may affect a few cell lines more than others within the same tumour.

treatments (e.g. hormonal therapy, see p. 338) act well on certain cell lines but not on others. The treatment may therefore only shrink the tumour (killing some cell lines) but not destroy the tumour completely (as other cell lines survive).

A classification of malignancy

New growths in the body can be classified in a manner based on the type of tissue the tumour arises from, even though the transformation from normal cell to tumour cell may involve varying degrees of changes in the tissue (Figure 1.16). The two major basic tissue classes found in the body are **epithelium** and **connective** tissues (see p. 15), and these form the basis of a classification for tumour growth. Epithelial-derived tumours are called **carcinomas**, and connective

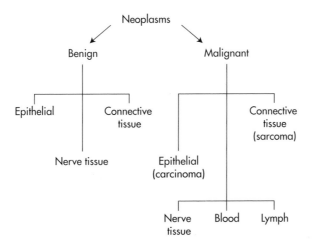

FIGURE 1.16 A classification of neoplasms. The benign and malignant divisions are both further divided according to their tissue of origin, i.e. epithelial and connective tissue, with some specialised tissues included.

tissue-derived tumours are **sarcomas**. Any tumour that arises from tissues other than epithelial or connective tissue (e.g. nerve tissue or blood) is added on as an extension of the classification (see Figure 1.16). Another consideration is the division of tumours into benign and malignant forms, the characteristics of which can be seen in Table 1.2 (p. 24). A complete classification therefore has to take into account both benign and malignant tumour types in epithelial, connective and other tissue origins (see Figure 1.16).

Key points

Cells

- Cells are the functional unit of life.
- Cells have organelles which carry out the metabolic processes of life.
- Cells form tissues, and there are two main structural tissues in the body, epithelial and connective tissues, plus tissues of the nervous system, blood, bone and lymphatic system.
- Many cells go around a cycle of events, the cell cycle which involves cell division (mitosis) and the period between two successive divisions (interphase).

Mitosis

- Mitosis is the division of the cell nucleus, and consists of prophase, metaphase, anaphase and telophase.
- Cytokinesis follows on from mitosis, and is the division of the cytoplasm

Cell cycle

- The stages of interphase are G_0, G_1, S and G_2.
- Certain genes control the movement of the cell around the cell cycle, and therefore control cell growth.
- The genes involved in stopping the cell in G_0 are *TP53*, *CDKN2A* and *RB1*.

Cancer

- Hyperplasia means an increase in cell growth leading to increased tissue mass.
- Dysplasia (atypical hyperplasia) means the cells have changed appearance and orientation and the tissues have disrupted architecture. It is called pre-malignancy.
- When the mass is within the basement membrane, with no metastases, it is called carcinoma *in situ.*
- If the tumour breaks through the basement membrane and sheds metastases it becomes an invasive carcinoma.
- Beneath the basement membrane the malignant tumour has access to blood and lymph and can therefore spread.
- Many cells in a tumour are dividing to form different cell lines, i.e. cell colonies all derived from the same parent cell and having the same characteristics.
- The word cancer must only be used in the context of a malignant infiltrative tumour, but never used for tumours that are non-malignant and non-infiltrative.
- Benign tumours are common, the cells are the same as the tissue of origin, they grow slowly by expansion, the tumour is encapsulated and does not produce metastases.
- Malignant tumours are rarer, but more common in the elderly. The cells are different from the tissue of origin, they grow fast by infiltration and metastases and the tumour has no capsule.

References

Blows W. T. (2001) *The Biological Basis of Nursing: Clinical Observations*, Routledge, London.

Blows W. T. (2003) *The Biological Basis of Nursing: Mental Health*, Routledge, London.

King R. J. B. (2000) *Cancer Biology* (2nd edn), Prentice Hall, London.

Kumar V., Cotran R. S. and Robbins S. L. (1997) *Basic Pathology* (6th edn), W. B. Saunders Company, Philadelphia.

Martini F. H. (2004) *Fundamentals of Anatomy and Physiology* (6th edn), Benjamin Cummings, Pearson Education International, San Francisco.

Strachan T. S. and Read A. P. (2001) *Human Molecular Genetics* (2nd edn), Bios Scientific Publishers, Oxford.

Chapter 2

The causes of cancer

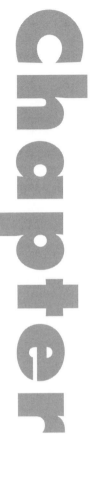

- Introduction
- The hormones and genetics of growth and cancer
- Environmental factors: carcinogens
- Key points

Introduction

Whilst it is true that the cause of cancer is unknown, it is also true to say that a lot of information has been gathered on the cause of cancer and the question now remains 'how does it all fit together?' The most significant information so far accumulated is presented in this chapter. The root cause of cancer lies at the molecular genetic level, that much is clear, but the problem however is trying to understand how the changes needed for the cell to become malignant occur, and what exactly happens after that.

Gene changes (or the development of a gene **mutation**) occur as a result of either errors in **mitosis** (or cell division, see p. 8) or as a result of an insult (or injury) caused by some kind of external agent, either viral, chemical or radiation. The terms used in this book include **carcinogen** [noun] (adjective = *carcinogenic*) (any substance that initiates and promotes cancer formation); **mutagen** [noun] (adjective = *mutagenic*) (any substance that promotes the formation of potentially dangerous changes called mutations in genes) and **teratogen** [noun] (adjective = *teratogenic*) (any substance that crosses the placenta from mother to child during pregnancy and harms the foetus).

The hormones and genetics of growth and cancer

One very vital cellular function that must be controlled by genes is growth. Cells grow both in size (**auxetic** growth, otherwise known as **hypertrophy**) and in numbers (**multiplicative** growth, otherwise known as **hyperplasia**, see p. 26). But the overriding consideration is that cellular growth satisfies the body's needs, and no more. This requires sophisticated signalling to instruct cells when growth is needed, and when it is not. The body needs two main forms of growth:

1 Growth from child to adult, i.e. growing in both size and sophistication.
2 Growth for replacing old dead cells; i.e. making good for wear and tear but not involving size or developmental changes.

Outside of these areas, any further forms of growth are not going to be required and will need to be *switched off* by genes. Cancer is a process where the growth is not only unwanted (i.e. it is not related to the body's needs), but it cannot be switched off, i.e. growth in the tumour has gone out of control.

Hormones and cytokines

Outside the cell, growth is partly triggered by chemical agents, i.e. **hormones** and **cytokines** (Table 2.1), which lock onto cell surface receptors and signal the cell to grow or not to grow. Generally speaking, hormones travel in the blood to all parts of the body, but only affect the cells and organs that have receptors that can bind that hormone, i.e. the **target organs**. Cytokines are chemicals usually related to the immune system that tend to have a more localised effect from one cell to other cells near to where they are released (there are, however, notable exceptions to this). Again, cytokines must bind to cell surface receptors and therefore target only those cells that have the appropriate receptors. **Autocrine** cytokines stimulate growth by binding to receptors on exactly the same cell as the one that produced it. **Paracrine** cytokines stimulate growth in cells other than the cell that produced it. The binding of a growth hormone or cytokine to its surface receptor activates the receptor and causes a signal within the cell that needs to pass to the nucleus to activate the genes (and thus the protein production) that is required for growth (Table 2.1).

Genetics

Within the cell, two types of genes control growth; the **proto-oncogenes**, which are sometimes called a '**c-onc**', a shorthand for the normal cellular version of the gene (see also 'v-onc' on p. 48), and the **tumour suppressor (TS) genes**. The proto-oncogenes code for proteins that are essential for transmitting the growth signal from the activated cell surface receptor to the nucleus. The hormone-bound receptor in turn activates these proteins inside the cell membrane, notably the **G-protein** (Figure 2.1) which then binds **guanosine triphosphate (GTP)**, a high-energy molecule similar to ATP (adenosine triphosphate). These proto-oncogenes (and their protein products) are therefore ultimately responsible for activating other genes in the nucleus that are needed for growth when the external hormone or cytokine signal binds (Figure 2.1). Tumour suppressor genes on the other hand code for proteins responsible for sending signals to the nucleus which block growth gene activation, thus

TABLE 2.1 The hormones, factors and cytokines related to growth in humans

	Origin	*Function*
Hormone		
Growth hormone	Anterior pituitary	Promotes growth and anabolism in normal cells
Thyroid hormones	Thyroid gland	Promotes metabolism essential for normal growth
Insulin	Pancreatic islet (beta-cells)	Promotes glucose uptake by cells (energy source for growth) and promotes protein synthesis
Parathyroid hormone	Parathyroid gland	Regulates bone growth (together with calcitonin) by controlling calcium levels in blood
Calcitonin (or calcitriol)	Thyroid gland	Regulates blood calcium levels (with parathyroid hormone) controlling bone growth
Female oestrogen and male testosterone	Female ovary and male testes	Promotes bone and muscle growth and reproductive development
Cytokine		
Interleukin-2 (Il-2)	T cells	Promotes growth and activates T cells and NK cells
Interleukin-8 (Il-8)	Monocytes	Promotes blood vessel growth
Tumour necrosis factor (TNF)	Macrophages and cytotoxic T cells	Kills tumour cells and slows tumour growth
Fibroblast growth factor (FGF)	Variety of cells	A family of factors stimulating growth in many tissues
Transforming growth factor-β (TGF-β)	Platelets, T cells, endothelium and macrophages	Promotes protein synthesis and thus growth in connective tissues
Growth factor		
Epidermal growth factor (EGF)	Duodenal glands	Promotes stem cell growth and epithelial growth
Insulin-like growth factor	Liver cells	Promotes bone and soft tissue growth
Platelet-derived growth factor (PDGF)	Platelets, smooth muscle cells and macrophages	Promotes growth in fibroblasts, smooth muscle and monocytes

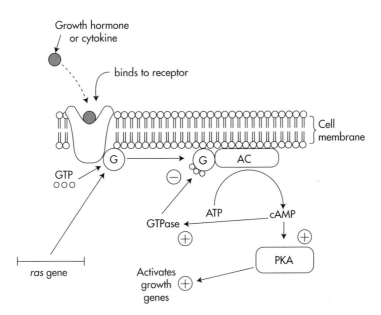

FIGURE 2.1 Growth hormone binding to a receptor on the cell surface activates a G protein on the inside of the membrane. The G protein binds GTP and moves along the membrane and activates the membrane-bound enzyme, adenylyl cyclase (AC). This enzyme creates the secondary messenger cAMP from ATP. cAMP activates (+) GTPase, an enzyme that removes GTP from the G protein, thus deactivating (−) the G protein. cAMP also activates (+) PKA (phosphokinase A) which can cause growth by activating (+) growth genes. G protein is coded for by the *ras* proto-oncogene.

preventing growth from spiralling out of control. Tumour suppressor gene proteins convey signals from surface receptors activated by growth inhibitor hormones or cytokines. It is very much like a car, which needs both an accelerator (to increase speed) and a brake (to decrease speed). Between them the car's speed can be controlled and fine-tuned to meet the demands of the road. Similarly, between proto-oncogenes (the growth accelerator) and tumour suppressor genes (the growth braking system) the cell's growth can be controlled and fine-tuned to meet the demands of the body, as dictated by the hormones and cytokines.

Cancer cells grow beyond the limitations set for normal cells because of serious changes that have occurred in these two gene systems. Genes are, unfortunately, prone to damage and disruption (i.e. damage to the DNA), and genes may then code for abnormal protein products that do not function properly, or, if the damage is extensive enough, they can fail to code for anything, and the protein function is then lost entirely. The cause of DNA damage is discussed later in this chapter (see p. 49), but here we consider the consequence of this damage. First, some DNA changes are called **mutations** (i.e. changes which still allow the gene to function albeit in an abnormal or different manner). Factors that cause mutations are called **mutagens**, or are said to be **mutagenic factors**. Such factors are likely to affect the genes controlling growth and therefore promote cellular changes leading to cancer. Mutations within proto-oncogenes can create highly active genes called **oncogenes**, which accelerate growth in that cell beyond anything the body requires. Mutations within tumour suppressor genes on the other hand can cause the genes to fail, and thus their control over growth is lost. This is the car with the accelerator jammed on and with the brake broken. In this case, the car would accelerate out of control with no opportunity to slow it down. Cellular growth does the same.

Mutation of genes

Changes in gene structure (**mutations**) lead to changes in the structure of the proteins that the genes code for, and these proteins will therefore either malfunction or fail altogether. The simplest mutation that can occur is a **point mutation** (see Figure 2.2A), where one base on the DNA is lost and replaced by a different base. An example of this might be where a DNA base sequence was normally AAT (i.e. adenine, adenine and thymine, which codes for the amino acid **leucine**) then suffered a point mutation, which may lead to the same sequence being changed to AAA (i.e. three adenines, which codes for the amino acid **phenylalanine**). This is often called a **missense mutation** because the original 'sense' of the codon has been altered to code for a different amino acid. The presence of this different amino acid in the protein causes the protein to malfunction or fail.

Other mutations include:

1 **Translocations**, where parts of two chromosomes are dislodged and swapped to each other's place (see Figure 2.2B), the resulting unions possibly creating an oncogene.
2 **Deletions**, where some DNA is lost entirely causing an incomplete chromosome (see Figure 2.2C), and incomplete or absent protein synthesis related to the missing genes.
3 **Inversions**, where a section of DNA is turned upside down and therefore coded and read backwards, causing disruption of the protein (Figure 2.2D).

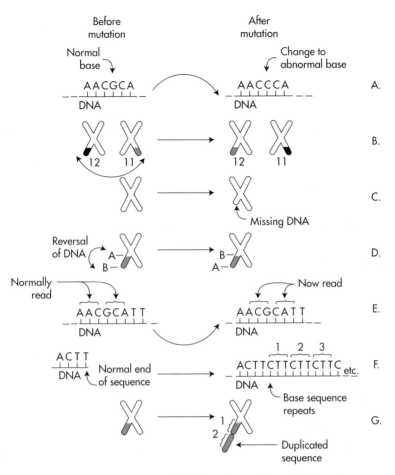

FIGURE 2.2 Genetic mutations. The left column shows before the mutation, the right column shows after the mutation. They are: (A) point mutation (one base replaced by another), (B) translocation (i.e. swapping DNA between two chromosomes), (C) deletion of a DNA sequence, (D) inversion, or reversing DNA backwards, (E) frame shift, where DNA is read incorrectly, (F) base sequence repeat, i.e. the same base repeated over again, (G) duplication, i.e. copying a DNA sequence and adding in on the end. (From Blows 2003, Figure 5.6.)

4 **Frame shifts**, where a gene is read one base out of alignment. For example a sequence like AACGTTCGGA would normally be read as the codons AAC, then GTT, then CGG and so on. In a frame shift to the right it would be read ACG, TTC, GGA and so on. This would mean that each codon is different from the original, and since each codon codes for an amino acid, the resulting protein would have all the wrong amino acids and would therefore fail (Figure 2.2E).

5 **Base sequence repeats** (known as a **stuttering gene**, Figure 2.2F), where the same sequence of three bases (i.e. each codon) is repeated over and over again, perhaps in some cases more than one hundred times (e.g. CTT, CTT, CTT, CTT etc.). The result is a protein with a long chain of the same amino acids in place. There is significant importance attached to this error in some disorders (Blows 2003), but its role in cancer is not fully evaluated.

6 **Duplications**, where some DNA is copied and added on the end of a chromosome (see Figure 2.2G); or **amplification** where there are many additional copies of a DNA stretch found in the cell. Amplification is particularly important as a cause of several human cancers because it often involves extra copies of proto-oncogenes which stimulate cell growth beyond normal or prevent apoptosis (see p. 35).

Many mutations can be repaired, and in Chapter 1 there is discussion about DNA repair in relation to the cell cycle (see p. 12). Chapter 1 also shows what happens to a cell when the damage is irreparable, a process called **apoptosis** (see p. 13). Sometimes, however, a cell survives even when the damage could not be repaired, and it continues to pass round the cell cycle, including mitosis. All the future daughter cells derived from this original cell will then carry copies of the mutation, and this gene error will be added to the accumulation over time of a number of gene errors within a single cell. This is even more likely to happen if the gene mutation occurs in any of the three tumour suppressor genes that help to control the cell cycle, i.e. the *TP53* gene, *RB1* gene and *CDKN2A* gene (see p. 12). It is necessary for at least two of these genes to be inactivated before the cell grows out of control.

TP53 is a tumour suppressor gene that is found on chromosome 17 (location 17p13.1). It codes for the protein **p53** which has some control over the process of monitoring DNA for its integrity and initiates repair if needed (see p. 13). If any mutation occurs within the gene *TP53* itself, this monitoring and repair process fails to function properly, and the cell may survive when it should not. The result is that the cell will carry that gene mutation into the subsequent cell populations that are formed from it by mitosis. Estimates put the number of human cancers that have a *TP53* genetic error in tumour cells as being 50 to 70%, including sporadic (i.e. not restricted to particular families) cases of breast, cervical, colorectal, skin, lung, bladder, ovarian, liver and bone cancers.

A similar tumour suppressor gene (called the *RB1* gene found on chromosome 13 at 13q14) codes for the **pRb** protein, a powerful growth inhibitory molecule (see p. 13). As seen in Chapter 1, the pRB protein halts the cell in G_1 of the cell cycle, and this controls any further growth. Mutation of the *RB1* gene causes failure of pRB protein which then allows growth to continue out of control. The primary tumour involved in *RB1* mutations is a malignancy of the eye called **retinoblastoma** from which RB is an abbreviation.

The *CDKN2A* gene is on chromosome 9 (at 9p21) and codes for two proteins both of which are involved in cell cycle control; **p16**^{INK4A} and **p19**^{ARF} (see p. 13). Deletion or mutations of this gene can and often do lead to inactivation of the cell cycle control resulting in an increase in mitosis and tumour development.

Major oncogenes

The following are some of the most important proto-oncogenes and their oncogene equivalents (after mutation) that affect the development of human cancers.

The *ras* group of proto-oncogenes

These normally code for proteins that convey growth signals from receptors on the cell surface to the nucleus. On arrival at the nucleus the signal increases gene activation leading to greater protein synthesis, and therefore growth. Hormones from the cell's environment that have bound on to the receptors are the trigger for the signal. About 40% of human cancers have *ras* gene mutations, i.e. the oncogenes **ki-ras** and **N-ras**.

1 *ki-ras* signals excessive growth stimulation across the cell cytoplasm, it is important in various forms of lung, ovarian, colon and pancreatic cancers.
2 *N-ras* does the same as *ki-ras*, and is involved in various forms of leukaemia.

The *myc* group of proto-oncogenes

The *myc* genes code for proteins that act as **transcription factors**. Transcription is the process of producing an RNA copy of the DNA in the nucleus of the cell (the first step for protein synthesis), and transcription factors are proteins which regulate this activity by binding to various sites of the DNA close to the gene being copied. These proteins then promote and accelerate transcription. They mutate to *c-myc*, *N-myc* and *L-myc* oncogenes:

1 The *c-myc* oncogene promotes growth in cells to excess, and is important in leukaemia, breast, stomach and lung cancers.
2 The *N-myc* oncogene is involved in leukaemia, and amplification of *N-myc* is important in childhood **neuroblastoma**.
3 The *L-myc* gene is a factor in human lung cancers.

The *erb-B* proto-oncogene gene family (*erb-B1*, *erb-B2*, *erb-B3* and *erb-B4*)

These code for cell surface receptors which bind growth hormones called **epidermal growth factors** to the cell surface. The *erb-B2* gene (on chromosome 7) is often overexpressed owing to amplification in breast cancers.

The *abl* (or *ABL1*) proto-oncogene (found on chromosome 9 at 9q34.1)

This codes for a protein called a **tyrosine kinase** which is important for activating certain intracellular proteins. These proteins are part of the cell signalling system for growth. The receptor component of the tyrosine kinase on the cell surface binds some growth hormones and cytokines.

It is the deletion of the **SH3 domain** of the *abl* gene (i.e. that part which normally inhibits the tyrosine kinase function) that causes it to become an oncogene. The tyrosine kinase then becomes increasingly active, leading towards malignancy in that cell. The *abl* gene's **SH2 domain** also helps to regulate tyrosine kinase activity, and mutations in this part of the gene cause abnormal tyrosine function.

The *abl* gene is also involved in a particularly well-understood translocation called the **Philadelphia chromosome** (or **Ph¹**). The defect is a 9:22 translocation, i.e. parts of chromosomes 9 and 22 break off and swap places, so a short section of 9 attaches to 22, and part of 22 attaches to 9 (see Figure 4.3, Ph¹ on p. 103 and translocations on p. 38). It is the addition of most of the *abl* gene from chromosome 9 to part of the chromosome 22 known as the *BCR* (**break cluster region**) that creates the Ph¹. Chromosomes break more easily at specific sites (more than 150 breaking sites that can result in malignancy in cells are now known across all the 46 chromosomes). The resulting 9:22

abl–BCR translocation is an oncogene found in 90% of patients with **chronic myeloid leukaemia** (see p. 102).

In addition to those listed here, there are other oncogenes known to be active in cancer development, and almost certainly more to be found.

Gene inheritance

Genes are inherited from one generation to the next through either a dominant or a recessive mechanism. New offspring carry 50% of their genes from their mother, and 50% of their genes from their father. This is why the karyotype (see p. 7) has chromosome *pairs*, one chromosome in each pair from the female parent, the other from the male parent. So the offspring has two copies of each gene, or **alleles** (see p. 6). Which copy will be used to provide the characteristics of the offspring, mum's or dad's (or put in genetic terms, which allele will be expressed into the **phenotype**)? First, phenotype means the body. When you look at another person you see their phenotype (their body characteristics, like hair colour). The genes responsible for the phenotype are decided by which genes are **dominant** (i.e. always contribute to the phenotype when present at one or both alleles) or **recessive** (i.e. they only contribute to the phenotype when present at *both* alleles, meaning no dominant gene is present). The inheritance patterns for dominant and recessive genes (and therefore genetic disorders like some cancers) can be seen in Figure 2.3.

Chromosomal abnormalities

Abnormalities in malignant cells are not confined to the genetic level. As the Philadelphia chromosome (Ph[1]) demonstrates, chromosomes can be abnormal as well, and such abnormality therefore involves many genes. The normal **karyotype** (see p. 7) consists of 46 chromosomes, but malignant cells can have very different, and grossly abnormal karyotypes, i.e. the numbers and types of chromosomes are abnormal. A normal karyotype has 23 pairs of chromosomes, one of each pair inherited from the mother, the other pair from the father. **Aneuploidy** means an abnormal number of chromosomes, either too many (47 or more) or more rarely too few (45 or less). Too many chromosomes is usually caused by a **trisomy** (i.e. three chromosomes instead of the two in a pair), and too few chromosomes is usually caused by a **monosomy** (i.e. one chromosome

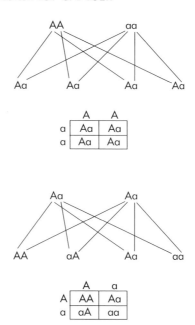

FIGURE 2.3 (Above) Dominant gene inheritance pattern in cross-over and punnet square. One parent has both dominant genes (AA), the other has both recessive genes (aa) and all the four offspring have at least one dominant gene. (Below) Recessive gene inheritance pattern in cross-over and punnet square. The parents are both mixed dominant and recessive genes (Aa). The four offspring are split, three with at least one dominant gene, but one with both recessive genes (aa). (From Blows 2003, Figures 5.2 and 5.3).

instead of the two in a pair). **Euploidy** means that the karyotype number is exactly a multiple of the normal 46 chromosomes. These 46 chromosomes are known as the **diploid** condition (also abbreviated to **2n**, where **n** is the normal **haploid** state of 23 chromosomes found in ova or sperm). Multiples of **n** would be **3n** (**triploid**, with 69 chromosomes) or **4n** (**tetraploid**, with 92 chromosomes). Triploid and tetraploid are grossly abnormal states and are often associated with malignancy in a cell. These abnormal states indicate a general instability of chromosomes occurring as part of the onset of malignancy, so that chromosome division during mitosis is unpredictable and results in these gross errors, including excessive DNA production.

As an example, Table 2.2 lists the grossly abnormal karyotype seen in one particular cervical cancer cell (chromosomes 8 to 18 shown)(Weinberg 1996).

TABLE 2.2 An example of chromosomal (8 to 18) abnormalities in a cancer cell

Chromosome number	Normal cell chromosomes	One particular cancer cell chromosomes
8	2	5
9	2	5
10	2	2
11	2	2
12	2	4
13	2	1
14	2	3
15	2	3
16	2	3
17	2	4
18	2	4
Total	22 chromosomes	36 chromosomes

Environmental factors: carcinogens

Carcinogens are anything that both initiates and promotes changes in the cell leading to cancer. Both **initiation** and **promotion** are necessary to cause cancerous changes (known as **malignancy**) to occur. Initiation is the original DNA damage (or gene mutation) that occurs, but this alone is not enough to turn the cell malignant. The cell may be able to correct the problem (using DNA repair enzymes), or even die rather than perpetuate the problem. Cell death in these circumstances is called **apoptosis** (see p. 13), and this ensures survival of only those cells with normal intact and viable DNA. It is quite possible that we produce many cells each day that have genetic mutations but they do not go on to become malignant cells because the problem is corrected or the cell dies. In cases like this, initiation has failed due to the lack of *promotion*.

Promotion is the second effect of the carcinogen. Here, the original damage is sustained by repeating the damage many times, over a period of time, until the cell can no longer cope with the onslaught, and the DNA mutation is allowed to persist, causing a permanent change in that cell. That cell now stands a good chance of becoming malignant. Promotion takes time to achieve, often years, and this is why repeated exposure to the carcinogen is needed throughout that time span to sustain the damage and therefore cause the cancer. Just one or a few exposures to the carcinogen are usually not enough to sustain promotion, and thus will not cause cancer. This is one reason why smoking is such a disastrous habit to acquire. Smokers are deliberately exposing themselves to the same carcinogens each and every day, over and over again, usually for years, ensuring both initiation and promotion of malignancy in their lung and other cells. They are doing exactly what is needed to cause cancer.

So what are these carcinogens that are damaging our DNA? Many factors in the human environment have the potential to promote the onset of malignancy in a cell. Such factors can be classified into:

1 Living organisms, usually **viruses**, which can infect tissues and cells and leave their own genetic 'fingerprints' behind, affecting the way the cells' genetics function.
2 **Chemicals** of many types can provoke genetic changes by irritation or direct damage to the cell, thus becoming carcinogens.
3 **Radiation** of various forms which can disrupt the DNA and thus seriously disturb gene function.

Living organisms: the virion

A **virion** is a completely intact virus, just as it would exist in the environment. Basically, virions consist of a protein outer shell surrounding a core of nucleic acid, either **deoxyribonucleic acid (DNA)** or **ribonucleic acid (RNA)**, never both together. This makes a useful means of classifying viruses, i.e. into DNA viruses and RNA viruses. The lack of a true cellular structure and the absence of the typical features of living organisms make it difficult to place the virus as something that is alive in the full sense of the word. Yet it can replicate and perform other functions, but only within the confines of a living host cell where it uses the cell's enzymes and raw materials to produce new virions.

Viruses can cause cancer (Figure 2.4) although the majority of human cancers have not been demonstrated to have a viral origin. Of the two viral groups, the RNA virions have very little effect on human cancers (although they are involved to a greater extent in animal tumours), except for the **human immunodeficiency virus (HIV)** and the **human T-cell lymphotropic virus (HTLV)**. However, a wider range of DNA virions are involved in the cause of human cancers. Examples of those virions that do have a role to play in the cause of human cancers are:

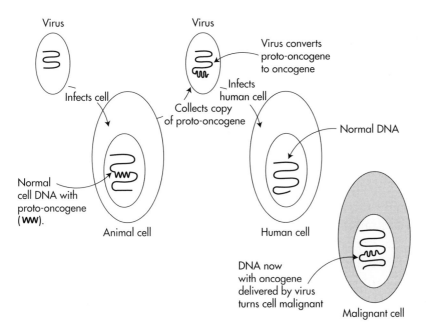

FIGURE 2.4 A virus causes cancer by first infecting an animal cell. The new virions produced there pick up one of the animal proto-oncogenes and incorporate it into the viral genetic material. The virus then converts the proto-oncogene to an oncogene (mutation), and then infects a human cell. The oncogene is implanted into the human DNA and it triggers malignancy in that cell.

1 *Epstein–Barr virus* (*Human herpes virus 4, HHV4,* a DNA virus) causes **Burkitt lymphoma** (a tumour of the lower jaw) and may be involved in **Hodgkin's disease** (see p. 107);

2 *Human papillomavirus* (HPV, a DNA virus) causes cervical and skin cancers.

3 *Hepatitis B* (*HBV*, a DNA virus) causes liver cancer (Murray *et al.* 2002).

4 *Human herpes virus 8* (*HHV8*, a DNA virus) causes **Kaposi's sarcoma**, a rare skin neoplasm that can spread to become a lymphoma (see also HIV below).

5 *Human T-cell lymphotropic virus-1* and *-2* (*HTLV-1*; *HTLV-2*, both RNA viruses) are retroviruses capable of causing leukaemia (see p. 98).

6 *Human immunodeficiency virus* (*HIV*, an RNA virus) weakens the immune system, and this increases the risk of malignancies caused by other viruses in association with the onset of **acquired immunodeficiency syndrome** (**AIDS**); notably in relation to

Kaposi's sarcoma (HHV8, see above), **non-Hodgkin's lymphoma** (see p. 108) and **Epstein–Barr virus-related lymphoma** (see above).

7 *Herpes simplex virus type-2* (*Human herpesvirus 2*, *HHV2*, a DNA virus) causes cervical cancer (Atlas 1994).

This list identifies different human herpes virus (HHV) by a number system (e.g. HHV2, HHV4 etc.), the numbers not shown are those types not involved in human cancers.

For a virus to cause cancer the infection has to be prolonged because the immune system was unable to eliminate the organism. Viruses fall into two main groups, the **DNA** viruses (those with DNA at their core) and the **RNA** viruses (those with RNA at their core). Chronic unresolved infections that may cause cells to become malignant are associated mostly with the DNA viruses and the *retroviruses*. Retroviruses are so called because they have RNA cores that are used by the virus to create a DNA copy, a process that is backward to the normal process of generating an RNA copy from DNA (*retro* = backward).

Virions cause cancer by first invading a cell, a process which usually requires the virion to lock onto a receptor on the host cell surface. At some point here, either before cell entry, or immediately after, the virion must de-coat, i.e. strip off the outer protein coat and release the nucleic acid core into the cell's cytoplasm. A number of DNA viruses then proceed to copy their core DNA (or the retrovirus copies its core RNA to form DNA) and incorporate this copy into the host cell's own DNA. The host cell now has a stretch of viral DNA (i.e. all the viral genes, now called a **provirus**) within the cell's own genes (Figure 2.5). When activated by the cell's mechanisms of replication, the provirus will code for viral proteins, which are then assembled inside the cell as new virions. This is how many viral infections happen, but here we are asking the question how does that cause cancer. Occasionally, the new virions produced may take on board a copy of a gene from the host cell that controls growth, i.e. a gene called a **proto-oncogene** (see p. 35). These genes control growth in the cell, but the copy taken by the virion can be altered (or mutated) to a form called an **oncogene** (in a virus this is known as a **v-onc**, or viral oncogene) (see p. 41 for an explanation of how oncogenes cause cancer). The virion is not only responsible for this change, but it can also be spread by the virus through cross-infection to other people, and lodge in the new host cell. The provirus will

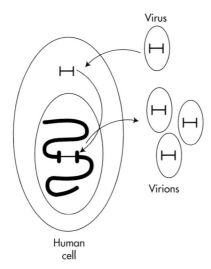

Virus

Virions

Human
cell

FIGURE 2.5 The creation of a viral provirus. The virion infects the cell and releases the viral genetic material. Only DNA can be inserted into DNA, so if the viral genetic material is RNA, a DNA copy is made first. The viral DNA is incorporated into the host DNA within the nucleus of the cell. Here it is called a provirus. Activation of this provirus causes production of new virions and these leave the cell, taking copies of the viral genetic material with them.

then introduce a potentially cancer-causing oncogene (the v-onc) into the new host. Examples of this process have also been recorded where a virion has introduced oncogenes into human cells which were originally animal proto-oncogenes, as a result of cross-infection from non-humans to humans.

Chemical agents

Chemicals are everywhere about us; i.e. they are in our food, in the air we breathe, in the cosmetics and cleansing agents we use, in the soil and food-growing agents we use (like pesticides), in our drugs and medicines, in our building materials, and so on. The list is endless, and that is because everything around us, including ourselves, is made of chemicals.

Most of these chemicals are totally harmless, many are even essential for our existence (like food, see p. 286), but a number of chemicals are harmful, and some actually promote cancer formation in living cells. Some are **free radicals**, highly reactive chemicals that can damage our cells.

Pollutants in our atmosphere are responsible more for respiratory diseases like asthma and bronchitis, and heart disease than cancer, but there are pollutants that may provoke malignant changes in the lungs or elsewhere.

Benzene

This is released from both burnt and unburned fuels and is one of the top ten carcinogenic agents. About 78% comes from petrol exhaust, another 9% from diesel exhaust, and another 7% from the evaporation of fuel from vehicles. Air pollution levels in heavy traffic areas rise to peak values between 8 am and midday, then again from 4 pm to 8 pm (corresponding to rush hour traffic volumes), especially during the winter months. It is also a component of tar in tobacco (see p. 51).

Particulates

These are tiny particles of matter than can react with other gases to form obnoxious compounds, and can penetrate deeply into the lungs when inhaled. Many particulates are **polycyclic aromatic hydro-carbons (PAH)**, which are known mutagenic agents (i.e. they cause gene mutations), or **nitrated polycyclic aromatic hydrocarbons (nitro-PAH)**, which are even worse mutagenic agents. Particulates come in several sizes, e.g. PM10s are particulates 10 micrometres (μm, or one thousandth of a millimetre) or smaller, down to PM2.5s which are one-quarter of the size of PM10s. Obviously, the smaller the particle the deeper it can get into the lung, and therefore the more cellular damage it can do. Diesel exhaust is the source of two powerful cancer-causing particulates, **1,8-dinitropyrene** and **3-nitrobenzanthrone**, the latter of the two being a nitro-PAH produced in much larger quantities when the diesel engine is working under a heavy load (Pearce 1997). Both these substances cause mutations in genes that can lead to malignancy.

Of course, air pollution is considered mostly to be a problem derived from vehicular exhaust and industry, but in cities where aircraft fly over the jet engines also cause very large amounts of pollution. An example is London, where jets dump 2 million tons of carbon dioxide, 13 thousand tons of nitrogen and 159 tons of particulates every year.

Smoking

Cigarette smoke contains **tar** that causes lung irritation and ultimately lung cancer. Tar is deposited in the lungs and paralyses the
cilia, the delicate hair-like structures that protect the lungs from
inhaled particles. Its sticky nature allows others dangerous chemicals
to stick to it and thus accumulate in the lungs.

Smoking in women is increasing, and there is a corresponding rise
in lung cancer in women. Mortality rates for women with lung cancer
as the cause of death rose dramatically across the world between
1960 and 1980; increasing by 100% in Japan, Norway, Poland, Sweden
and the UK, by more than 200% in Australia, Denmark and New
Zealand, and by more than 300% in the USA and Canada. Passive
smoking also increases the risk of lung cancer in non-smokers by
26%, to the tune of about 600 cases every year in the UK. Passive
smokers absorb a chemical called **4-(methylnitrosamino)-1-(3-
pyridyl)-1-butanone** (known as **NNK**), which is the by-product of
burning nicotine, and therefore only found in cigarettes. It causes a
type of lung cancer called an **adenocarcinoma** (see p. 157), which is
common in passive smokers. And mothers who smoke near their
babies put the infants' lives at risk. Approximately 80 cot deaths per
year in the UK are caused by the infants' passive smoking from their
parents' cigarettes.

About 30% of all deaths per year are caused by smoking-related
diseases, compared with 2% of deaths caused by air pollution.
Lung cancer has reached epidemic proportions worldwide, with
about 660,000 new cases of lung cancer occurring each year, which
corresponds to the world's increased tobacco usage. Smoking
causes the presence of activated receptors on the surface of lung
cells that bind various growth hormones, including **gastrin-
releasing peptide** (**GRP**). These receptors are normally active
during lung development in foetal life, and are not expected to be
active after that. Long-term heavy smoking reactivates these receptors and this may increase the risk of lung cancer. It appears that
once re-activated, these receptors remain active years after giving
up the habit, indicating permanent changes in the lung.

And it is not just lung cancer that is the problem, smoking has now
been directly linked as a cause of cancers of the mouth, pharynx, larynx, tongue, oesophagus, urinary bladder, cervix, stomach, pancreas,
breast and kidney. It also causes a range of non-cancer diseases such
as heart disease, strokes, bronchitis, asthma and vascular diseases.

Table 2.3 shows the major carcinogenic agents found in tobacco smoke.

In all, cigarettes contain a deadly cocktail of over 4,000 toxic substances (Figure 2.6). In addition to those noted above, the list includes **arsenic**, **hydrogen cyanide**, **toluene** and **acrolein** (all in the tar), **acetone**, **ammonia**, **carbon monoxide** (a gas that deprives blood of its oxygen), **lead** and **mercury** (two highly toxic metals), and of course **nicotine** (the agent that causes the addiction to cigarettes). Smoking is now known to be the biggest avoidable cause of disease and early death in humans. Globally, around 4 million people die from smoking each year (that is one person every eight seconds), and if this trend continues the figure will rise to over 6 million smoking-related deaths per year by 2030. Unless this problem is tackled head on it is difficult to see how any progress can be made in conquering cancer.

TABLE 2.3 Carcinogenic agents found in tobacco smoke

Carcinogenic agent	Notes
Benzo(*a*)pyrene	A PAH component of tar in tobacco (PAH see p. 50)
Dibenza(*a*)anthracene	Another PAH component of tar in tobacco
Nickel	A metal linked to lung cancer
Cadmium	A poisonous metal, dangerous when inhaled. It causes kidney damage and increased risk of cancers
Radioactive polonium	A breakdown product of radium with its own radioactive half-life of 138 days. Most sources of radioactivity are linked to cancer
Hydrazine	A toxic compound and possible carcinogen. Hydrazine sulphate may reverse the effects of cachexia, but this remains controversial (cachexia, see p. 308)
Ethyl carbamate (urethane)	Used in the plastics industry, this is a known carcinogen
Formaldehyde	A component of the tar in tobacco. It is used to preserve dead bodies and organs. It is a carcinogen
Nitrogen oxides (or oxides of nitrogen)	Nitric oxide (NO) and nitrogen dioxide (NO_2), collectively known at NO_x (or NOX), both respiratory irritants now linked to cancer
Nitrosodimethylamine	Poison when inhaled, carcinogenic and teratogenic (i.e. it crosses the placenta and harms the foetus)

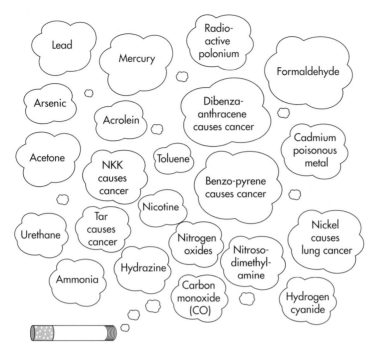

FIGURE 2.6 What the smoker is inhaling.

A recently reported British study (Anon. 2004) of nearly 34,500 males (possibly one of the biggest research sample sizes ever !) that was conducted over 50 years beginning in 1951 (and one of the longest) shows quite clearly the following:

1 That half of all smokers will die from their habit.
2 That smoking *shortens your life expectancy by 10 years*.
3 That stopping smoking at any age improves health and life expectancy.
4 That smoking is now recognised as the *top health hazard in the world*.

Surely, the case for *not* smoking is now overwhelming (Anon. 2002).

Radiation

Radiation is another environmental factor which we cannot escape, but we do have some power to reduce exposure to a minimum. We are constantly subject to what is termed **background radiation** (Figure 2.7), i.e. natural radiation sources which between them provide a constant level of radiation to which we are all unwittingly

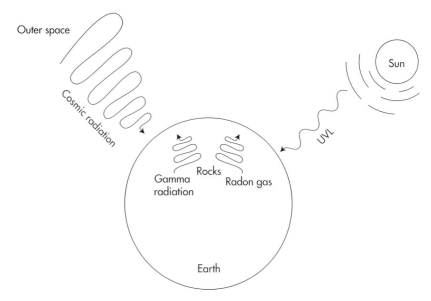

FIGURE 2.7 Sources of natural (background) radiation. UVL = ultraviolet light.

exposed. The main sources of background radiation are sunlight (i.e. *ultraviolet light* from sunshine), radiation from the *rocks* beneath us, *radon gas* and *cosmic radiation*. Radiation comes in four main forms.

Alpha (α) radiation

Alpha particles are two neutrons and two protons combined. Such 'large' particles (by atomic standards) are weak and relatively slow, and are incapable of penetrating skin. Therefore, alpha particle radiation is only considered to be dangerous to people if it is eaten. An example of alpha particle radiation is that given off by the radioactive material used in smoke alarms.

Beta (β) radiation

These are high-energy electrons, which are much smaller than alpha particles and are very much faster moving. They are therefore harder to stop than alpha. Unlike alpha particles, electrons technically have no mass, and are therefore capable of deep penetration of human tissues. This makes them more dangerous to health when people are exposed to them.

Electrons, the outer components of atoms, are capable of gaining or losing energy. The more energy electrons gain the faster and more excited they become, moving rapidly into positions further away from the nucleus of the atom. Eventually the electron gains enough energy to fly off the atom and become a free entity. It is these free electrons, travelling at great speeds, that are beta radiation. With high speeds and high energy, coupled with no mass, the electrons have considerable penetration and damage ability.

Electromagnetic radiation

This is part of the **electromagnetic spectrum** (Figure 2.8), which is a way of classifying a particular group of energies that occur in a waveform rather than particles. Many forms of these energies exist, as shown by the spectrum, including *light*, *X-rays* and *radio waves*. Being a wave means that it has a pattern of peaks and troughs (or ups and downs), in the same way that ripples on a pond have high points (the peaks of water) and low points (the troughs of water). And like pond ripples, electromagnetic waves move outward from the source, but at much greater speeds than pond ripples. The distance measured from the top of one peak to the top of the next peak is the **wavelength**. Obviously, the shorter the wavelength the more waves will be able to pack into a metre. This is the **frequency**, the shorter the wavelength the greater is the frequency (i.e. each peak arrives at its destination more frequently if the wavelength is short). Conversely, the longer the wavelength the lower the frequency (each peak arrives far less frequently if the wavelength is long). It is the difference in the wavelengths (and thus in the frequency) that distinguishes one waveform from the next (Figure 2.9). In this spectrum different forms of waves are presented according to their *wavelengths* (measured in

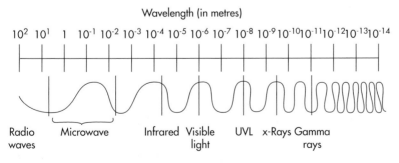

FIGURE 2.8 The electromagnetic spectrum.

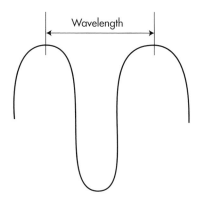

FIGURE 2.9 The measurement of a wavelength is the distance from one peak to the next.

metres [**m**] or subdivisions of a metre, like **centimetres** [**cm**]), or the *frequency* (measured in **hertz** [**Hz**], or variables of this, e.g. **mega-hertz** [**MHz**]) with high frequency at one end of the spectrum, low frequency at the other. Long wavelength (low frequency) waves include radio waves, followed by radar waves. The frequency increases considerably as we pass through infrared and visible light. Very high frequency waves include ultraviolet light, X-rays and gamma rays (notice the different wavelengths between, for example, radio waves, visible light and X-rays in Figure 2.8). Along with increasing frequency we also see an increase in the levels of energy. The high frequency of the ultraviolet light, and even higher frequencies of X-rays and gamma rays, means that these waves have very high energies compared with radio waves, and this means greater penetration of tissues and potential tissue damage.

Gamma radiation (or **gamma rays**) has an extremely high frequency, (10^{-10} cm, or 10^{-12} m), i.e. a wavelength of only 1/10,000,000,000 cm long (one ten thousand millionth of a centimetre from one peak to the next !), and therefore it has extremely high energy, which is what makes it dangerous to cells and tissues. It has the high level of energy required to dislodge electrons from atoms making it a source of *ionising radiation* (see p. 57), which is what happens inside the cells when exposed to this source. Such ionising radiation causes damage to DNA and therefore increases the cell's risk of turning malignant. Gamma radiation is found naturally coming from rocks and soil, from radon gas and as cosmic radiation from the sun and outer space.

All these are natural background sources of radiation to which we are all subjected (see p. 54). Man-made sources of gamma radiation include X-rays and nuclear contamination from atomic energy plants or nuclear weapons. Fortunately we can avoid X-rays unless absolutely necessary (see p. 61), and nuclear fallout is extremely rare (nuclear fallout accounts for less than 1% of a typical human lifetime exposure to gamma rays).

X-rays have a wavelength that is longer than gamma rays, but between 10^{-9} to 10^{-10} m it is still very short, and is thus a high-energy ionising radiation. This makes exposure dangerous, and should be kept to a minimum (see Figure 2.8, and medical X-rays on p. 61). **Ultraviolet light (UVL)** is a longer wavelength still (10^{-8} m) but is also part of the more hazardous forms of ionising radiation, and again exposure to it should be strictly limited. Sunlight is the most important natural source of UVL but man-made sources, like sun-beds, are also potentially dangerous if used for too long. The big danger is skin cancer since it is the skin that receives the main dosage (see p. 247), but UVL also causes premature ageing of the skin. Protective skin lotions and wearing protective clothing helps to filter out the harmful UVL when exposure is inevitable, but deliberate sun bathing or use of the sun-bed should be avoided or limited. Sun exposure should be restricted to those parts of the day when sunshine is less intense.

Visible and **infrared light** are forms of non-ionising radiation, having not enough energy to release electrons from atoms. Visible light has a wavelength of 10^{-6} m, and infrared between 10^{-4} and 10^{-5} m (Figure 2.8).

Electromagnetic radiation with a wavelength between 10^{-2} m (or 1 cm) and 10 m is called **microwave** radiation (Figure 2.8). Microwaves are produced inside a **magnetron**, and this can be another potential source of radiation. Microwave ovens (wavelength of about $10^{-2} \times 20$ m, or 20 cm,) and mobile phones (wavelengths from 22 cm up to about 3 m or more) both use microwaves. These wavelength values fall into the non-ionising category for radiation, which means that they are less damaging to cellular structures, but are still a potential health hazard and should be used with caution. Microwaves heat water by increasing the energy of the water molecules, and this is the basis by which the microwave oven works to heat food. It is also the reason why mobile phones have received a great deal of interest in terms of their health hazard potential. The brain contains water and extensive use of the mobile phone may raise the temperature of this water. Whilst mobile phone manufacturers and distributors support their product as safe for human use the reports of brain tumours associated with extensive mobile phone use cannot be ignored. Claims that radiation levels used in mobile phones are well below radiation guidelines should be treated with caution, because it very much depends on the length of exposure, and ultimately the only really safe level of radiation is zero. *Anything* above this carries some degree of risk, and should not be considered as totally safe.

Some people spend long periods talking on their mobile phone, and clearly this excessive exposure to microwave radiation can only be bad for the brain cells adjacent to the transmitter. Some people claim to have suffered memory losses, dizziness, fatigue and headaches, even fits, when they use their mobile phone for long periods. This shows that the radiation is having some adverse affect on the brain, and it is a warning sign that further brain exposure to mobile phone radiation could lead to more serious consequences, like malignancy. Limiting the use of the mobile phone to an absolute minimum is clearly a sensible precaution, and some people do keep mobile phones for emergencies only. One group of people who should *never* use mobile phones, other than in extreme emergencies, are children. The growing and developing brain is more prone to potential radiation effects that the adult mature brain. And adverse effects on the developing brain may be permanent, so again a sensible precaution would be not to issue children with mobile phones as routine. Given that children do not need the phone at school, and that the vast majority of calls that are made (by adults and children alike) are actually not necessary (i.e. they are made solely because the phone is conveniently there), it makes sense to avoid this form of radiation. However, with the continuing growth of sales in the mobile phone industry, it would appear that most people are prepared to take the risk, and we are therefore likely to see increased problems, like brain tumours, as a consequence.

Some people can be seen both smoking and talking on the mobile phone at the same time. This **'fag-fone folly'** seems to be courting double dangers, the twin carcinogenic hazards of cigarette tar and mobile phone radiation, at the same time. This is throwing all caution to the wind, and shows that these individuals appear to have no regard for their future health at all. It is a classic example of the reference made to biology identified in the Preface to this book, i.e. not being seen as applicable to our daily lives (see p. xiv).

Neutron radiation

This is a stream of high-energy neutrons, i.e. particles from the nucleus of an atom that have no charge (neither positive nor negative). To obtain such particles the nucleus must be split (called **fission**, or 'splitting the atom'), an event that happens in nuclear reactors or nuclear explosions. This makes exposure for most people remote. Neutron radiation is more penetrating that alpha or beta radiation, but less penetrating than gamma radiation. However, because the neutron particle has a large mass (in atomic terms) it is considerably damaging.

The natural sources of background radiation (see p. 54) are made up of these different types of radiation. The *soil* and *rocks* are both a source of generally low levels of gamma radiation; the amount depends entirely on the nature of the rocks beneath you. Granite, and other forms of igneous (fire-formed) rocks, may yield a slightly higher proportion of radiation than sedimentary rocks like clay, which may yield none at all. Some rocks may test for higher levels of radiation if they have been contaminated with radioactive elements during the time they were deposited. Soil is derived from the underlying rocks (with organic matter mixed in) and is therefore also a potential source of radiation, particularly if the soil is derived from subterranean igneous rocks.

  Radon gas is a radioactive product of the decay process of **uranium** (Figure 2.10). Radioactive decay means the breakdown of

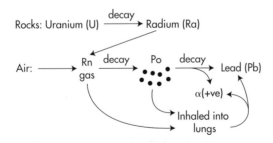

FIGURE 2.10 Uranium (U) is found in certain rocks. Over time it decays (i.e. loses parts of the nucleus of the atom) and changes to radium (Ra). Radium does not remain as such in rock since further decay causes it to change to radon (Rn), a gas that leaks from the earth into the atmosphere. Radon can be inhaled into the lungs in an enclosed space. Further decay of radon leads to polonium (Po) which can attach to dust, water vapour or air particles, and can also be inhaled. Decay of polonium releases positively charged alpha (α) particles, resulting, ultimately in the formation of lead (Pb).

atoms, releasing sub-atomic particles, i.e. **α** (**alpha**) and **β** (**beta**) as part of the process. These released particles become the radiation (see p. 54). Radon gas comes from the soil, and thus ultimately from the uranium in rocks, particularly concentrating in volcanic rocks (e.g. granite), or limestones and sandstones. When liberated into the open-air, radon gas disperses with no harmful effects. In fact radon gas itself causes no health risk to humans from the outside of the body. However, in enclosed spaces, such as in a house, it is potentially more harmful as it is then breathed in. Radon itself decays to form radioactive 'daughters' which release alpha particles. Again these are not harmful from outside the body, but if the radon daughters are inhaled directly into the lung it increases the risk of lung cancers. The UK national average of radon activity in houses is 20 becquerels per cubic metre, causing a lifetime risk of lung cancer of 1 in 300 people. Action is needed if the level in a house rises to 200 becquerels per cubic metre; the equivalent to a lifetime lung cancer risk of 1 person in 30. One of the radioactive daughters of radon gas (a solid particle called **polonium**)(see Figure 2.10) attaches itself to dust, water or smoke particles in the air, and this facilitates its inhalation into the lungs.

Cosmic radiation comes from outer space. This term includes several different elements contributing to an overall radiation effect. These elements include atomic particle matter (made up from approximately 2% electrons, 85% protons, 12% helium nuclei and 1% heavier nuclei), photons (packages of electromagnetic light energy, particularly ultraviolet light which is shorter wavelength than visible or infrared, and therefore has more energy)(Figure 2.11), and higher energy particles of various kinds including microwaves (see p. 57) and X-rays (see p. 57). At ground level cosmic radiation accounts for about 10% of the background radiation, but it increases in intensity with altitude because the atmosphere (which affords some protection) gets thinner as altitude is increased and thus provides less protection. This causes an increased risk of radiation exposure to flight crew of aircraft who are exposed to this increase on a daily basis, and those who fly long distances regularly. The odd flight here or there is not a problem, but regular air travellers are warned that they are exposing themselves to greater radiation levels (sometimes 100 to 300 times more than that encountered at sea level), therefore, the more you fly, or the higher you fly, the greater the risks. Aircraft are not built to protect the occupants against this important radiation source for very practical reasons. Lead shielding

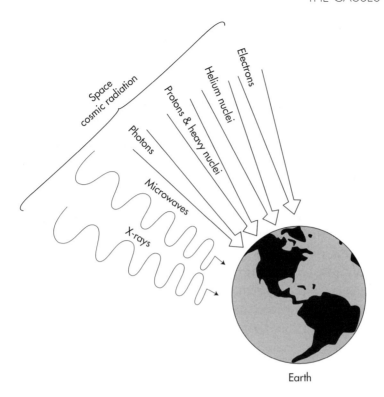

Earth

FIGURE 2.11 Cosmic radiation is a collection of atomic particles, photons, microwaves and X-rays.

is the only truly effective protection and the weight of lead makes this economically impossible. Because this radiation is ionising (see p. 57), exposure to it causes damage to deoxyribonucleic acid (DNA), which makes up our genes (see p. 4), and this predisposes the cell to increased risk of malignancy, especially those cells that reproduce rapidly like blood cells, sperm and ova. Some studies have shown air-crew to have higher than average numbers of cancers, including cancer of the brain, prostate, skin, breast, colon and leukaemia (Kahn 1999). This is also a major problem for astronauts, who are likely to suffer the greatest risks of all, and one that needs addressing before any long manned space flights are attempted.

Artificial sources of radiation are very important to consider because exposure to these sources should, at least in theory, be able to be reduced to a minimum or eliminated entirely. What humans produce humans should be able to avoid. In practical terms this is not always possible, and so artificial sources of radiation must be part of the equation when calculating risks. The use of X-rays in medicine has proven extremely valuable in the diagnostics of many disorders, both in the standard X-ray form seen in hospitals associated with departments like accident and emergency, and as the newer forms of X-ray equipment, such as **computerised axial tomography** (**CAT** or **CT**) scans (Coutts 2002). Whatever their form, medical X-rays should be used only when essential, and then with great caution (Blows 2002). X-rays are measured using a unit called the **rad** (which stands for radiation absorbed dose), whilst the **standard international** (**SI**) equivalent of this is the **Gray** (**Gy**), the unit for measuring the X-ray energy absorbed per unit mass of body tissue. This is the energy that causes the tissue damage, one Gray being one joule of absorbed energy per kilogram of body tissue. One standard chest X-ray delivers about as much energy to the tissues as does background radiation over ten days or so.

All electrical equipment produces electromagnetic radiation to some extent, particularly televisions and visual display units (VDU), and sitting in front of these for too long, or too close, is not good for the health.

Key points

Genes

- Mutations are errors in genes caused by an external agent called a carcinogen, e.g. viral, chemical or radiation.
- A teratogen is any substance that crosses the placenta from mother to child during pregnancy and harms the foetus.
- Cells grow both in size (hypertrophy) and in numbers (hyperplasia).
- Cellular growth must satisfy the body's needs, and no more.
- Growth is normally required from child to adult and for replacing old dead cells.
- Outside the cell, growth is partly triggered by hormones and cytokines.
- Two types of genes control growth; the proto-oncogenes ('c-onc') and tumour suppressor (TS) genes.
- Proto-oncogenes code for proteins essential for transmitting the growth signal to the nucleus.
- Tumour suppressor genes code for proteins that send signals to the nucleus to block growth.

- Mutations in proto-oncogenes create oncogenes which accelerate growth in that cell.
- *ras, erb, myc* and *abl* are all proto-oncogenes that mutate in various cancers.
- The gene mutation may occur in any of the three tumour suppressor genes that control the cell cycle, i.e. the *TP53* gene, *RB1* gene and *CDKN2A* gene.
- Aneuploidy is an abnormal number of chromosomes (often seen in cancer cells). This is usually caused by a trisomy (three chromosomes replace two) or by a monosomy (one chromosome replaces two).
- Both initiation and promotion are necessary to cause cancerous changes in a cell.

Carcinogenesis

- Carcinogens are anything that both initiates and promotes changes in the cell leading to cancer.
- Viruses, chemicals of many types and radiation can be carcinogens.
- The virus can mutate a cell proto-oncogene (c-onc) to form a viral oncogene (v-onc).
- A number of chemicals promote cancer formation in living cells by damaging DNA.
- Cigarette smoke contains tar that causes lung irritation and lung cancer.
- Cigarettes contain a deadly cocktail of over 4,000 toxic substances.

Radiation

- Radiation comes in four main forms, alpha (α) (two neutrons and two protons combined), beta (β) (high-energy electrons), electromagnetic (wave form) and neutron (high-energy neutrons).
- X-rays have a longer wavelength than gamma rays, but are still high-energy ionising radiation.
- X-rays are measured in units called the rad (radiation absorbed dose).
- The standard international (SI) equivalent of this is the Gray (Gy), the unit for measuring the X-ray energy absorbed per unit mass of body tissue.
- Radiation and chemicals are carcinogenic because they damage DNA and thus cause mutations in the genes.

References

Anon. (2002) Smoking Statistics. **www.wpro.who.int/tfi/docs/wntd02/18FS%20smoking%20stats.doc**

Anon. (2004) Smoking shortens life span 10 years, British study finds. **http://www.sfgate.com/cgi-bin/article.cgi?**

Atlas R. M. (1994) *Micro-organisms in our World*, Mosby, Kentucky.

Blows W. T. (2002) X-ray examination. *Nursing Times*, Diagnostic Procedures supplement, 44–7.

Blows W. T. (2003) *The Biological Basis of Nursing: Mental Health*, Routledge, London.

Coutts A. (2002) Diagnostic investigations part 2: Computerised tomography, *Nursing Times*, 98 (37): 41

Kahn F. (1999) Cosmic radiation: high altitudes may be bad for your health, *Financial Times*, Monday April 12th 1999. (Also at **www.aviation-health.org/cosmic_radiation.html**)

Murray P. R., Resenthal K. S., Kobayashi G. S. and Pfaller M. A. (2002) *Medical Microbiology*, Mosby, St Louis.

Pearce F. (1997) Devil in the diesel, *New Scientist*, 25th October 1997, 4.

Weinberg R. A. (1996) How cancer arises, *In* What You Need to Know About Cancer, *Scientific American* (Special Issue), 275 (3): 32–40.

Chapter 3

Body defences against cancer

- Introduction
- The immune system
- The chemical defences
- Immunity and cancer
- Key points

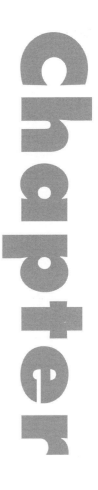

Introduction

The body must defend itself against potential harm, both from the *outside* environment around us, and from the *inside* environment within us. Chapter 2 identified a wide range of outside agents that can cause damage to DNA (see p. 48), and as such they are capable of inflicting health-destroying changes to our cells, like the mutations listed in Chapter 2 (see p. 38). If cellular DNA is damaged the cell could become malignant (see p. 24), and the body must defend itself against abnormal cells like these. The defence strategy of the body is known as **immunity**.

Immunity involves the interaction of multiple cells, many being the white cells of the blood, and the chemical agents produced by these cells. These white blood cells (WBCs) are reviewed in Chapter 4.

The immune system

Immunity can be divided into two main types: **non-specific immunity** and **specific immunity**. The difference between these two forms is fundamental to our understanding of how our defences work.

Non-specific immunity

This is a system which defends the body against *entry* of unwanted agents. As such it does not require the agents themselves to be recognised by the system, it just needs to know that these agents are not part of the individual (i.e. they are **non-self**, or *foreign*). The system then keeps them out of the body (as best as it can under quite difficult circumstances). There are four categories of non-specific immunity: physical barriers, chemical barriers, cellular barriers and species differentiation.

Physical barriers

These are structures like the skin and mucous membranes. They are therefore mostly on the outside of the body and form an impenetrable layer. **Skin** has an outer layer that consists of keratinised stratified epithelium (see p. 16). The very outer layer of this is dead tissue (its difficult to think that when looking at another person you are seeing dead tissue!) and as such it is difficult for most organisms to get through this layer. This is despite many organisms living on the surface as **commensals** (i.e. organisms that live on or in the body but cause it no harm). Very few organisms are capable of penetrating intact skin. However, if that outer dead layer of the skin is broken the barrier defence is lost and the surface commensals would gain entry to deeper layers where they may possibly become a **pathogen** (i.e. a disease-causing organism) and begin the process of setting up an infection. Skin covers about 98% of the body surface, and the gaps caused by various natural openings (the mouth, nose and others) are similarly protected by mucous membrane.

Unlike the very outer layers of skin, mucous membrane is living tissue, and is therefore more suitable for lining surfaces inside the body that are daily subjected to outside environmental agents. The best examples of these are the lining of the digestive tract (subject to environmental agents in food and drink) and the lining of the respiratory tract (subject to environmental agents in the air). Mucous membrane produces the sticky substance **mucus** which traps these foreign agents and takes steps to eliminate them back to the environment again. The lungs are particularly difficult to keep clean from unwanted agents in the air (as in air pollution). The mucous membrane of the respiratory tract traps the inhaled agents on the sticky mucus. The cells of the membrane have developed tiny hair-like structures called **cilia** and these beat repeatedly backwards and forwards, giving a brush-like action, sweeping the mucus (and its trapped agents) upwards towards the throat and out of the lungs. It is known as the **muco-ciliary escalator**, and it delivers the contaminated mucus to a point in the throat where it can be swallowed. In the stomach the unwanted agents can be destroyed by the acid conditions there. Smoking paralyses this muco-ciliary action, and the mucus (laden with the harmful agents) drains by gravity further down into the lungs where it can accumulate and cause harm.

Chemical barriers

These include **hydrochloric acid** in the stomach, which has a very low **pH** (i.e. a strong acid), and therefore any unwanted environmental agent that is swallowed, as may be found in food or drink, will be destroyed by the acid before entering the body. It is tempting to think of something that has arrived in the stomach as having already entered the body. This is not strictly true. Contents of the digestive tract are not *inside* the body until they have been absorbed through the gut wall into the cells and blood. For example, dietary fibre (previously called roughage) does not strictly enter the body, but it passes through without being absorbed. So, the *inside* of the lumen of the digestive tract from mouth to anus is therefore part of the *outside* of the body.

Cellular barriers

These are cells that destroy any unwanted foreign agent that gets into the body. **Phagocytes** fall into this category. These are cells that engulf and destroy the foreign agent. Do not refer to these cells as *eating* foreign substances, because eating implies that these cells have a digestive tract of their own, which they most certainly do not. Engulf is a better term, and this involves the phagocytes surrounding the foreign agent and taking it into their cytoplasm encased in a membrane. Inside the cytoplasm of the phagocyte are other membrane-bound organelles (see p. 5) called **lysosomes** that contain digestive enzymes. By merging the membrane-bound foreign agent with the lysosomes the agent is destroyed. **Macrophages** are a major phagocytic cell in both blood and body tissues; and **neutrophils** also have phagocytic activity.

Species differentiation

This means that certain diseases are suffered by a particular species and not by others. Consider for a moment if you have ever encountered a dog suffering from measles. Probably not; and the reason is that dogs do not catch measles, it's a human disease. The question is why? Science puzzled over this for years, but may now have the answer, or at least part of the answer. To catch a disease it is necessary first for the organisms to **colonise** the body. But, this is not enough as they can be removed, e.g. by hand washing, which is an excellent way of removing colonised organisms on the hands. To overcome the removal process the organisms must be able to stick to the cells and tissues, a process called **adhesion**. If they can stick to the tissues they then stand a chance of invading the body and causing disease. In species differentiation a particular species is immune from the disease simply because the organisms have no means of sticking to the cells of that species; i.e. they are unable to demonstrate adhesion in that species.

The term *foreign agent* indicates something from the environment that is not part of the body, but not all foreign agents are harmful. Food, for example, is a foreign agent that is both valuable and essential to the body. Another term is **antigen**, which is also a foreign agent to the body, but one that causes a reaction from the immune system. In fact, the term **immune response** means the reaction between the body's immune system and an antigen. This immune response, or reaction, is designed to eliminate the antigen from the body as it is seen by the immune system as potentially harmful and must be removed. Antigens are mostly proteins (like bacteria, viruses and pollen), but sometimes they are other substances (like dust particles). It is the nature of the immune response to antigens that is the role of specific immunity.

Specific immunity

This is where some cells of the blood plasma and the lymphatic system, called **lymphocytes** (one of our types of **leucocytes** or **white blood cells, WBC**) (see p. 94) are genetically triggered to respond to a particular antigen, and not to any others. One lymphocyte, for example, may be triggered to respond to the flu virus, but will not respond to anything else. One particular type of lymphocyte learns this specificity in the **thymus gland** (they are called **T-cells**, where T stands for thymus). The gland is just above the heart (Figure 3.1). During human childhood, immature T-lymphocytes migrate from bone marrow, where they were created, to the thymus gland. Here they take on a specificity, learning to respond only to one particular antigen (see p. 79). They then spend their existence in the blood, the tissues or the lymph nodes, waiting to contact that particular antigen. When they meet with this antigen they will react in a manner that is designed to destroy that antigen. The thymus gland is like a finishing school for lymphocytes, where they will learn their most important lesson, i.e. which antigen should they destroy. Those

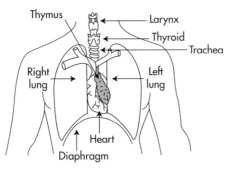

FIGURE 3.1 The thymus gland is in the chest immediately above the heart. (Redrawn from Martini 2004.)

that fail this process and do not acquire a specificity will pay the ultimate price and be destroyed themselves. This is the harsh reality for those lymphocytes who drop out of thymic school. The gland is most active during human childhood, after which most lymphocytes are enriched with a specificity to one of the full array of harmful antigens the body is likely to encounter. So after puberty, since the thymus gland has less students, it gradually reduces in size and function, but never entirely disappears.

The T lymphocytes are only one of two types of lymphocytes, the **B-cells** and **T-cells**. They basically look the same through a microscope, but they behave, when activated by their specific antigen, in very different ways, as identified below. Both are formed originally in bone marrow, but whilst B-cells stay there until fully mature the T-cells migrate to the thymus. All lymphocytes remain dormant until they are activated by the presence of the particular antigen to which they have specificity.

B-cells and antibodies

B-cell lymphocytes are activated by contact with the antigen to which they are specific. Usually one B-cell will be activated in this way, but many more are needed, and will be obtained by multiple divisions of the original cell into a colony of many thousands of cells, all active against the same specific antigen. Activation of B-cell lymphocytes results in B-cells being converted into **plasma cells** (Figure 3.2), which then start to release proteins called **antibodies**. These antibodies carry the same specificity as the parent B-cell and the activated plasma cell, i.e. they will bind to the same antigen that the original B-cell was active against. This type of immune reaction (i.e. using antibodies) is known as **humoral immunity**. By binding to the antigens, antibodies provide a wide range of valuable functions, all of which are important in the fight against the antigens. However, in the case of living antigens (e.g. bacteria) they do not actually kill the antigens. This task is left to cells who are dedicated to the role of killing antigens.

Antibodies carry out the following functions against their specific antigens:

1 They can render many antigens harmless, especially viruses and some **protozoans** (single cell animals that can sometimes enter the body as an antigen).

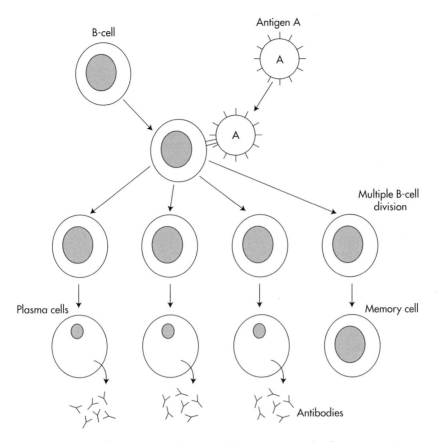

FIGURE 3.2 B-cell activation. The B-cell shown is specific for antigen A. On meeting with antigen A the B-cell goes through multiplication. The daughter cells mostly become plasma cells that produce antibodies. These antibodies are also specific for antigen A. Some activated B-cells will become memory cells.

2 They can neutralise some toxins, e.g. **tetanus toxin** (a dangerous poison that causes the disease **tetanus**; the toxin is released by the bacterial organism *clostridium*).

3 They can prevent adhesion of some organisms, and thus prevent tissue invasion (see p. 68).

4 They can immobilise certain antigens, especially bacteria that use tail-like structures called **flagella** to move.

5 They can activate the complement system (see p. 81).

6 They can form complexes with antigens, and these complexes become the targets for phagocytosis (see p. 68).

Being proteins, antibodies are also known by the form of the protein they are made from, namely **immunoglobulins** (**Ig**)(the word means *globular proteins of the immune system*). There are five main classes (or types) of immunoglobulins; IgA, IgD, IgE, IgG and IgM.

Immunoglobulin A (**IgA**) (Figure 3.3) (15–20% of the total blood plasma immunoglobulins) is an important antibody for the protection of surfaces against antigen invasion. It is found in various secretions that bathe surfaces, such as lachrymal fluid (bathing the surface of the eye), mucus (covering the surface of the digestive and respiratory systems), saliva (protecting the mouth), breast milk (where it protects the surface of the infant's digestive tract), sweat (protecting the skin surface) and bile.

Immunoglobulin D (**IgD**) (Figure 3.3) (only a trace quantity of the total blood plasma immunoglobulins) is the least understood of the antibodies. It is found on the surface of many B-cell lymphocytes and may have a role in the activation of these B-cells.

Immunoglobulin E (**IgE**) (Figure 3.3) is normally only a trace quantity of the total blood plasma immunoglobulins, but the level is often raised in individuals who suffer from allergies. IgE is different in having the ability to bind not only to antigens but also to **mast cells** at the same time (Figure 3.4). Mast cells are found in many tissue types, and they contain a cocktail of chemicals which induce **inflammation** when released, particularly a chemical called **histamine**. It seems strange that we have chemicals that cause inflammation, after all, we do not like inflammation because it causes us pain and discomfort. Histamine, and other similar chemicals, induces inflammation because it is through inflammation that the immune

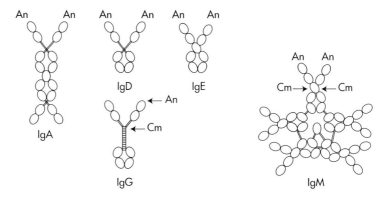

FIGURE 3.3 The five classes of immunoglobulins (antibodies). The antigen binding sites (An) occur at the ends of the molecule, and the complement binding sites (Cm) are at the hinge area (a few examples of each are shown). (Redrawn from Roitt *et al.* 2001.)

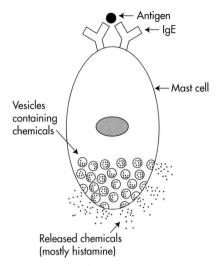

Antigen
IgE
Mast cell
Vesicles
containing
chemicals
Released chemicals
(mostly histamine)

FIGURE 3.4 Two IgE molecules are cross-linked by a binding antigen on the surface of a mast cell. This causes the release of chemicals, particularly histamine, from the mast cell.

system works properly. A lack of inflammation would put the immune system at a serious disadvantage. By binding to mast cells IgE can effect the release of the inflammatory chemicals at that moment when the antigen also binds to the IgE (Figure 3.4). In this way the inflammation caused coincides with the presence of an unwanted antigen. Increased amounts of IgE lead to an inappropriate amount of mast cell activation and inflammation, as seen in allergic disorders such as hay fever, contact dermatitis and asthma.

Immunoglobulin G (IgG) (Figure 3.3) (70–75% of the total blood plasma immunoglobulins) is the second antibody to respond to infections getting into the body, but is the most important of the antibodies in the fight against infection. It is mostly found in blood plasma and tissue fluids. It crosses the placenta and provides immunity for the unborn child during pregnancy, and remains in the child's blood providing up to nine months immunity following birth.

Immunoglobulin M (IgM) (Figure 3.3) (10% of the total blood plasma immunoglobulins) is the first antibody to respond to an infection, but being a large molecule it is confined to the blood. It therefore is unable to fight the infection in tissue fluid, which then becomes a job for IgG. The initial surge in IgM at the start of an infection usually gives way to IgG when levels of this secondary antibody are raised enough. IgM is, however, the best antibody for activating **complement** (see p. 81); a process known as **complement fixation**.

Antibodies are 'Y'-shaped proteins with an antigen-binding site at the end of the two 'arms' and a site at the junction of the 'arms' for activating complement (Figure 3.5). IgE, in addition, has a mast cell-binding site at the 'foot' end of the molecule. IgA is two molecules joined (as shown in Figure 3.3) and IgM is five molecules joined (as shown in Figure 3.3), a structure known as a **pentomer**.

There are two types of B-cells known, i.e. B1 and B2. B2 cells are produced and mature in bone marrow and on activation they will manufacture IgG, IgA and IgE. B1 are also produced in bone marrow but mature outside of bone marrow, and when activated they pro-duce mostly IgM. The body's ability to produce and use antibodies is determined by various factors. **Active immunity** is a term used when the body produces its own antibodies in response to antigens. **Passive immunity** is the term used when the body uses antibodies from an outside source (i.e. they are not produced by the body that uses

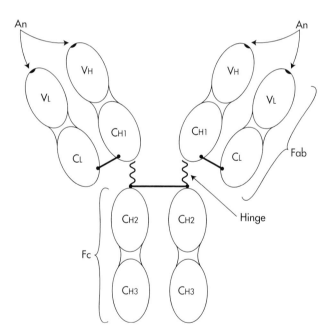

FIGURE 3.5 The simplified structure of an antibody. The domains are V (vari-able) and C (constant). The chains are L (light) and H (heavy). The heavy chain has four domains, one is variable and three are constant. The light chain has two domains, one variable and one constant. The Fab segment is the antigen-binding fragment, the Fc segment is the crystallisable fragment. The antigen-binding site (An) is at the end of the Fab segment. A hinge region in the middle allows movement of the two Fab arms. The molecule is held together by bonds shown as cross-bridges.

TABLE 3.1 The mechanisms of active/passive and natural/artificial immunity

	Active immunity	*Passive immunity*
Natural	Catch the disease and recover	Breastfeeding (IgA) and through the placenta (IgG)
Artificial	Vaccination	Injection of antibodies

them). If you read back over the last few paragraphs you should discover a classic example of passive immunity.

Natural immunity occurs when the cause of the antibody production is purely natural (i.e. by the hand of nature). If you read back over the last few paragraphs you should discover a classic example of natural immunity. **Artificial immunity** is when antibody production is caused by human intervention. Table 3.1 shows the combination of active or passive with natural or artificial immunity.

From Table 3.1 it can be seen that the *passive natural immunity* mentioned in an earlier paragraph was IgG crossing the placenta. Vaccination has become a major mechanism for *active artificial immunity* against infections, and it seems likely that anti-cancer vaccines will become an important way of fighting cancers (see p. 341). Another way for the future is likely to be with the injection of specific anti-cancer antibodies (an *artificial passive immunity*) (see p. 339).

T-cells

The specific immunity related to T-cell activation is known as **cell-mediated immunity**. T-cells do not activate so easily as B-cells, even when coming face to face with the antigen to which they are specific. Follow this scenario in combination with the Figure 3.6:

1 If the T-cell meets up with the same antigen to which it is specific, nothing happens . . .
2 So it is necessary first for the antigen to be engulfed by a particular phagocyte (see p. 68) called an **antigen-presenting cell (APC)**.
3 The APC destroys the antigen and expresses (exposes) some of the antigen proteins onto its surface.
4 When the APC shows these exposed antigen proteins to the same T-cell, nothing happens . . .

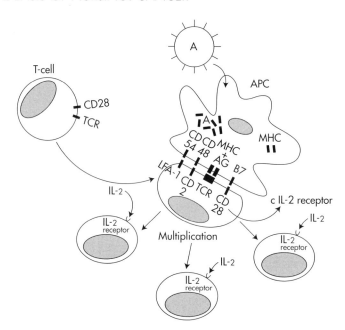

FIGURE 3.6 Activation of a T-cell. The antigen (A) is engulfed and broken up by an antigen-presenting cell (APC). Antigen proteins will be expressed on the APC surface in combination with major histocompatability complex (MHC) proteins produced by the APC. The T-cell binds to the APC using the binding molecules LFA-1 (binds to CD54), CD2 (binds to CD48), TCR (binds to the MHC/antigen protein complex), CD28 (binds to B7). Production of Il-2 is important as a stimulation for the process. After activation, the T-cell will multiply to form larger numbers which will include memory cells. TCR = T-cell antigen receptor; IL = interleukin; LFA = lymphocyte function antigen; MHC = major histocompatibility complex.

5 So what the APC must do next is to produce some of its own proteins to expose on its surface *in combination* with the antigen proteins. These 'home grown' proteins are one of the classes of proteins known as **major histocompatibility complex (MHC)**. There are three classes of MHC proteins: class I, class II and class III. Class I and II proteins are specifically for exposing onto the surface of a cell, and in the correct combinations they act as cell markers, to identify 'self' (those cells that belong to the body) from 'non-self' (foreign cells). This is similar to name badges worn by individuals to identify those who belong to that particular institution from those who do not.

6 Once produced, the correct combination of MHC class proteins with the antigen proteins is exposed to the T-cell, which is then activated.

From this it can be seen that B-cells and T-cells, as identified earlier, behave in very different ways, and that includes activation. Once activated, the single T-cell needs to divide many thousands of times to form a colony of activated T-cells, all with the same specificity, i.e. multiple divisions similar to what the B-cells did (see p. 70).

There are two major types of activated T-cells developed in the thymus gland; the **T helper** and **T cytotoxic** cells.

The T_H **cell** (**T helper cell**) falls into two main forms, T_H1 which produce chemicals (called **cytokines**) (see p. 36) that are important for killing intracellular organisms (i.e. those inside the cell), and for the generation of T_C cells (see below), and T_H2 which also produce cytokines that are important for B-cell multiplication (see p. 70). T_H cells do not directly kill antigens, but they provide a much greater opportunity for the other type of T-cell lymphocytes, the T_C cell, to kill the antigens.

The T_C **cell** (the **T cytotoxic cell**) is the cell that actually kills the antigen. They do this by developing close contact with the antigen followed by a lethal disruption of the antigen membranes, and the antigen then dies. T_C cells produce proteins called **perforins** which are stored in granules within the cytoplasm. On close contact with the antigen the perforins are released from the granules into a confined space formed between the two cells. The perforins become incorporated into the membrane of the antigen, forming holes which lead to the disruption of the membrane and the death of the antigen. This close contact is essential because release of the perforins from a distance would not be effective. Close contact is achieved largely through the role of the T_H cells which therefore increase the kill rate of the T_C cells enormously.

In addition, two other types of T-cells have been identified. The T_S **cell** (**T suppressor cell**) reduces the immune response and restores the immune system to normal after the response is no longer required. The T_D **cell** (**T delayed hypersensitivity cell**) launches a prolonged defence against persistent antigens when an acute response has failed.

Both B-cell and T-cell lymphocytes produce **memory cells** when they are activated by antigen exposure. Memory cells created after a first exposure to the antigen persist in the circulation and lymphatic system and provide a rapid and stronger defence should the same antigen return and a second exposure occur. Memory T-cells rapidly convert to T_C cytotoxic cells and attack the antigen, while memory B-cells convert to plasma cells rapidly and secrete antibodies when faced with a second or subsequent exposure to their specific antigen. In this way, memory cells provide rapid removal of antigens when they return after the first exposure. This is why '*we cannot catch*' certain diseases more than once. In reality we probably do catch these diseases many times, but whilst the first exposure causes symptoms it also creates the memory cells. After that, the memory cells eliminate all subsequent exposures to the antigen before any symptoms arise.

Natural killer cells

Natural killer cells (**NK cells**) are another form of lymphocyte also called a **large granular lymphocyte** (**LGL**), and these are important to our defences against cancer. As the name suggests they are bigger than the average lymphocyte and contain many dark granules. Like other white cells, NK cells are derived from bone marrow and occupy most body tissues, forming for example, 5–15% of the total lymphocytes in blood plasma. They kill two things, virus-infected cells and tumour cells. They do this by the same mechanism as that used by T-cells when they kill antigens (see p. 77). The NK cell's granular contents (enzymes called **perforins** and **granzymes**) are liberated when in close contact with the antigen membrane. Perforin acts like the lytic complex (see p. 83) in making a hole in the membrane through which granzymes can then enter. Granzymes are proteolytic (protein digesting) enzymes which cause the antigen cell to die.

NK cells exposed to the cytokine **interleukin-2** (**Il-2**)(see p. 36) become **lymphokine-activated killer** (**LAK**) cells. These cells have been used in clinical trials to kill malignant cells.

The approximate percentages of the different lymphocytes in circulation are: T helper cells 55%, T cytotoxic cells 25%, B-cells 10% and NK cells 10%.

Lymphocyte surface molecules

Proteins on the cell surface act as **markers**, as **adhesion molecules**, as **antigen-binding sites** and as **activation molecules**.

Adhesion molecules allow two cells to stick together, a vital process for several reasons including cell activation and the killing of antigens. Antigen-binding sites allow lymphocytes to recognise and bind only their specific antigens and activation molecules to facilitate the switching on of inactive cells (i.e. inactive cells are said to be in the *resting state*). One important group of surface molecules is called the **CD system**. CD stands for **clusters of differentiation** (or **cluster differentiation**). Surface markers develop on T-cells at various stages of their development in the thymus gland (see p. 69) (Figure 3.7). All T-cells have the following surface molecules:

1 **CD3** (a vital marker for activation).
2 **TCR** (their specific antigen-binding site).
3 **CD2**, an adhesion molecule that binds another molecule called **LAF-3** (where LAF means leucocyte function antigen, LAF-3 is also known as **CD58**).
4 **CD28** (an activation molecule which binds **CD80** and **CD86**).
5 **CD154** (another activation molecule which binds **CD40**) (Lydyard *et al.* 2004, Roitt *et al.* 2001).

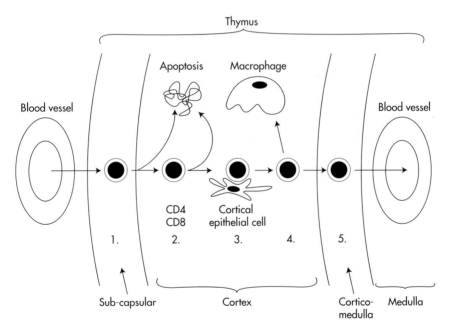

FIGURE 3.7 T-cell lymphocyte maturation through the thymus. (1) The immature T-cell enters the gland from the blood into the sub-capsular region. (2) In the cortex it gains its CD4 or CD8 status. If there are problems at this stage the cell will go to apoptosis (cell death). (3) The T-cell gains its specificity and learns to not respond to 'self' (the body's own cells). Failure to learn this causes it to go to be phagocytosed by macrophages. (4) Final adjustments to the T-cell receptor (TCR) are made before entry into the medullary blood supply as a mature T-cell. (Redrawn from Roitt *et al.* 2001.)

In addition the specialised T-cells have the following surface molecules:

1 T helper cells have **CD4** which binds to MHC class II proteins.
2 T cytotoxic cells have **CD8** which binds to MHC class I proteins (Figure 3.8).

B-cells produce antibodies, and use antibodies as part of their cell surface receptors and markers. B-cell receptors (BCR) are IgM and IgD (see p. 72) plus **CD79,** a receptor similar to CD3, i.e. it is important for B-cell lymphocyte activation. Other co-receptors that modulate B-cell activation are **CD19, CD20, CD21** (CD21 also binds a complement protein called **C3**, see p. 81), **CD32, CD40, CD80** and **CD86**. B-cell adhesion molecules are **CD22, ICAM-1** (ICAM means **intracellular adhesion molecule**) and **LFA-3**. This last molecule facilitates B-cell binding to T-cells which is necessary for co-operation between the two lymphocyte systems.

It is worth noting that, for the interested reader, the entire CD system is listed in Roitt *et al.* (2001, pp. 437–40).

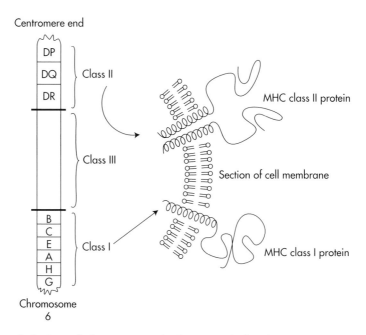

FIGURE 3.8 Part of chromosome 6. Genes code for the MHC proteins, class I, II and III. Class I and II are cell surface transmembranous receptor proteins. Class III genes code for complement proteins. (Redrawn from Roitt *et al.* 2001.)

The chemical defences

The complement system

The binding of antibodies to the antigen allows the activation of a chemical chain reaction called the **complement system** (Figure 3.9). This consists of a series of nine proteins that must be activated in a particular sequence in order to function. In the absence of such activation they remain dormant in the blood plasma. The complement system is activated either via the **classical pathway** or the **alternative pathway** (see Figure 3.9 for details). Complement proteins are identified by the letter 'C', so the nine proteins are labelled C1, C2, C3 and so on to C9. Some are split in the process into two components 'a' and 'b', notably C3 becomes C3a and C3b, and C5 becomes C5a and C5b. Some of these protein combinations are enzymes called **convertases** which continue the process by converting a specific protein into the next. Other proteins are also involved. The full details of this reaction are shown in Figure 3.9. The important points to consider are the resulting products and their functions. There are four main products of complement activation (the complement proteins involved are shown in brackets, see also Figure 3.9).

Chemotaxins (C3a, C5a)

These are chemicals which attract white cells of most kinds to the scene of the antigen invasion (e.g. the site of infection). The advantage of this is the concentration of body defensive cells at the site where they are needed most.

Opsonins (C3b)

These are chemicals that label antigens for phagocytosis by coating the surface (see p. 68). Macrophages need to know what cells to destroy by phagocytosis at the scene, so they are labelled by a coating of opsonins. This often means that macrophages will engulf and destroy a complex of antigens with antibodies attached (known as the **immune complex**).

Anaphylotoxins (C3a, C5a)

These are chemicals that cause inflammation to occur. C3a and C5a have a dual role (see chemotaxins above). How C3a and C5a cause

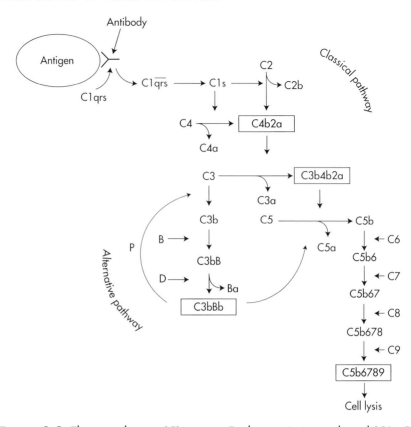

FIGURE 3.9 The complement (C) system. Each protein is numbered (C1, C2 etc), and combinations in boxes indicate enzymes (called convertases). C proteins can be split by convertases into two portions, a and b. C1qrs is first activated by the binding of an antibody to an antigen. The activated C1s component splits off and converts C2 and C4 to their respective a and b parts. C4b combines with 2a to form C3 convertase that splits C3 into C3a and C3b. The cascade follows either the classical or alternative pathways, both of which split C5 to C5a and C5b. Combining C5b with C6, C7, C8 and C9 forms the lytic complex (C5b6789) that can lyse (breakdown) antigen cell membranes. B, D and P are additional factors needed for the alternative pathway, and c3bBb is an alternative C3 convertase.

inflammation is shown in Figure 3.10. **Inflammation** is vital for the function of the immune response, even though it may produce unpleasant symptoms for us. This is because inflammation results in dilation of blood vessels (called **vasodilation**), which brings more blood and therefore more white cells to the scene of the antigen invasion, and it causes greater permeability of the capillary wall. This last function allows white cells like macrophages to pass from the blood into the tissues where antigens are likely to be. Inflammation

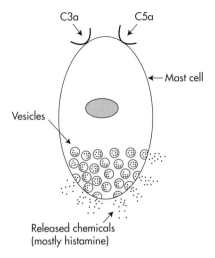

FIGURE 3.10 The complement components C3a and C5a are anaphylo-toxins, i.e. they can cause inflammation by degranulation of mast cells (similar to IgE, see Figure 3.4).

increases the efficiency of the immune system considerably, and is therefore a necessary evil in our fight against invading organisms.

Lytic complex (a combination of C3b, C5b, C6, C7, C8 and C9 called MAC, or membrane attack complex)

This is a chemical complex that is capable of killing the antigen by breaking down the antigen membranes (the word *lytic* comes from *lysis* that means 'breakdown').

The acute phase proteins

These are a collection of liver-produced proteins which are normally in low quantities but increase rapidly following the introduction of an antigen in the body. Their purpose is to activate the complement system, to increase the ability of the body to opsonise organisms (see p. 81) and to limit the tissue damage during infection. They are also important in tissue repair. A major protein in this group is **C-reactive protein (CRP)** which directly interferes with bacterial metabolism, activates the complement system (via the **alternative pathway**, see Figure 3.9) and acts as an opsonin (see p. 81). The main activity of acute phase proteins is against bacterial infections, so they do not play a big role in the body's fight against cancer.

The cytokines, chemokines and other chemicals

Cytokines are chemicals of small molecular size produced by a wide variety of cells in response to stimulation of some kind (King 2000). They are cell-signalling agents, binding to either themselves (**autocrine activity**) or to other cells nearby (**paracrine activity**). As such they induce a wide variety of cellular responses, including growth (protein synthesis), cell differentiation (see p. 2), chemotaxis (see p. 81) and cellular activation. Some are causes of inflammation (see p. 82), and these are the **pro-inflammatory cytokines** (e.g. Il-2, TNFα, IFNγ), while others reduce inflammation, the **anti-inflammatory cytokines** (e.g. Il-4, Il-10, Il-13). Cytokines occur in several types.

Interleukins (Il)

These are cell-signalling agents between lymphocytes and co-ordinate immune cell activity. They bind to specific receptors on T_C cells and NK cells, and LAK cells (see p. 78). They work in combination with other cytokines in a cascade effect. There are several kinds called **Il-1**, **Il-2**, **Il-3** and so on. When these are produced by lymphocytes they are often referred to as **lymphokines**, or **monokines** if produced by monocytes. Some of these are growth factors (see Table 2.1, p. 36). Table 3.2 states the functions of the major interleukins:

The role of interleukins in anticancer therapy is discussed in Chapter 12 (see p. 340).

Interferons (IFN)

These are a group of **glycoproteins** (proteins with sugars attached), of which there are two types: **type I** (comprising **IFNα** and **IFNβ**, both binding to the same receptors), and **type II** (comprising **IFNγ**, which binds to its own receptor). Interferons are pro-inflammatory cytokines which are antiviral in nature, which means they are secreted by many cells when they are virally infected.

IFNα is coded for by more than 20 genes on chromosome 9. It is antiviral, reduces growth in both normal and malignant cells, increases NK cell activity and influences cell differentiation.

IFNβ is coded for by one gene on chromosome 9. It is very similar to IFNα in that it is also antiviral, reduces growth of both normal and malignant cells, and increases NK cell activity. The paracrine

TABLE 3.2 The major interleukins

Interleukin	Notes and function
Il-1α and 1β	Derived from macrophages and many other cells, they cause fever, activate lymphocytes, induces acute phase protein production, activate vascular endothelium, cause cells to produce Il-6 and mobilise neutrophils
Il-2	Derived from activated T_H and NK cells, it increases proliferation and efficiency of T cells, B cells and NK cells, and increases the formation of immunoglobulins
Il-3	Causes increased proliferation of bone marrow cells (to increase WBC production)
Il-4	Derived from activated T cells it activates B cells, increases T cell proliferation and increases IgG and IgE immunoglobulin proliferation
Il-5	Growth of eosinophils, B cell activation and increases IgA response
Il-6	Derived from fibroblasts, B cells and T cells, macrophages and bone marrow cells, it activates T-cell lymphocytes, causes fever, and increases acute phase protein production
Il-8	Chemotaxis of neutrophils
Il-10	Activates B cells, reduces macrophage activity and induces activity of T_H1 cells
Il-12	Activates NK cells and induces activity of T_H1 cells

effect of IFNα and IFNβ (see p. 84) on surrounded cells causes a reduction in protein synthesis which helps to shut down virus replication in those cells.

IFNγ is coded for by one gene on chromosome 12. It has a similar antiviral role but also has a part to play in the activation of immune cells such as macrophages, and the development of specific immunity. It also causes reduction of growth in both normal and malignant cells.

The role of interferons in anti-cancer treatment can be found in Chapter 12 (see p. 340).

Tumour necrosis factors (TNF)

There are several kinds called **TNFα, TNFβ, TNFγ** and so on. TNFα activates vascular endothelium and macrophages, it causes fever and it can cause shock, and it increases vascular permeability, i.e. the capillaries become more permeable, as in inflammation (see p. 82).

Leukotrienes, thromboxanes, prostaglandins and prostacyclins

These are chemical groups derived from the **phospholipids** that make up part of the cell membrane (Figure 3.11). This is an interesting secondary function for the fatty components of cell membranes, i.e. acting as a reserve for the production of these substances. The enzyme **phospholipase A$_2$** acts to convert the phospholipid from the membrane to **arachidonic acid**, which is then acted on by another enzyme called **cyclo-oxygenase** (**COX**) to produce **thromboxanes** and **prostaglandins** (identified as **PG**, and classed as **PGA** to **PGI**). This last prostaglandin (i.e. PGI) is also known as **prostacyclin**. Alternatively, arachidonic acid can be converted to **leukotrienes** if acted on by the enzyme **lipoxygenase**. Thromboxanes, prostaglandins and leukotrienes are inflammatory mediators, i.e. causing inflammation, which is essential for the efficient function of the immune system (see p. 82) (Clemens 1991). Thromboxane is an important mediator in the process of blood clotting (i.e. it promotes blood clotting) and in normal circulation this must be constantly opposed by the production of prostacyclin.

Prostacyclin is also produced from arachidonic acid in endothelial cells (those lining blood vessels). Here these chemicals help to prevent platelet aggregation (and thus prevent blood clotting) during normal circulation of blood (see p. 97 for platelets), and prostacyclin can cause vasodilation (Germann and Stanfield 2002).

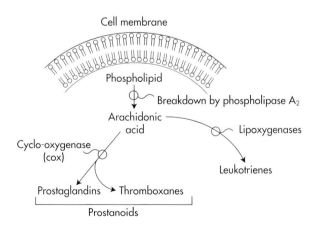

FIGURE 3.11 The production of arachidonic acid from cell membrane phospholipids, and the subsequent production of prostanoids and leukotrienes from arachidonic acid.

In addition, there are other chemical agents related to cellular growth and these are listed in Table 2.1 (p. 36).

Chemokines are small molecules (over fifty of them are known) which are chemoattractants (i.e. involved in chemotaxis, see p. 81) for various leucocytes including lymphocytes, monocytes, NK cells, neutrophils and memory cells (see p. 77). They are produced by a wide variety of cells such as platelets, T-cells and macrophages.

Immunity and cancer

In the fight against cancer the immune system has an important role to play, although the efficiency of the immune system in attacking and destroying tumours was considered greater in the past than it is today. This is because as knowledge grows in both tumour biology and the mechanisms of immunity it has become apparent that our defence system is not as good as it was first thought in fighting new growths. A better defence is launched against the viruses that can cause some tumours (see p. 46) rather than against the tumour itself. This is not to say that our immune system does nothing to kill malignant cells, because it does, and using our knowledge of cancer and the immune system it is becoming a viable proposition to manipulate our immunity to do more in fighting the tumour cells (see also Chapter 12, p. 339). Surveillance by the immune cells and their products (antibodies) is directed mainly against incoming foreign agents (antigens), like viruses and bacteria, and since malignant cells are not from the outside environment, i.e. they are transformed by genetic manipulation from normal tissue cells, they are not technically antigens in themselves, but they can produce surface antigens that provoke an immune response. Virally infected cells will attract the attention of the immune surveillance, but in chapter 2 we saw how few tumours were actually caused by viruses (see p. 46), and so our immune surveillance is not the best as a mechanism against the majority of human cancers.

Malignant cells can and do create abnormal products, mostly proteins known as tumour-associated antigens, which then occur on the cell surface or even leave the cell, and these act like any other antigen in that they cause an immune response. Table 3.3 lists the important tumour antigens found in human cancer cells. Again, these products may be of viral origin (from a virally infected cell), or caused by genetic mutation (see p. 39). However, attempts to identify

TABLE 3.3 Some of the known tumour antigens used in diagnosis (King 2000)

Tumour antigen	Found in association with
Prostate-specific antigen (PSA)	Prostate cancer
Melanoma antigen expression (MAGE)	Melanomas
Renal antigen expression (RAGE)	Melanomas, kidney tumours
Carcinoembryonic antigen (CEA)	Colon cancers
Common acute lymphoblastic leukaemia antigen (CALLA)	Leukaemia
Mucin	Breast and ovary cancer

antigens specific to malignant cells (i.e. not found in normal cells) have resulted in only a few being found (Table 3.3).

Some others are produced by both malignant and normal cells, but appear to be in much reduced quantities coming from the normal cell to those found coming from malignant cells, so it may not be a case of what is detected but how much (quantity rather than quality). Measuring the levels of these antigens may therefore be useful in **immunodiagnosis** (using an immune response to identify the presence of a tumour) or **immunotherapy** (using an immune response to help in the treatment of a tumour). Immunotherapy is considered in Chapter 12 in relation to cancer treatment (see p. 339). **Monoclonal antibodies** are used to identify these antigens. Monoclonal antibodies are artificially produced antibodies that can target very specific antigens; they can be purified and produced in large quantities for both laboratory and clinical use. They are becoming an important adjunct treatment for various cancers (see Chapter 12, p. 339, and also LeMone and Burke 2004, p. 223). Radiolabelled antibodies (i.e. those given a mild radioactive component which can be detected by a scanner) can sometimes be used in immunodiagnosis. These antibodies are against specific tumour antigens, and when bound to the tumour cells the cancer is highlighted on the scanner screen.

Although, as said here, the immune system is much better at detecting and destroying viruses than tumour cells, many cancer cells are detected naturally by the immune system and attacked by the patient's own antibodies, T-cells and NK cells.

Cytotoxic T-cells (T_C) bind to malignant cells which produce tumour antigen in association with MHC class I proteins on the cell surface. Since tumour cells produce MHC class I (see p. 80 for MHC

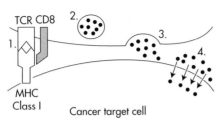

Cytotoxic T-Cell

FIGURE 3.12 The cytotoxic T-cell kills a cancer cell by (1) binding to it using the MHC class – TCR/CD8 receptors, (2) and (3) releasing perforins (shown as black blobs) from the storage site within vesicles in the T-cell (4). Perforins create holes in the cancer cell membrane and the cell dies.

proteins) the interaction is going to be with CD8 cells, which are the cytotoxic T-cell (T_C) type (see p. 80). Following this binding, the T_C cell will release vesicles containing **perforins**, which are proteins that cause a channel to form in the malignant cell membrane (see Figure 3.12). Through this channel water and ions can pass causing lysis (breakdown) and therefore death of the malignant cell. The cytotoxic T-cell is then free to attack other cells (King 2000).

NK cells (see p. 78) are similar in the way they kill malignant cells. They are effective in destroying isolated cancer cells in the blood but also good at penetrating the tissues and attacking clumps of malignant cells without harming normal cells. Receptors on the surface of NK cells recognise tumour antigens in association with MHC class I proteins, the receptors having adhesion and activation qualities. The killing of malignant cells by both T_C and NK cells is *antibody-independent* (meaning antibodies are not involved); but other cells called **K cells** (i.e. **killer cells**) attack those tumour cells that have a surface antigen associated with a bound antibody. They are therefore *antibody-dependent* (i.e. antibodies *must* be bound to the cancer cell surface before the K cell acts). This is not a major immune defence system since the antibodies needed for this interaction are rare, but if these antibodies can be supplied to the patient artificially as part of a treatment plan this will improve the kill rate of K cells. In addition to cell lysis, T_C cells also produce **tumour necrosis factor** (**TNF**) and **interferon** (**IFN**)(see p. 84), which can bind to malignant cell receptors and induce cancer cell death. These cytokines can also be used in treatment (see Chapter 12, p. 340).

Malignant cells can, and do, escape these killing mechanisms. If the cancer cell, for example, mutated in a manner that resulted in a loss of its ability to produce MHC class I proteins, then the colony of cancer cells derived from that mutated cell would escape from immune surveillance and attack, and therefore would survive. The few tumour specific antigens produced, as noted earlier on p. 88, are also a factor in allowing cancer cells to escape the immune system. In addition, the need for lymphocytes to recognise and bind to cancer cell surface receptors means that it becomes difficult for the immune cells to attack cancer cells that are deep in a mass where these immune cells are unable to reach.

Key points

Immunity

- There are two main types of immunity: non-specific and specific.
- Non-specific immunity defends against the entry of unwanted organisms, the agents themselves not being recognised by the system. It identifies only that these agents are non-self, or foreign.
- The four categories of non-specific immunity are physical barriers (e.g. the skin), chemical barriers (e.g. gastric acidity), cellular barriers (e.g. phagocytes, which engulf organisms) and species differentiation (i.e. some species cannot catch certain diseases).
- Antigens are foreign agents that invade the body, causing a reaction to occur in the immune system, i.e. an immune response.
- Antigens are mostly proteins (e.g. bacteria, viruses and pollen), but they can be other substances (like dust particles).
- Specific immunity involves lymphocytes which respond to a articular antigen, and not to any others.
- The lymphocytes come in two types: B-cells and T-cells.
- Activation of B-cell lymphocytes results in these cells being converted into plasma cells which then release proteins called antibodies.
- Activation of T-cell lymphocytes results in several forms of cells which are capable of killing antigens.

Antibodies

- Antibodies are also known as immunoglobulins (Ig) and occur in five classes: IgA, IgD, IgE, IgG and IgM.
- Antibodies are 'Y'-shaped proteins with antigen-binding sites at the end of the two 'arms' and a site lower down for activating complement.

- In active immunity, the body produces its own antibodies in response to antigens, but in passive immunity the body uses antibodies from an outside source (e.g. from mother to child through breast milk or the placenta).
- Natural immunity means the antibody production is purely natural (i.e. by the hand of nature), whilst artificial immunity is when antibody production is caused by human intervention.

Immune cells

- There are two major types of activated T-cells: the T helper (T_H) and the T cytotoxic (T_C) cells.
- Both B-cell and T-cell lymphocytes produce memory cells when they are activated by antigen exposure.
- Natural killer cells (NK cells) are lymphocytes (also called large granular lymphocytes, LGL) and these kill cancer cells.

Complement system

- The complement system consists of nine blood proteins that must be activated in a particular sequence in order to function.
- There are four main products of complement activation, chemotaxins (which attract immune cells to where they are needed), opsonins (which coat antigens for phagocytosis), anaphylotoxins (which cause inflammation) and the lytic complex (which can kill antigens).

Cytokines

- Cytokines are small chemical molecules produced by a variety of cells in response to stimulation. They are cell-signalling agents, binding to either themselves (autocrine activity) or to other cells nearby (paracrine activity).

Malignancy

- Surveillance by the immune system is better directed against viruses than against malignant cells.
- Malignant cells create abnormal proteins known as tumour-associated antigens on the cell surface.
- Both T_C and NK cells are antibody-independent but K cells (killer cells) are antibody-dependent.
- T_C cells produce tumour necrosis factor (TNF) and interferon (IFN) which cause cancer cell death.

- Malignant cells can escape if the cancer cell has mutated and lost its ability to produce MHC class I proteins.

References

Clemens M. J. (1991) *Cytokines*, BIOS scientific publishers, Oxford.

Germann W. J. and Stanfield C. L. (2002) *Principles of Human Physiology*, Benjamin Cummings, San Francisco.

King R. J. B. (2000) *Cancer Biology*, Prentice Hall, London.

LeMone P. and Burke K. (2004) *Medical-Surgical Nursing, Critical Thinking in Client Care* (3rd edn) Pearson Education International, Prentice Hall, New Jersey.

Lydyard P., Whelan A. and Fanger M. W. (2004) *Instant Notes: Immunology* (2nd Edn), BIOS Scientific Publishers, London.

Martini F. H. (2004) *Fundamentals of Anatomy and Physiology* (6th edn), Benjamin Cummings, Pearson Education International, San Francisco.

Roitt I., Brostoff J. and Male D. (2001) *Immunology* (6th edn), Mosby, Edinburgh.

Chapter 4

Blood and lymphatic cancers

- The biology of blood
- Bone marrow cancers
- The lymphatic system
- Lymphatic cancers
- Nursing skills: stem cell treatment and blood transfusion
- Key points

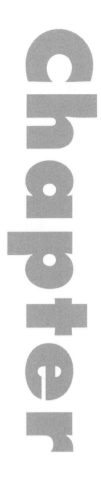

The biology of blood

Blood is the body's liquid tissue and major transport system. Tissues have a matrix in which cells are embedded, the matrix for blood being the liquid called **plasma**. Plasma is mostly water with dissolved substances in it, including minerals like sodium and calcium, nutrients like glucose and amino acids, and a range of different proteins. These proteins include clotting factors, hormones, antibodies, and the blood's own collection of proteins, like albumin and globulin. The cells (often referred to as **formed elements**) embedded in this liquid matrix are of three main types: **erythrocytes** (**red blood cells, RBC**), **leukocytes** (**white blood cells, WBC**) and **thrombocytes** (**platelets**). All of these are derived from the same cells found in **bone marrow** called **stem cells**, or more specifically **haemopoietic stem cells** (*haem* = blood, *poiesis* = forming).

Stem cells generally are **undifferentiated**, i.e. they are at the earliest stages of cell formation and have not yet, at that point, started to become a specific cell type. The move towards cell specialisation is called **differentiation**. It is useful to remember differentiation by the fact that specialised cells, like brain and muscle cells, are different to each other. They carry out very different functions and are incapable of reverting back to their former primitive condition. At much earlier stages of development all cells are derived from the same cell cluster, which is formed from the fertilised ovum. The terms **totipotent** (*potent* = able to do), **pluripotent** (*pluri* = more) and **multipotent** (*multi* = many) **stem cells** are often used to reflect the different stages of stem cell development (Figure 4.1), where totipotent cells are capable of becoming any one of the 216 different body cell types (i.e. they are cells of the very early cell mass after fertilisation). Cells then move on from totipotent to multipotent by *switching off* genes in the nucleus, leading to increasing specialisation (or differentiation). Ultimately, the stem cells remaining in adult life are only those there to replace the fully differentiated cells that are lost by depletion or damage, like blood cells.

Bone marrow cells (or haemopoietic stem cells) are a good example of these, where these stem cells are capable of forming into any one of four major types of blood cells (called **cell lineages**, or lines):

1 **Myeloid** (the granulocytes [polymorphonuclear cells] and mononuclear cells).
2 **Lymphoid** (the lymphocyte lineage).

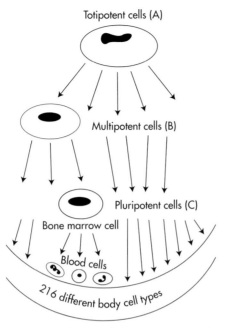

Totipotent cells (A)

Multipotent cells (B)

Pluripotent cells (C)

Bone marrow cell

Blood cells

216 different body cell types

Figure 4.1 (A) Totipotent cells are the starting point for 216 different cell types in the body, (B) multipotent cells have switched some genes off so they are more specialised, (C) pluripotent cells (e.g. bone marrow cells) are a further specialisation, by deactivating more genes they give rise to several types of highly specialised cells, e.g. blood cells.

3 **Erythroid** (the erythrocyte lineage).
4 **Megakaryocytes** (the platelet lineage).

Group 1 on this list, the myeloid lineage, includes the **polymorphonuclear cells**, or **polymorphs** for short (*poly* = many, *morph* = shape, i.e. the cells with many shaped nuclei). These same cells are also known as **granulocytes** because they also have granules in their cytoplasm (see p. 4). There are three types of granulocytes (polymorphs) called **neutrophils, basophils** and **eosinophils**.

Neutrophils are by far the commonest of the white blood cells in circulation (accounting for about 60–70% of adult WBCs), and the commonest of the granulocytes (over 95% of circulating granulocytes). They are short-lived phagocytes. A **phagocyte** is any cell that engulfs and destroys unwanted foreign substances (known as **antigens**), such as bacteria and viruses, that may enter the body, and these cells are therefore extremely valuable in our defences against infections. Neutrophils play an important part in the discussion of stem cell treatment (see p. 108).

Basophils are present in very small numbers in circulation (Table 4.1). Their granules contain inflammatory agents, such as histamine, and when these are released they trigger an inflammatory response. This is valuable in aiding the immune defence against certain antigens, but is also the cause of allergic responses (i.e. inappropriate immune responses).

Eosinophils occur in small numbers in blood (Table 4.1). They also have cytoplasmic granules, but this time the granules contain, amongst other things, antihistamine, and this helps to settle any inflammatory response down. These cells also appear to act in defence of the body against parasitic infections.

The other cells included in the myeloid lineage are the **mononuclear cells**, or **monocytes**. These are the largest white cells and are important phagocytes that are capable of migrating out of circulation into the tissue fluid (called **extracellular fluid**, or **ECF**). On moving from the blood to the ECF monocytes change their nature and are then known as **macrophages**. They are very important in our defences against bacterial and viral infections, and in lymphocyte activation.

Group 2 on the list, the lymphoid lineage, consists of two types of **lymphocytes**: the **T-cells** and the **B-cells**. Lymphocytes are the cells of our **specific immune system**, the T-cells being active against viral and tumour cells, while the activated B-cells (known as **plasma cells**) produce **antibodies**. Antibodies (otherwise known as **immunoglobulins**, or **Ig**) are proteins designed to interfere with and block many aspects of bacterial and viral infections, although they do not actually kill these antigens. They do, however, provoke chemical reactions that ultimately can kill antigens, as well as prevent antigen replication and spread. Activated T-cells kill antigens and are responsible for transplant rejection.

Group 3 on the list are **erythrocytes** (or **red blood cells**, **RBC**), which contain the **haemoglobin** necessary for oxygen transportation around the body. They have no nucleus, i.e. they are **anucleated** (*a* as a prefix = without, i.e. without a nucleus), and therefore only survive about 120 days, after which they are destroyed and must be replaced from bone marrow. They have a shape described as a *bi-concave disc*; in other words they are round with two flattened surfaces, both of which are dented slightly in. This shape allows for ease of passage through capillaries and provides the best possible surface area for the exchange of gases. Erythrocytes are more numerous than any other cell group (Table 4.1).

TABLE 4.1 Normal blood cell and haemoglobin values.

Blood cell	Cell count (in blood)
Erythrocytes	Male: 4.6–6.2 × 10⁶ / μl (SI = 4.6–6.2 × 10¹² / l) Female: 4.2–5.4 × 10⁶ / μl (SI = 4.2–5.4 × 10¹² / l)
Lymphocytes	1000–4800 / μl (SI = 1.0–4.8 × 10⁹ / l)
Monocytes	0–800 / μl (SI = 0.0–0.8 × 10⁹ / l)
Eosinophils	0–450 / μl (SI = 0–0.45 × 10⁹ / l)
Basophils	0–200 / μl (SI = 0–2 × 10⁹ / l)
Neutrophils	1800–7000 / μl (SI = 1.8–7.0 × 10⁹ / l)
Thrombocytes	150,000–400,000 / μl (SI = 0.15–0.4 × 10¹² / l)
Haemoglobin (in erythrocytes)	Male: 13.5–18.0 g / dl (SI = 2.09–2.79 mmol / l) Female: 12.0–16.0 g / dl (SI = 1.86–2.48 mmol / l)

Note: g = grams, dl = decilitre, SI = Système International, mmol = millimole, l = litre, μl = microlitre.

Group 4 on the list are platelets (thrombocytes). These are critical in preventing blood loss by two means. Small holes in capillaries can be physically blocked by platelets until a repair is complete. For larger damage to major vessels, platelets initiate the blood clotting mechanism. Platelets are the body's own method of **haemostasis**, or the control and prevention of blood loss (Blows 2001).

Blood cell formation

The development of mature blood cells from stem cells in bone marrow occupies several stages for each cell line. Figure 4.2 shows the cells involved at the various stages of development (or differentiation). We will use the same cell lineage list as seen before (see p. 94):

1 Myeloid cell lines develop first from haemopoietic stem cells to **myeloid stem cells**, and these can become either (a) **myeloblasts**, which then develop into **myelocytes** and finally any of the granulocytes; or (b) **monoblasts** and finally **monocytes**. Notice, the term *blast* indicates a primitive cell type.
2 Lymphoid cell lines develop first from haemopoietic stem cells to **lymphoid stem cells**, and these can become **lymphoblasts**, which then develop into lymphocytes.

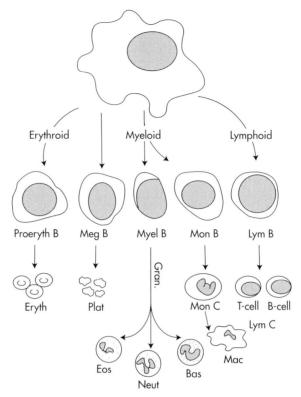

FIGURE 4.2 Blood cell lineages from bone marrow stem cells. The four lineages are erythroid (leading to red blood cells, or erythrocytes), megakaryocytes (leading to platelets), myeloid (splitting into two lines, one leading to granulocytes, the other leading to monocytes) and lymphoid (leading to lymphocytes). Bas = basophils; Eos = eosinophils; Eryth = erythrocytes; Lym B = lymphoblasts; Lym C = lymphocytes; Mac = macrophages; Meg B = megakaryoblasts; Mon B = monoblasts; Mon C = monocytes; Myel B = myeloblasts; Neut = neutrophils; Plat = platelets; Proeryth B = pro-erythroblasts. (Redrawn from Blows 2001, Figure 2.1.)

3 Erythroid cell lines develop first from haemopoietic stem cells to **pro-erythroblasts**, and these become **erythroblasts**, which then develop into erythocytes.
4 **Megakaryocytes** are the precursor of the thrombocytes (or platelets).

Bone marrow cancers

Bone marrow cancers are called the **leukaemias**. Basically, this group of diseases involves malignant changes to cells in the bone marrow.

The haemopoietic stem cells of the bone marrow show a lack of ability to differentiate normally into the range of blood cells expected. Instead, the bone marrow stem cells incline towards the production of white cells in large numbers, with a corresponding lack of red cells or platelets. Worse still, the white cells that are produced appear to enter circulation and exist at an immature stage of their production, i.e. 'blast' cells, and therefore do not function fully. The result is an abnormal blood picture showing a mix of excessive immature white cells with a lack of red cells and platelets, due to their abnormal development in the bone marrow.

Leukaemia exists in various forms depending on which cell lineage is predominant in the peripheral blood. Then each type can be further divided into a rapidly developing severe leukaemia with blast cells in peripheral blood (the *acute* form) or a slowly developing less severe leukaemia with some mature cells in peripheral blood (the *chronic* form).

The acute leukaemias are the result of two abnormal processes going on simultaneously. These are:

1 *Excessive growth expansion,* where the growth of new blood cells has accelerated well beyond the requirements of the blood, and
2 *Failure of differentiation and maturation,* where the stem cells have failed to become the normal range of mature red cells, white cells and platelets; instead becoming mostly of one immature type (i.e. white cells).

The chronic leukaemias tend to be less severe than the acute disorders partly because mature cells do appear in the blood, reducing the symptoms of the disease. They also mostly occur in the older age group.

The classification of the leukaemias is:

1 **Acute lymphocytic** (or **lymphoblastic**) **leukaemia** (**ALL**).
2 **Chronic lymphocytic leukaemia** (**CLL**).
3 **Acute myelocytic** (or **myeloblastic**) **leukaemia** (**AML**).
4 **Chronic myelocytic** (or **myeloid**) **leukaemia** (**CML**).

This classification is a little simplistic, but covers the majority of cases seen. The symptoms of both the acute and chronic leukaemias are found in Table 4.2.

TABLE 4.2 The symptoms of leukaemia

Acute leukaemias	Chronic lymphocytic leukaemia (CLL)	Chronic myeloid leukaemia (CML)
<ul><li>Rapid onset of symptoms</li><li>Fatigue, pallor and breathlessness (due to the anaemia, a lack of haemoglobin in circulation, caused by the low red cell count)</li><li>Infections and fever (due to low mature white cell count)</li><li>Bleeding (due to low platelet count), e.g. petechiae (dark red spots of bleeding into the skin or mucous membrane); ecchymoses (bruising due to bleeding into the skin); epistaxis (nose bleeds) or bleeding from the gums</li><li>Bone pain (due to bone marrow expansion)</li><li>Lymphadenopathy (disorder of lymph nodes), splenomegaly (enlarged spleen) and hepatomegaly (enlarged liver)(all due to spread of leukaemic cells to these organs)</li><li>Headache and vomiting (due to central nervous system involvement)</li></ul>	<ul><li>Often asymptomatic (*a* = without, i.e. no symptoms) especially at first</li><li>Vague symptoms of fatigue, weight loss and anorexia (loss of appetite)</li><li>Anaemia (see under acute leukaemias)</li><li>Increased risk of infections</li><li>Lymphadenopathy, hepatomegaly and splenomegaly (see under acute leukaemias)</li><li>Unlike CML, conversion to an acute form by 'blast crisis' is rare (see under CML)</li></ul>	<ul><li>Slow onset of symptoms and slow progress of the disease</li><li>Fatigue, weight loss, weakness</li><li>Anorexia (see under CLL)</li><li>Extreme splenomegaly (see under acute leukaemias), causing a dragging feeling in the abdomen</li><li>After an unpredictable period, half of the patients will enter a gradual *accelerated stage* with increased symptoms, especially anaemia. There is failure in response to treatment, and it leads to a 'blast crisis' (many immature cells in circulation, similar to acute myelocytic leukaemia, AML)</li><li>The other half develop 'blast crisis' quickly</li></ul>

Acute lymphocytic (or lymphoblastic) leukaemia (ALL)

This form of leukaemia is the most common cancer seen in children (it accounts for about 80% of childhood cancers), and is found in boys more than girls. Half of all cases have an age of onset from 2 to 5 years old, peaking between 3 and 4 years old. The other half of the cases occur at any age, but again the majority of these are before 15 years of age.

The white cells in this disease develop rapidly but do not progress to become mature cells (i.e. 60 to 100% of the WBCs remain as immature blasts; see p. 97). They accumulate in bone marrow and suppress the differentiation of any remaining normal stem cells. The result is a shortage of red cells (an anaemia), whilst normal mature white cells and platelets are also low, and this causes most of the symptoms and complications of the disease (Table 4.2).

Two terms may be used in clinical practice; **leukaemic leukaemia** (showing high levels of immature blast cells present in the blood with a corresponding raised WBC count), and **aleukaemic leukaemia** (*a* = without; showing low levels of immature blast cells with a corresponding low WBC count).

The treatment of ALL has improved enormously, and the prognosis is good for many children, although some children and particularly adults with this disease have a less favourable outcome.

Chronic lymphocytic leukaemia (CLL)

CLL accounts for about 30% of all leukaemias in the Western world, but remains rare in Asia. It affects mostly people over the age of 50 years. The cancer is that of B-cell lymphocytes in the majority of cases, only about 5% being T-cell lymphocyte in origin.

The B-cells involved do not respond to activation by antigens, causing a low antibody count in the blood and a corresponding increased risk of infection. About 15% of cases do, however, show antibody production against red cells, causing the RBCs to break down (i.e. a **haemolytic anaemia**, *haemo* = blood, *lysis* = break down). Abnormal B-cells migrate from the bone marrow into the blood and infiltrate many other tissues, including lymph nodes.

Half of the patients have abnormalities of their **karyotype** (i.e. the chromosomes in the cell nucleus, see p. 7), of which the most characteristic abnormality is **trisomy 12** (three number 12 chromosomes instead of the normal two). Unfortunately this karyotype abnormality carries a poor prognosis. They may also show abnormalities of chromosomes 11 or 14.

Acute myelocytic (or myeloblastic) leukaemia (AML)

This is actually a group of diseases affecting mostly adults, the incidence increasing with age. The group, also called the **acute non-lymphocytic leukaemias**, arises from various origins, including multipotent stem cells or monocyte–granulocyte precursor cells (Figure 4.2). Eight different disorders are recognised, classified by the **French–American–British (FAB)** system:

M0 class, slightly differentiated AML.
M1 class, AML with no differentiation.
M2 class, AML with differentiation.
M3 class, acute pro-myelocytic leukaemia.
M4 class, acute myelo-monocytic leukaemia.
M5 class, acute monocytic leukaemia.
M6 class, acute erythroleukaemia.
M7 class, acute megakaryocytic leukaemia.

The resulting blood picture is different in each case depending on which cell line is most affected, and that depends on which precursor or stem cell is involved in the malignancy. Classes M6 and M7 are odd since they involve erythrocyte and platelet cell lines, respectively. Hence the reason for the term *non-lymphocytic*, i.e. involving all the cells except lymphocytes. Class M3 involves a translocation between chromosomes 15 and 17, i.e. t (15:17) (see p. 38 and under CML below). The resulting combination involves the retinoic acid receptor gene. Retinoic acid itself is an active form of vitamin A (Devlin 2002), and the error on the gene for the retinoic acid receptor manages to block myeloid differentiation (although the mechanism is unclear). This can be treated with high doses of retinoic acid.

Chronic myelocytic leukaemia (CML)

This disorder affects mostly adults between the ages of 25 and 60 years, peaking in incidence between 40 and 50 years of age. It accounts for about 20% of all cases of leukaemia. The genetic basis for this disease lies with the formation of the **Ph[1]** (known as the **Philadelphia chromosome**)(see p. 42 and Figure 4.3). What happens is that a **translocation** (see p. 38) occurs between two chromosomes, numbers 9 and 22, i.e. t (9:22). In this case the translocation involves a large portion of the long arm of chromosome 22 (the long arm is referred to as **q**, thus 22q), which breaks off and swaps places with a tiny fragment from the long arm of chromosome 9 (i.e. a tiny fragment of 9q). The remains of chromosome 22 with the re-attached fragment from 9q form what is called the Philadelphia chromosome (Ph[1]) (Figure 4.3). The breaks occur in the *BCR* gene (short for *breaking point cluster*) on chromosome 22, and the *ABL* gene on chromosome 9. The new combination on chromosome 22 creates an **oncogene** (see p. 38) called **bcr-c-abl**, that leads to cancerous changes in the bone marrow since it causes uncontrolled cell growth in affected cells (Nussbaum 2001). However, discovery of the Ph[1] chromosome is not diagnostic by itself, since this genetic error is also sometimes seen in acute myeloblastic leukaemia (AML) and acute lymphoblastic leukaemia (ALL). The blood picture for CML shows a large increase in the numbers of leucocytes, which are mostly granulocytes of the neutrophil type, but also eosinophils and basophils.

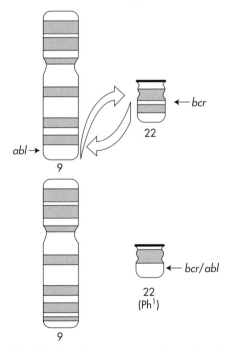

FIGURE 4.3 The Philadelphia chromosome (Ph[1]). The lowest parts of the long arm of two chromosomes (9 and 22) break off and swap places (a 9:22 translocation). The segment from 9 contains the *abl* gene, whilst the break point on 22 is close to the *bcr* gene. The recombination, called the Philadelphia chromosome (Ph[1]) creates the combined *bcr/abl* oncogene.

There appears to be no block to the maturation of these cells, so the cells in the blood are mature but mostly of the granulocyte type. The bone marrow shows a large increase in the myeloid stem cell mass.

The lymphatic system

The **lymphatic system** is a tissue fluid drainage system, which serves several functions, mainly to return excess tissue fluid to the blood and to filter and destroy unwanted **antigens** (e.g. bacteria or viruses). Lymph, the watery fluid medium of the system, is first derived from blood plasma as **tissue fluid** (also called **extracellular fluid**, or **ECF**)(Figure 4.4) which then drains away as lymph. Tissue fluid

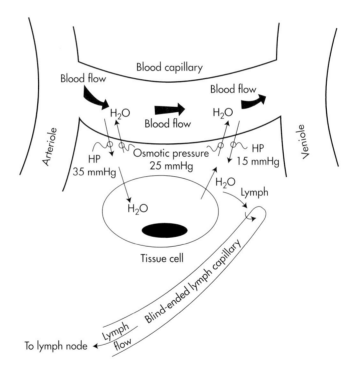

FIGURE 4.4 The formation of extracellular (tissue) fluid. The hydrostatic pressure (HP, the equivalent of blood pressure) forces water (H_2O) out of the capillary. This is higher at the arterial end of the capillary (35 mmHg) than at the venous end (15mmHg). The osmotic pressure is caused by plasma proteins in the blood attracting water back into the capillary at 25 mmHg pressure throughout. The net flow of water is 35 −25 (= 10 mmHg) *out* of the capillary at the arterial end, and 25 − 12 (= 13 mmHg) *in* to the capillary at the venous end of the capillary. Lymph is formed from the excess tissue fluid collected by the lymphatic capillaries.

enters blind-ended lymphatic capillaries in the tissues, and the fluid is now called lymph. This drains towards the **lymph nodes** in **afferent vessels** (*afferent* = towards), which have non-return valves.

Lymph nodes are usually small (most are less than 2.5 cm long) and they contain a number of compartments. In the **cortex** (or outer layer) of the node the compartments contain **follicles** of densely packed B-cell lymphocytes. Surrounding the B-cell core of these follicles are T-cells, which migrate in and out of the node and also extend into the inner layer of the node (the **medulla**). The medulla also has many macrophages and plasma cells present. Lymphocytes are originally derived from bone marrow (see p. 97) and they find their way into lymph nodes via the blood and ECF. T-cells spend some time in the **thymus gland** prior to relocating in the lymph nodes. The thymus gland (located in the chest, above the heart) is the site of T-cell maturation, where these cells gain their specificity. The lymph nodes are the site where many of these cells will reside and ultimately meet with the antigens which will trigger a specific response (i.e. activation of T-cells, and B-cell conversion to plasma cells for the production of antibodies, see p. 70). It is no wonder lymph glands become a hive of activity and swell up when infections occur. Macrophages, the phagocytic cells (see p. 68) also collect within the lymph nodes. There they remove and engulf any invading antigens such as bacteria and viruses that are passing through the gland.

Lymph glands are also the sites where many loose malignant cells (called **metastases**, see p. 229) become trapped as they drain from the malignant tumour, and these also provoke an immune response. Lymph nodes are often the first line of defence against metastases and they can become overwhelmed and heavily involved in the cancer. Surgical removal or radiation of lymph nodes involved in the cancer is usually an essential component of the therapy.

On leaving the nodes the lymph drains back towards the blood via **efferent vessels** (*efferent* = away from), which then empty into one of two main **lymphatic ducts**. The left lymphatic duct is the largest and extends from the abdomen to the left shoulder. This returns lymph from the legs, the left arm and most of the left side of the trunk and head to the blood of the left **subclavian vein**. The much smaller right lymphatic duct returns lymph drained from the right side of the head, right arm and right side of the chest to the blood in the right subclavian vein (Figure 4.5). When the lymph nodes become involved in cancer, and often when they are removed, the drainage of lymph becomes more problematic. It slows down,

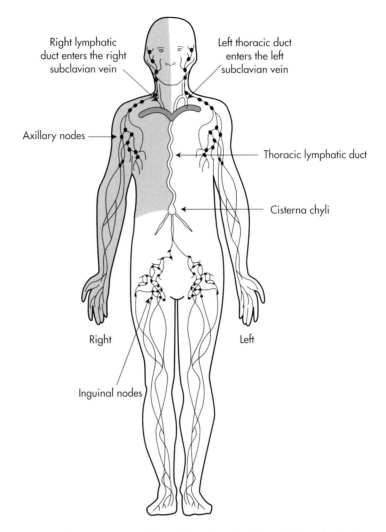

FIGURE 4.5 The drainage of lymph back to the blood. The shaded area on the right of the body is drained by the short right lymphatic duct into the right subclavian vein. The unshaded area on the left side and lower parts of the body is drained by the long thoracic duct, which starts at the cisterna chyli in the upper abdomen, and empties into the left subclavian vein. Some lymphatic nodes are shown. (Redrawn from Marieb 2001.)

with the potential for the pooling of lymph in the tissues causing swelling known as **lymphoedema** (see p. 306). Normally proteins do not easily escape the blood capillaries, so tissue fluid is usually low in proteins. When proteins do get into the tissue fluid the only way for them to get back into the blood is via the lymphatic drainage. Lymphoedema prevents the proteins from returning and the tissue fluid becomes richer in protein (sometimes up to 30 g/litre). These proteins attract more water out of the blood capillaries and the tissues swell further.

Some larger, specialised lymphatic nodes form organs with their own name. The **tonsils** (in the throat) and **adenoids** (in the nose), the **spleen** (in the abdomen) and **Peyer's patches** (associated with the digestive tract) are all important components of the lymphatic system.

The spleen is especially interesting. It acts like a giant lymph node but is attached to the blood circulation, not the lymphatic system (apart from its own lymphatic drainage of course). Whilst lymph nodes filter out antigens from lymph, so the spleen does the same from the blood, i.e. it filters particles, old red blood cells and bacteria directly from circulation. In the spleen, immune responses to blood-borne antigens are initiated, helping to keep the blood clean and sterile. Removal of the spleen is known as **splenectomy**, a surgical procedure done either as an emergency because of trauma to the spleen or more selectively because of splenic involvement in diseases like cancer. Whilst it is true that an individual can live without a spleen, the loss of the spleen is potentially a problem in the long term, and should be avoided if at all possible. Splenectomy patients may suffer more infections due to the presence of blood-borne bacteria, and they also show abnormally old red cells remaining in circulation as well as an increased platelet count.

Lymphatic cancers

Cancers of the lymphatic system fall into two categories, *primary* tumours that arise from the lymphatic system itself, and *secondary* tumours, which are delivered to the lymphatic nodes from primaries arising elsewhere.

Lymphomas are primary tumours of lymph nodes. Thomas Hodgkin was a pathologist at Guys Hospital, London, who first described lymphomas in the early 1800s, and now lymphomas are classified into either **Hodgkin's disease** or **non-Hodgkin's disease**, depending on the tissue pathology of the tumour. Lymphocytes are residential cells in lymph tissue (see p. 105), and most lymphomas arise from malignancy of one of the lymphocyte types (i.e. either B-cells or T-cells)(see p. 70).

Hodgkin's disease results in swollen, often painless lymph nodes usually at restricted sites close to the axis of the body (i.e. the trunk). These frequently start in the cervical (neck) region and go on to involve the axillary and inguinal nodes, spreading by *contiguity* (i.e. by

TABLE 4.3 The principal forms of non-Hodgkin's disease

Non-Hodgkin's lymphoma	Where seen
Burkitt's lymphoma	Usually in African children
Mantell cell lymphoma	Mostly in older men
Follicular lymphoma	Mostly in the elderly
Small lymphocytic lymphoma (SLL)	Mostly in the elderly
Diffuse large cell lymphoma	Children and the elderly
Lymphoblastic lymphoma	Mostly in children

contact with neighbouring cells). Tissues outside the nodes are not often involved. The cause of the disease is unknown. It can spread to the nodes serving other tissues, including the liver, lungs, spleen and bone marrow. As Hodgkin's disease progresses it causes anorexia, weight loss, anaemia and weakness. A fever (known as **Pel-Ebstein fever**) is also seen, where the temperature rises and falls in a cyclic manner. Hodgkin's disease is characterised by the presence of large cells called **Reed-Sternberg cells** seen on microscopy in the tumour. Reed-Sternberg cells are giant malignant cells derived from T-cell lymphocytes. The disease occurs twice as often in men as in women and peaks in incidence between the ages of 15 and 35 years, then again between 55 and 75 years.

Non-Hodgkin's disease is a term used to describe a collection of lymphatic tumours including lymphomas, all of which show an *absence* of Reed-Sternberg cells. The highest incidences occur between the ages of 50 and 70 years, with men more frequently affected than women. Non-Hodgkin's disease involves peripheral nodes (i.e. arms and legs) more than Hodgkin's disease, and spreads by *non-contiguity* (i.e. not directly to neighbour cells but spreads over distance). It also spreads more to tissues outside the nodes than Hodgkin's disease does. Table 4.3 shows the major forms of non-Hodgkin's disease.

Nursing skills: stem cell treatment and blood transfusion

Autologous and allogenic transplantation

Bone marrow stem cells are undifferentiated cells which are capable of becoming any of the blood cell types; red cells, white cells or platelets (see p. 94). Treatment using stem cells involves first the collection (or harvesting) of these cells from the patient (for an autologous transplantation) or from another person (for an allogeneic transplantation). The patient's bone marrow is then destroyed to kill any remaining malignant cells and is replaced with the harvested cells. The concept is based on the idea that collecting and preserving the stem cells allows the opportunity to destroy remaining diseased bone marrow cells and then replace them by new bone marrow formed from the harvested cells. Forming bone marrow from stem cells collected *from the patient* is called an **autograft** (i.e. a bone marrow tissue graft taken from themselves). Autograft cells are primarily used to treat lymphoma (Hodgkin's and non-Hodgkin's) and myeloma. A graft of stem cells taken *from a different donor* and given to a patent is called an **allograft** (or an **allogeneic** transplant). Such allogeneic grafts are often used to treat acute and chronic myeloid leukaemias and acute lymphoblastic leukaemia. In order to do this, the cells used have to be carefully matched to the patient. A much more rigorous matching process is required than that seen in a straightforward blood transfusion. Close relatives (usually full siblings, parents or children of the patient) are likely to have a greater chance of matching the patient than cells taken from more distant relatives or strangers, because close relatives will share many more genes in common with the patient than anyone else. However, national and even international data banks of stem cell types are held on computers in order to find matches quickly for those who need urgent treatment but do not have a suitable close relative. It is often a slow process, so it is not really suitable for those needing urgent treatment.

The procedure for harvesting, storage and use of stem cells is likely to vary from unit to unit, and perhaps from one consultant to the next. Nurses will need to become familiarised with local procedures and policies, particularly with regards to checks and safety precautions. As an example, the following procedure is likely to be similar to most, and is used here to illustrate the nature of the treatment and to highlight a number of points.

The patient is first likely to be treated for 3 to 5 days with a growth hormone called **G-CSF (granulocyte colony-stimulating factor)**. This promotes the growth of neutrophils by stimulating development of the myeloid lineage of cells (Figure 4.2). In some patients G-CSF is given after intensive chemotherapy, in other patients it may be given with low dose chemotherapy, or on its own. Obviously G-CSF will be used on its own in relatives if the cells are collected for an allograft. In addition to promoting neutrophil production, G-CSF will speed up the self-replication of the bone marrow stem cells, and many more of these will find their way into peripheral blood (i.e. increased stem cell mobilisation). Chemotherapy is used to reduce the patient's disease to a minimum before stem cell collection begins. Ideally, the patient should be in remission for this procedure, or at least have minimal residual disease.

Stem cells are then collected (or harvested) from the patient after around 3 or 4 days of G-CSF treatment. Harvesting is done by a machine that collects stem cells from whole peripheral blood, the blood then being returned to the patient. This takes 3 to 4 hours per session, with one session carried out each day for several days, or sometimes it can be completed in one session. Some units may still collect stem cells from bone marrow directly, taking the bone marrow from a puncture site made in the pelvis. However, it is now generally recognised that the collection of stem cells from peripheral blood is not only simpler, it is less invasive and can be done as an out-patient procedure. Peripheral blood harvesting also shows better results than bone marrow collection, with patients undergoing the former procedure getting faster recovery of bone marrow function, i.e. they spend less time in a neutropenic state (**neutropenia** = lack of neutrophils, *penia* = lack of), and therefore they have less risk of infection, and they consequently go home sooner (Anon. 1998). Harvested blood cells are checked by the laboratory and stored by freezing until they are required.

The patient is then given a combination of chemotherapy and radiotherapy to destroy all the remaining bone marrow, which should then eliminate the malignancy completely. If used, the radiotherapy component is likely to be **total body irradiation** (**TBI**) to destroy bone marrow within the entire skeleton. This will, of course, leave the patient vulnerable to infections, due to their very low white cell counts, and they are likely to require **isolation**, with full nursing precautions against infections. Infection is linked to the severity and length of time **immunosuppression** (i.e. reduced immunity due to low white cell count) occurs. As neutrophil numbers fall the infection risk increases. Antibiotic cover will be necessary to help to protect them against bacterial infections, but there is little protection, other than careful isolation, to offer against viral infections. Protection of the patient against infection could involve anything from the simplest measures such as hand washing through to single room isolation occupancy, or sometimes even the use of positive pressure air filtration systems to remove organisms from the air that the patient breathes.

The stored stem cells (from autografts) are defrosted in a water bath and returned to the patient via a peripheral blood line. Allograft cells are usually delivered to the patient fresh. The day the cells are given to the patient is known as *Day 0*. Return of the stem cells is usually through a **Hickman line**, but may be through a **peripheral inserted cannula** (**PIC**). The Hickman line (or Hickman catheter) is a tube usually inserted in the subclavian vein in the neck, and this allows the administration of drugs or repeated blood sampling without further puncturing of the veins. Tunnelling of the catheter below the skin of the chest for some distance helps to prevent infection from reaching the circulation. Stem cells returned to the venous blood in this manner will find their way to the interior of bones to form new bone marrow. Meanwhile, the peripheral blood may be supported by transfusions of whole blood or transfusions of the separate cellular components of blood depending on what the patient is short of. For example, if they are short of platelets (i.e. **thrombocytopenia**, *penia* = lack of), they will receive a platelet transfusion.

Blood transfusion

The giving of blood from one person to another has been tried for hundreds, if not for thousands of years, since it was recognised early that some people's lives can be saved by blood from a donor. However, many also died from the reactions that often followed. Today we recognise the reasons for these dangerous reactions and careful tests and checks are carried out to avoid them. There are several different ways for the grouping of blood, but two methods are of particular importance; the **ABO system** and the **rhesus system**. In the *ABO system* the red blood cells have any combination of two **antigens** (i.e. proteins capable of provoking an immune reaction) on their surface; **antigen A** and **antigen B**. If the red cells have only antigen A, this is **blood group A**; cells with only antigen B produce **blood group B**; antigens A and B together produce **blood group AB**, and no antigen A or B on the red blood cell surface is called **blood group O**. Present in the plasma are **antibodies** (immune proteins that react with antigens) (Blows 2001). Table 4.4 indicates which antibody is in each blood group. From this it can be seen that each individual does not have the antibodies to react with their own antigen. However, they do have the antibodies that are capable of reacting with antigens of a different blood to their own.

TABLE 4.4 The ABO blood group system

Blood group	Antigen on RBC	Antibodies in plasma
A	A	Anti-B (reacts with B antigen)
B	B	Anti-A (reacts with A antigen)
AB	A and B	Neither anti-A nor anti-B are present
O	Neither A nor B	Anti-A + anti-B (reacts with both)

In the *rhesus system* a second type of RBC surface antigen, the D-factor, gives rise to the **Rhesus factor**. If the D-factor is present, the blood is **rhesus (Rh) positive**, and the plasma has no **anti-D antibody**. If the D-factor is absent, the blood is **rhesus (Rh) negative**, but the plasma has anti-D antibody. Any of the four ABO groups can be either Rh positive or negative: i.e. eight blood groups in all. In all these cases the plasma antigens cannot react with their own red cells, but **transfusion** of blood from one person to another creates the conditions in which a reaction could occur, and this must be avoided. Figure 4.6 shows which blood groups can be used safely between the different donors and recipients. Any reactions that may occur would be between the *donor antigen* and the *recipient antibody*, and it is these combinations that must be compatible in any transfusion. Incompatible transfusions will lead to reactions which may even be fatal. **Haemolysis** is one type of reaction where red cells are destroyed, haemoglobin is released and the patient can suffer severe **anaemia** with **jaundice**. **Agglutination** is another type of reaction where red cells clump together in large lumps, which can then block smaller vessels, like the arterioles within the kidneys, causing kidney failure.

Recipient blood

Donor blood	A Anti-B antibody	B Anti-A antibody	AB None	O Anti-A + Anti-B antibodies
A	✔	✘	✔	✘
B	✘	✔	✔	✘
AB	✘	✘	✔	✘
O	✔	✔	✔	✔

FIGURE 4.6 Blood group compatibility. The antibodies of the recipient (top) are matched against the antigen of the donor (left). ✔ = compatible (no reaction), ✘ = incompatible (reaction). (From Blows 2001, Figure 2.2.)

These are **mismatched** transfusions, and must be avoided. Careful checking that the correct blood group is given to the correct patient is vital to prevent a possible fatal reaction (Nichol *et al.* 2000).

Key points

Blood

- Plasma is water with minerals, nutrients and different proteins, including clotting factors, hormones, antibodies, albumin and globulin dissolved in it.
- The cells in blood are erythrocytes (red blood cells), leukocytes (white blood cells) and thrombocytes (platelets), all derived from bone marrow cells called haemopoietic stem cells.
- Stem cells are undifferentiated, meaning they have not yet become a specific cell type, and are capable of becoming RBCs, WBCs or platelets.
- The four major types of blood cell lineages are myeloid (the granulocytes or polymorphonuclear cells, and the mononuclear cells); lymphoid (the lymphocyte lineage); erythroid (the erythrocyte lineage) and megakaryocytes (the platelet lineage).
- Three types of granulocytes (polymorphs) exist, called neutrophils, basophils and eosinophils.
- Neutrophils are the commonest of the white blood cells in circulation.
- Neutrophils are phagocytes, i.e. a cell that engulfs and destroys antigens.
- Monocytes are large phagocytic cells that can migrate out of circulation into the tissue fluid where they change their nature and are known as macrophages.
- Two types of lymphocytes occur, T-cells and B-cells.
- Lymphocytes are the cells of our specific immune system.
- T-cells are active against viral and tumour cells.
- Activated B-cells are called plasma cells and they produce antibodies.
- Antibodies are also called immunoglobulins (Ig).
- Erythrocytes are red blood cells (RBCs) containing haemoglobin, which carries oxygen around the body.
- Platelets are the body's own method of haemostasis, i.e. the control and prevention of blood loss.

Blood cell formation

- Myeloid cell lines develop first to myeloid stem cells, which can become either myeloblasts (becoming myelocytes and finally granulocytes); or monoblasts (becoming monocytes).
- 'Blast' indicates a primitive cell type.
- Lymphoid cell lines develop first to lymphoid stem cells, becoming lymphoblasts, then lymphocytes.
- Erythroid cell lines develop first to pro-erythroblasts, becoming erythroblasts, then erythocytes.
- Megakaryocytes become thrombocytes (platelets).

Blood cancers

- Leukaemia is a group of diseases involving malignant changes to bone marrow cells.
- The types of leukaemia are acute lymphocytic (or lymphoblastic) leukaemia (ALL), chronic lymphocytic leukaemia (CLL), acute myelocytic (or myeloblastic) leukaemia (AML) and chronic myelocytic leukaemia (CML).
- Acute leukaemia causes abnormal blood with excessive immature white cells and a lack of red cells and platelets.
- Chronic leukaemia has more normal mature cells in circulation and affects the elderly more than the young.

Lymphatic system

- The lymphatic system returns excess tissue fluid back to the blood, and filters out and destroys bacteria or viruses.
- Lymph is derived from blood plasma which first forms extracellular fluid then lymph.
- Lymph nodes have compartments in the cortex containing follicles of densely packed B-cell lymphocytes with T-cells surrounding.
- The inner layer of the node is the medulla, with macrophages and plasma cells.
- Lymph nodes are the sites where many malignant cells (metastases) from the malignant tumour become trapped, and these provoke an immune response.
- Removal of lymph nodes involved in cancer often makes the drainage of lymph more problematic, i.e. it slows down, causing pooling of lymph in the tissues and swelling (lymphoedema).
- The spleen acts like a lymph node attached to the blood circulation.

- Splenectomy (removal of the spleen) may result in more infections due to blood-borne bacteria, and abnormally old red cells remaining in circulation with an increased platelet count.

Lymphatic cancers

- Lymphomas are primary tumours of lymph nodes and are classified into either Hodgkin's disease or non-Hodgkin's disease.
- Hodgkin's disease causes swollen, painless lymph nodes, anorexia, weight loss, anaemia, fever and weakness and is characterised by the presence of large Reed-Sternberg cells seen on microscopy in the tumour.
- Non-Hodgkin's disease is a term used to describe a collection of lymphomas, all of which show an absence of Reed-Sternberg cells.

Treatment of blood cancers

- Treatment of bone marrow cancers using stem cells involves the collection of these cells from the patient or a donor (stem cell harvesting, or leukapheresis).
- The patient is treated to destroy the remaining bone marrow, followed by replacement of the harvested cells.
- During this time the patient is vulnerable to infections and should be isolated.

Blood transfusion

- In the ABO blood grouping system the red blood cells have combinations of two antigens, A and B.
- Only antigen A on the RBC surface is blood group A; only antigen B is blood group B; antigens A and B together form blood group AB, and no antigen A or B on the red blood cell surface is blood group O.
- The rhesus system means the D-factor is either on the RBC surface (Rh positive) or is missing (Rh negative).
- The plasma of Rh positive blood has no anti-D antibody.
- The plasma of Rh negative blood has anti-D antibody.
- Incompatible transfusions will lead to possibly fatal reactions.
- Haemolysis is where red cells are destroyed, haemoglobin is released and the patient can suffer severe anaemia with jaundice.
- Agglutination is another reaction where red cells clump together in large lumps, blocking smaller blood vessels, causing problems like kidney failure.

- Mismatched transfusions must be avoided by careful checking that the correct blood group is given to the correct patient.

References

Anonymous (1998) *Bone Marrow and Stem Cell Transplantation*, Leukaemia Research Fund, London.

Blows W. T. (2001) *The Biological Basis of Nursing: Clinical Observations*, Routledge, London.

Devlin T. M. (ed) 2002 *Textbook of Biochemistry with Clinical Correlations* (5th edn), Wiley-Liss (John Wiley & Sons, Inc), New York.

Marieb E. N. (2001) *Human Anatomy and Physiology* (5th edn), Benjamin Cummings, San Francisco.

Nichol M., Bavin C., Bedford-Turner S., Cronin P. and Rawlings-Anderson K. (2000) *Essential Nursing Skills*, Mosby, Edinburgh.

Nussbaum R. L. (2001) *Thompson and Thompson Genetics in Medicine.* (6th edn), W.B. Saunders Company, Philadelphia.

Chapter 5

Cancers of the digestive tract

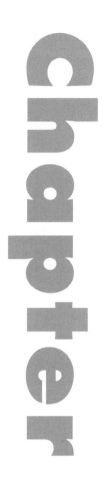

Introduction

Apart from the pain and fear associated with all cancers and their treatment, malignancy of the digestive tract carries with it one particular additional problem, **malnutrition**. Poor nutrition is a huge subject, and is expanded in detail in a separate chapter (Chapter 11, p. 286), so this chapter should be read in conjunction with Chapter 11. Nutritional problems in digestive cancers stem from several factors. Chief among these factors are that these cancers specifically can cause malabsorption of nutrients by obstructing the digestive tract, and they also cause **anorexia** (poor or no appetite) by inducing nausea and vomiting. Maintaining nutrition in patients with digestive disorders of this kind becomes a major challenge for nurses and other health-care professionals.

The digestive system

The digestive tract is essentially a muscular tube, the muscle being of the **smooth muscle** type which functions automatically (i.e. without conscious control). It is very different to the muscle that we use to move (see p. 20). The purpose of this muscle is to contract and push food along the tube. A wave-like contraction, called **peristalsis**, moves food along the tube, and other muscular contractions ensure that food is broken down and well mixed with the digestive chemicals. The inner lining of the tract is **mucous membrane** (see p. 15), and this is important because not only does it prevent digestion of the muscle layer by the chemicals, but it contains many glandular structures which are the site where most tumours of the digestive tract arise.

The digestion of food (see Figure 5.1) begins in the mouth with the twin mechanical actions of chewing and churning, using the teeth and tongue to mix food with the saliva to form a **bolus**, which is then swallowed. Saliva has the enzyme **amylase** which breaks down **starch**, a complex carbohydrate, into sugars called **disaccharides**. So the mix of mechanical with chemical digestion begins immediately.

A swallowed bolus enters the **oesophagus**, a muscular tube that drives food towards the stomach. Like all the digestive tract, the oesophagus is lined by mucous membrane. In the stomach more mechanical churning of food is also accompanied by chemical activity (Figure 5.2). About 1 to 3 litres per day of **hydrochloric acid** (**HCl**) is produced by **parietal** (also called **oxyntic**) cells in the stom-

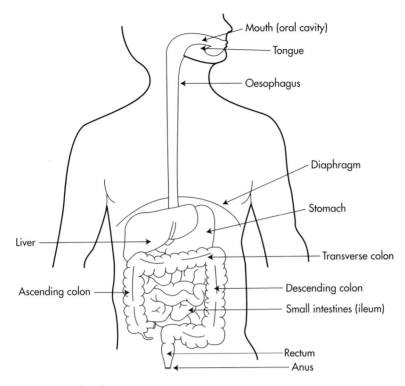

Mouth (oral cavity)

Tongue

Oesophagus

Diaphragm

Stomach

Liver

Transverse colon

Ascending colon

Descending colon

Small intestines (ileum)

Rectum

Anus

FIGURE 5.1 The digestive system.

ach mucosal wall lining. HCl is acidic, having a **pH** value of about 1.5 (the acid end of the **pH scale** which is a measure of **hydrogen ion concentration** in a liquid)(Blows 2001, p. 109). The low pH of HCl is essential for the activation of the protein-digesting enzyme **pepsinogen** to a functional state called **pepsin**, and this can then start the process of protein breakdown to **peptides** (small proteins). Pepsinogen comes from the **chief** (or **zymogenic**) cells of the mucosal stomach wall lining. HCl production is increased by the action of **histamine** (from **ECL,** or **enterochromaffin-like** cells of the mucosal wall lining) and by **gastrin** (from **G cells** also in the mucosal lining).

What leaves the stomach is **chyme,** an acidic mix of broken down food particles and chemicals. This enters the **duodenum** through the **pyloric sphincter** (see Figures 5.2 and 5.3). In the duodenum further products and enzymes act on the contents, as shown in Table 5.1. The duodenum is a vital step in the digestive process. Here bile enters from the liver via the biliary apparatus, i.e. two hepatic ducts beneath the liver join to form a common bile duct which joins the duodenum.

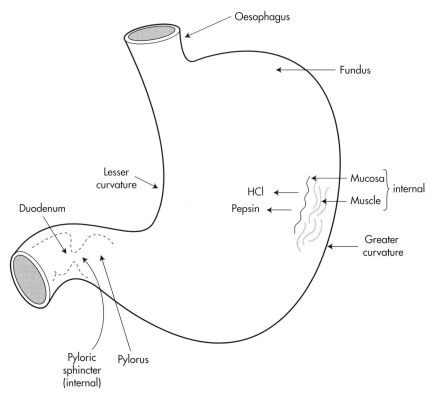

FIGURE 5.2 The stomach. The internal wall structure consists of multiple layers of smooth muscle, providing mechanical movement, and mucosa, secreting hydrochloric acid (HCl) and the enzyme pepsin.

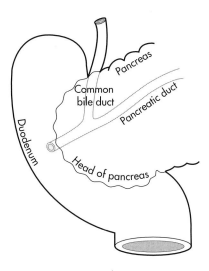

FIGURE 5.3 The duodenum with the head of the pancreas. The pancreatic and common bile ducts join just prior to entry into the duodenum.

TABLE 5.1 The main substances and their actions in the duodenum

Substance	From	Function	Notes
Bile	The liver	Emulsifies fats (i.e. combines fats with water) and changes the acid conditions from the stomach back to base (alkaline)	Drains into the duodenum from the bile duct, part of the biliary apparatus from the liver
Pancreatic amylase (an enzyme)	The pancreas	Continues the conversion of starch to sugars	Salivary amylase is destroyed by the stomach acid, but in the alkaline of the duodenum (see bile), pancreatic amylase continues this function
Lipase (an enzyme)	The pancreas	Breaks down fats from triglyceride form to fatty acids and monoglyceride	Fats must be emulsified by bile
Trypsinogen (a pro-enzyme, i.e. not yet activated)	The pancreas	As trypsin it breaks down proteins to amino acids	Must be converted to the active form trypsin in the duodenum
Chymotrypsinogen (a pro-enzyme, i.e. not yet activated)	The pancreas	Chymotrypsin breaks down proteins to amino acids	Must be converted to the active form chymotrypsin in the duodenum

In addition, a cystic duct leads to the gall bladder which stores and concentrates bile (see Figure 5.4). Bile is a little like washing-up liquid, it acts to emulsify fats, i.e. it makes fats able to blend with water, a vital step for lipase activity (and for washing-up) (see Table 5.1). Bile also converts the acidity of chyme back to alkaline (as it was in the mouth), a vital step for amylase activity. Also joining the duodenum is the pancreatic duct, bringing enzymes that will continue the digestive process (see Table 5.1). Both ducts, the bile duct and the pancreatic duct, join together at a point called the **ampulla of Vater**. An ampulla is a small nipple-like protrusion that extends a short way into the lumen of the bowel. The arrival of bile and pancreatic enzymes together at this one point is not by chance since the pancreatic enzymes are dependent on bile. Bile, which consists largely of

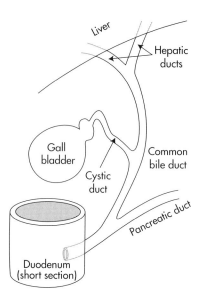

FIGURE 5.4 The biliary system. The common bile duct joins the liver to the duodenum. Bile can be stored in the gall bladder that connects with the common bile duct via the cystic duct.

bile salts, bile pigments and water, is also an important excretory mechanism from the liver. Substances arriving in the bowel via the bile can either be recycled or become incorporated into the faeces for excretion.

The **jejunum** is a continuation of the duodenum leading to the small bowel (the **ileum**). In the ileum the final stages of digestion take place followed by absorption of nutrients into the blood. Table 5.2 identifies the events and the enzymes involved. Lipids are also absorbed from the ileum in fatty acid and monoglyceride form, only to be reconstructed as triglycerides again (see Table 5.1). Minerals, vitamins and water are all absorbed without prior digestion.

After passage through the ileum and absorption is complete the bowel contents consist mostly of the indigestible fibre content of the diet and water. This enters first the **caecum** (also the site of the **appendix**), then the **colon** (the large bowel). The colon is divided into several sections, first the **ascending colon**, then the **transverse colon**, the **descending colon** and finally the **sigmoid colon**. The whole digestive system ends at the **rectum** and the **anus**. The colon acts like a spin dryer in that it absorbs water making the contents dryer and more solid. Here also are bacteria (called the **intestinal flora**) that act to produce some vitamins which can be absorbed (the so-called 'good' bacteria of the advertisements).

TABLE 5.2 The main enzymes and their products active in the ileum

Nutrient from duodenum	Acted on by (enzyme)	End product for absorption
Maltose	Maltase	Two glucose molecules per single maltose molecule
Sucrose	Sucrase	One glucose and one fructose per single sucrose molecule
Lactose	Lactase	One glucose and one galactose per single lactose molecule
Peptides	Aminopeptidase	Amino acids
Peptides	Carboxypeptidase	Amino acids
Peptides	Dipeptidase	Amino acids
Peptides	Tripeptidase	Amino acids

Note that the subject of nutrition is reviewed in more detail in Chapter 11.

Cancers of the mouth

Smoking and alcohol are often major contributors to oral cancers, i.e. cancers involving the mouth, tongue and lips, and of cancers of the jaw. Smokers have two to four times greater risk of oral cancers than non-smokers, and if smoking is combined with regular alcohol consumption the risk rises to 6 to 15 times that of the non-smoker and non-drinker. Tobacco is the most important factor, with higher incidence of the disease in individuals who chew tobacco and those who smoke a pipe. South-East Asia has a greater incidence of oral cancer because of the social habit of chewing tobacco.

Males appear to be more often affected than females, especially in relation to cancer of the lip (which is where cigarettes and pipes are held), which is as much as ten times as common in men. Oral cancer affects the elderly more, being rare before 40 years of age but with a sharp increase in cases over 70 years of age. Genetic changes also occur in many cases, including loss of several chromosome regions (notably **18q, 10p, 8p** and **3p**, where p = the short arm and q = the long arm of the chromosome, see also p. 7). In addition there are short arm deletions in chromosomes 13, 14, 15, 21 and 22 in 70% of cases, and extra copies of the short arm of chromosome 7 (7p) in 90% of cases. The **erb-B** gene family amplification (see p. 42) and others have been identified in oral cancer cells. All this suggests a vital role for gene mutations in the cause of this disease.

About 95% of cases of mouth cancers are **squamous cell carcinomas** (see p. 15 for squamous cells)(Kumar *et al.* 1997; Woolf 1998). Over 50% of the cancers of the mouth occur on the under surface of the tongue and floor of the mouth. Spread can be local, into the deeper tissues of the jaw, creating a major problem for complete surgical removal, and resulting in extensive disfigurement if the jaw and tongue are removed (see also Chapter 12, p. 321). Lymph node spread is also a problem, and is often present already at first consultation. The **submandibular** (under the **mandible**, or lower jaw) lymph node group is usually the first involved, followed by more distal spread to the lungs, bone or the liver.

Cell markers can be measured and this gives a good indication as to the degree of cell differentiation there is in the tumour. Such markers are the **cytokeratins**, where poorly differentiated cells express **cytokeratins 8** and **9**, and well-differentiated cells express **cytokeratins 1** and **10**. The cytokeratins are markers produced by keratinising cells, i.e. cells that produce keratin in the cytoplasm (see p. 16).

Treatment is likely to begin with some form of surgery to excise as much of the tumour as is possible, and this step causes enormous physical and psychological stress for the patient. This form of radical surgery, often resulting in the loss of the tongue and lower jaw, is going to leave the patient with great difficulties in feeding and speaking, as well as overwhelming embarrassment about the way they look to others. They may become isolated and depressed, and hide their face, even from their family. This is a major problem for all concerned with the patient, and the nurses must do what they can to give support to the patient and their family. It is going to take time for the patient, and even the family, to come to terms with the disfigurement, and reconstruction is a long and painful process, with no guarantee of a satisfactory result. It is times like this that makes oncology nursing such a challenging career, and good nurses can make a major difference to the patient's life.

Oesophageal cancer

The oesophagus is a muscular tube with a mucosal lining, connecting the pharynx (at the back of the mouth) to the stomach, and it conveys the swallowed food into the stomach entrance (see Figure 5.1).

Most cancers of the oesophagus are squamous cell carcinomas (about 90% of cancers, arising from squamous epithelium) or adenocarcinomas (about 5% of cancers, arising from the glandular components of the mucous membrane), but other types do occur far less frequently. Factors influencing the onset of squamous cell carcinoma are chronic inflammation of the oesophagus (a feature seen throughout the bowel, see colon on p. 133), alcohol and tobacco use, retarded passage of food through the oesophagus and dietary factors, such as vitamin or mineral deficiency (see p. 291) and high nitrate content of food.

Close to 50% of sqamous cell carcinomas involve the genetic error of the *p53* gene (see p. 40). About 50% of them arise in the central one-third of the oesophagus, 30% in the lower (distal) third and 20% in the upper (proximal) third. Three main types are seen: (1) **crateriform**, a raised type (i.e. protruding out from the level of the mucosa) with a central ulceration forming a crater; (2) **polypoid**, a soft bulky mass projecting into the tube lumen; and (3) **stenosing**, a strongly infiltrative form extending into the oesophageal wall.

In adenocarcinoma, the cancer may arise from what is called **Barrett's oesophagus**, which is a change of the normal squamous epithelium to columnar epithelium (see p. 16) which shows a dysplasia (see p. 27) in at least 3 cm of the distal (stomach) end of the oesophagus. Oesophageal cancers can spread locally into the wall and beyond into the lower respiratory tract, the lung itself and the **mediastinum** (the space between the lungs that contains the heart). The heart and aorta are rarely involved. Because the disease comes on insidiously (gradually and with few or no early symptoms), it is often the case that spread has occurred before diagnosis is made, making treatment more difficult and the **prognosis** (the future outlook for the patient) is poorer. Symptoms are **dysphagia** (difficulty or pain in swallowing), **anorexia** (poor appetite), weight loss and fatigue as the oesophagus begins to become obstructed by the tumour. Pain also occurs associated with the passage of food. If the tumour can be detected early enough before spread occurs, surgical excision and the replacement by an artificial tube is an option.

Gastric cancer

Cancer of the stomach (**gastric carcinoma**) occurs in two forms: intestinal and diffuse.

The **intestinal form** is the commonest type seen in high-risk areas of the world, i.e. Japan especially, but also Iceland, Columbia, China,

Chile, Brazil, Hungary, Spain and Costa Rica. Intestinal means that the cancer arises from gastric mucosa that has first undergone chronic inflammation (**chronic gastritis**), followed by changes in the stomach cell type to that resembling cells of the small or large intestines. This change of cell appearance is called **intestinal metaplasia**. An important risk factor in the cause of intestinal carcinoma is nitrites in the diet (derived from nitrates in food, and may be changed to **nitrosamines** and **nitrosamides**, see Figure 5.5). Other risk factors include the eating of smoked foods (the smoking of foods puts carcinogenic agents on the food, see p. 45), eating pickled vegetables and a *high* salt diet, a *low* intake of green vegetables (see p. 134), chronic gastritis (especially with the organism *Helicobacter pylori*) (Cottrill 1996), **pernicious anaemia** (deficiency of vitamin B_{12}, see p. 293), and after some forms of partial **gastrectomy** (removal of part of the stomach). The intestinal form of stomach cancer occurs most

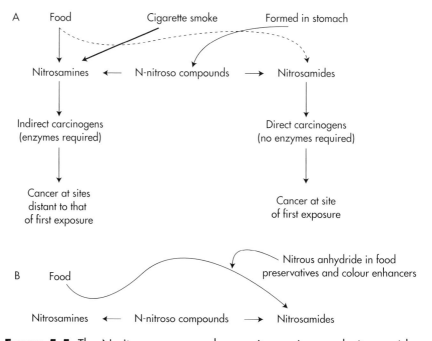

FIGURE 5.5 The N-nitroso compounds are nitrosamines and nitrosamides. (A) Most nitrosamines come from smoking or chewing tobacco, with far less coming from food or produced in the stomach. There is very little nitrosamide normally in food. Nitrosamines are indirect carcinogens (they need enzymes), so they cause cancers beyond the first site of exposure. Nitrosamides are direct carcinogens (no enzymes needed) so they cause cancer directly at the site of first exposure. (B) The addition of nitrous anhydride in food preservatives or food colour enhancers converts nitrosamines to nitrosamides.

after the age of 50 in twice as many men as women. There is a gradual decline in the incidence of this disease, notably in the USA.

The **diffuse form** shows particular geographical or sex dominance. It arises from the native stomach mucosa and is not associated with chronic gastritis. This form is linked to having **blood group A** (see p. 111) with about 50% of the patients having this blood type. The risk factors for this form of stomach cancer are not well determined but may include those listed for the intestinal form. The onset of the disease is often before 50 years of age, and the incidence appears to remain unchanged in the USA.

Gastric carcinoma therefore appears to be in two distinct forms, or as some would say, two distinct diseases. The main sites for gastric carcinoma are 50 to 60% in the *pylorus* and *antrum,* 25% in the *cardiac area*, and the rest are in the *fundus* and *body* of the organ. The *lesser curvature* bears about 40% of cases, the *greater curvature* about 12% of cases (see Figure 5.2 for all these locations, and explanations of these terms). The degree by which the cancer has infiltrated into the stomach wall is the important factor (i.e. the *depth of invasion*) as it determines how advanced the disease is and the likelihood of spread outside of the organ, and thus the potential outcome. Growth occurs in three main types: (1) **exophytic**, where the tumour extends out from the wall and into the stomach lumen; (2) **flat** (or **depressed**) where the tumour is not easily identified within the mucosa; and (3) **excavated** where the tumour erodes into a crater extending into the stomach wall. Eventually, the tumour will spread to lymph nodes and other organs.

Gastric carcinoma usually begins insidiously and may show vague, obscure symptoms, or even be asymptomatic (without symptoms) at first. This makes early detection very difficult, and those persons at high risk (see risk factors) should be screened regularly for signs of the disease. The screening consists of a **barium meal** and **endoscopy**. A barium meal involves the patient swallowing the compound barium, which is radio-opaque (i.e. it shows up on X-ray films) and the cancer can be identified as an elevated irregular lesion often with a central crater. Endoscopy means the passage of a scope into the patient's stomach under sedation, and this allows not only for the surgeon to view the stomach wall but also to take tissue samples (called **biopsies**) of suspect lesions for analysis in the laboratory. At the same time gastric washing samples can be obtained through the scope to examine for malignant cells. Even quite advanced disease can be asymptomatic, or may present with weight loss and abdominal discomfort.

Therefore, many patients are not seen until the disease is at a later stage, and the prognosis is therefore that much poorer.

Other symptoms include nausea and vomiting, **anorexia** (see p. 308), **dysphagia** (difficulty with swallowing) and gastric bleeding, associated with **iron deficiency anaemia**. Treatment of gastric cancer must be, at first, surgery to remove as much of the tumour as is possible. This means an operation called a **gastrectomy**, i.e. removal of part (partial gastrectomy) or all (total gastrectomy) of the stomach will be carried out. Postoperatively the patient may find a particular complication occurs when they eat. It is called **dumping syndrome**, and occurs most often after partial gastrectomy of the distal portion of the stomach and joining (**anastamosis**) of the stomach stump with the **jejunum** or **duodenum** (see Figure 5.6). Dumping syndrome occurs when a food **bolus** (a swallowed ball of food mixed with saliva) passes too quickly from the stomach into the duodenum or jejunum. The bolus attracts water from the blood into the intestines which then become dilated with fluid. The blood volume is decreased and movements of the bowel (known as bowel **motility**) are increased. The symptoms of dumping syndrome occur about 5 to 30 minutes after eating and include nausea and vomiting, cramping pain in the stomach (**epigastric**) area, and loud active bowel sounds (called **borborygmi**). Later symptoms are those associated with disturbance of blood glucose levels. The blood sugar rises and this triggers a large insulin release, which in turn results in a **hypoglycaemia** (low blood sugar level). The corresponding lower blood volume may

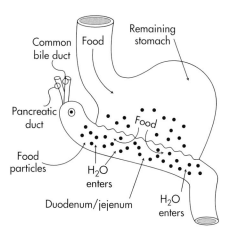

FIGURE 5.6 Dumping syndrome. After a gastrointestinal anastomosis, food passes quickly into the intestine causing water to enter and swell the bowel.

cause a **tachycardia** (fast pulse rate) and a degree of **hypotension** (low blood pressure), with corresponding dizzy spells. Dumping syndrome will eventually correct itself after a year or so following surgery, but it is unpleasant. The symptoms can be reduced by eating smaller, more frequent meals, and by allowing more time to eat the meal. The patient should be encouraged to break up the food into small portions and to swallow smaller boluses. It may also help to separate the consumption of fluids from food (i.e. they are given at different times), and to increase the fats and protein in the diet, and reduce carbohydrates, especially the sugar content of the food. Resting after the meal in a **semi-recumbent** (partly upright) position for 30 minutes after the meal can help.

Gastrectomy can also cause **pernicious anaemia** due to the loss of **intrinsic factor** in the formation of vitamin B_{12} (see Figure 5.7). *Intrinsic* factor is produced by the stomach in response to the consumption of *extrinsic* factor in the diet. The combination of the two factors results in B_{12} **complex**, which is then absorbed into the **terminal ileum** (where the small intestine joins the large intestine). Removal of the stomach means that B_{12} complex cannot be formed or absorbed. Vitamin B_{12}, which is needed for the formation of **haemoglobin** (see p. 293) is normally stored in the liver, and will now need to be given by injection for life to keep the liver stores topped up.

Also, following gastrectomy, the patient may develop poor absorption of **folic acid, calcium** and **vitamin D**. Weight loss, seen in

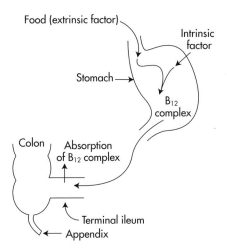

FIGURE 5.7 Vitamin B_{12} synthesis and absorption. Extrinsic factor in the diet meets intrinsic factor in the stomach to form the B_{12} complex. This complex is absorbed in the terminal ileum.

nearly 50% of gastrectomy patients, is due to the combination of reduced meal size (involving poor calorie intake) with nutrient mal-absorption. Dietary adjustments involving the advice of the dietician are needed to improve the patient's nutritional status (LeMone and Burke 2004)(see also Chapter 11).

Cancer of the small bowel

Small bowel cancers, i.e. those of the duodenum and ileum, are uncommon, being 40 to 60 times *less frequently* encountered than those of the colon. In total they account for only 5% of tumours of the digestive tract. About 45% of them are **adenocarcinomas**, about 30% are **carcinoid tumours** and a further 10% are small bowel **lymphomas**. The remainder are of connective tissue origin, i.e. **sarcomas** (see p. 29).

Adenocarcinomas arise from the internal mucosal lining. Approximately 40% occur in the duodenum around the **ampulla of Vater** (see p. 121). Many of these tumours are found in association with **Crohn's disease** (sometimes called **regional ileitis**), a chronic inflammatory condition of the bowel (mostly the small bowel). This is one example of a recognised trend that digestive cancers are often linked to chronic inflammatory diseases of the mucosa (see also **ulcerative colitis** on p. 133) (Anon. 2004). Adenocarcinomas often produce mucin (mucus). One variant is the **small cell carcinoma** (also called **oat cell**, and is similar to the small cell carcinoma of the lung, see p. 157) that consists of small round or oval cells producing and secreting small peptides (tiny proteins). These tumours are prone to invasion and spread widely from the point of origin, making the prognosis rather poor.

Carcinoid tumours occur most frequently in the appendix (see p. 138) and then the ileum (together these account for about 60 to 80% of the carcinoid total, and are considered to be of *mid-gut* origin), less frequently in the colon and rectum (10 to 20% of the total, and considered to be of *hind-gut* origin) and the least frequently seen sites are the oesophagus, stomach and duodenum (considered to be of *fore-gut* origin). The references to fore-, mid- and hind-gut relate to the way the digestive system develops as an embryo. The most frequent site, the appendix, appears also to be the least important, since the carcinoid tumours here are rarely aggressive and often discovered on routine appendicectomy (removal of the appendix). The ileum and the colon are the sites of the more aggressive tumours that invade and spread easily. Generally these aggressive tumours are slow-growing but highly invasive, and produce metastases which spread to the liver and local lymph nodes. They can be the cause of **carcinoid syndrome**, a systemic reaction to a massive release of active compounds from tumour cells into the circulation. The effects of carcinoid syndrome include wheezing, **hypertension** (high blood pressure), palpitations, flushing of the face and chest, watery diarrhoea and right-sided heart failure.

Small bowel **lymphomas** account for only about 10% of the total of small bowel tumours (see also lymphomas in Chapter 4, on p. 107). They are diffuse and poorly differentiated, and are important particularly in children as non-Hodgkin's lymphomas (see p. 107). Small bowel lymphomas are often derived from B-cells of the lymph node tissue that occur in the mucosa, i.e. **mucosa-associated lymphoid tissue** (**MALT**). Again, the activation of this lymph tissue is a result of inflammation (see p. 82).

Sarcomas of the small bowel are relatively rare and are mainly **leiomyosarcomas**, which are malignancies of the smooth muscle wall of the bowel (see p. 21) (Souhami and Tobias 2003).

Cancer of the pancreas

Pancreatic cancer is one of the most difficult cancers to diagnose early, remaining asymptomatic until quite advanced. By then it is often only amenable to palliative treatment (see p. 322), making the prognosis very poor. The disease is on the increase, particularly in the elderly population, being the fourth (male) and fifth (female) leading causes of death from malignancy in the western world (Woolf 1998). Most cases are sporadic, with only a few familial episodes recorded.

Pancreatic cancers are mostly adenocarcinomas derived from glandular epithelium. Two forms are recognised, the **ductal** and the **non-ductal** types. The ductal type accounts for most of the pancreatic tumours and two-thirds of them arise from the head of the gland. They are more often associated with genetic mutations than the non-ductal type. Point mutations in the *k-ras* gene (a proto-oncogene, the locus is 12p)(see p. 41) and *c-erb-B2* (a proto-oncogene on 7p) are known to exist as promoters of ductal pancreatic cancers. Other causative factors include smoking (now known to be a strong link) and perhaps viral infections. The disease starts mostly in the seventh decade of life with a slow-growing asymptomatic tumour that is not detected until a late stage. About 60% of the tumours arise in the head end of the gland, which is the site for entry of both the pancreatic and biliary ducts into the duodenum, and a tumour here can obstruct either or both ducts. Biliary duct obstruction blocks bile flow from the liver and causes **jaundice** (a yellow skin colour due to bile pigment deposits in the tissues). Pain is a feature of later stage disease, often when surgery in no longer an option. Spread of the disease into the local lymph nodes and then the liver occurs. Survival rate measured at 5 years is very poor, only around 2% of patients are alive after 5 years.

Neoplasms of the colon and rectum

The **colorectal cancers** are a very important group of malignant diseases, with many health authorities and hospitals creating specialised units to tackle the problem, and a growing number of nurses becoming **advanced nurse practitioners** (**ANPs**) in colorectal nursing.

Polyps

Non-malignant (benign) and *non-neoplastic* (no malignant potential) **polyps** of the large bowel are growths arising from the mucosal or submucosal lining of the gut wall, and they extend into the lumen of the bowel. Although they are benign (see p. 24), they are problematic in themselves because they can obstruct the lumen and prevent normal bowel function. About 35 to 50% of adults have benign polyps in their colon.

These polyps can be classified into various types. The **hyperplastic polyps** are commonly found in more than 50% of the over 60 age group. They are *not* **pre-malignant**, i.e. they do not become a malignant tumour, and consist of hyperplasia (see p. 26) of normal mucosal

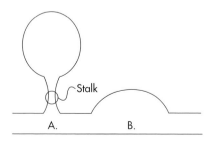

Figure 5.8 Polyps. (A) Pedunculated (on a stalk), (B) sessile (no stalk).

cells. They are mostly small (up to 5 mm in diameter) and mostly asymptomatic (without symptoms). **Juvenile polyps** are sporadic polyps most frequently found near the rectum in children under 5 years of age. They range from 1 to 3 cm in diameter and are pedunculated. Polyps generally may be **pedunculated** (i.e. on a stalk) or **sessile** (i.e. having no stalk)(see Figure 5.8). **Papillary** is another term that means benign epithelial growths consisting of mucosal glandular tissue. Other types include **inflammatory polyps** found in association with **inflammatory bowel disease** (**IBD**). IBD is essentially two disorders, **Crohn's disease** (mostly of the small bowel) and **ulcerative colitis** (of the large bowel). The presence of inflammation of the digestive mucosa increases the risk of neoplastic disease at that site (see p. 130).

Adenomas

Adenomas are *neoplastic* tumours (new growths with malignant potential) derived from the glandular epithelial components of the mucous membrane lining of the bowel. The new growth of tissue is a benign dysplasia (see p. 27), but as such it can become malignant. Such a move to malignancy results in an **adenocarcinoma**. Adenomas may be **villous** (1%, slow growing, soft, spongy, large sessile growths with frond-like projections and potentially malignant) or **tubular** (5 to 10%, made from tubular glands, small, becoming pedunculated) or **tubulovillous** (over 90%, a mix of the previous two)(see Figure 5.9). The potential for malignancy in adenomas is based on (1) tumour size, i.e. the large adenomas carry the greatest risk, and (2) the **histology**, the nature of the tissue from which the tumour is made, i.e. the greater the degree of dysplasia present the

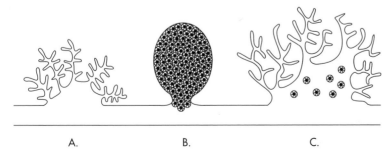

A.   B.   C.

FIGURE 5.9 Adenoma polyps: (A) villous, (B) tubular, (C) mixed tubulovillous. (Redrawn from Woolf 1998.)

higher is the risk. Because adenomas have a long pre-invasive phase and they grow slowly (i.e. they double their size in about 10 years in most cases), there is an opportunity for early detection and removal, which is the only real safe treatment option. They may be asymptomatic for long periods (making routine screening for 'at risk' individuals the only means of detection), or patients may present with **anaemia** (low **haemoglobin** level in circulation due to bleeding at the adenoma site), **occult blood** in the faeces (occult means 'hidden', because the blood cannot be seen in the stool, and must be detected by chemical tests), or they develop a partial obstruction of the bowel.

Adenocarcinomas

Adenocarcinoma is the malignant growth of the bowel (i.e. cancer of the small or large bowel). Adenocarcinoma was discussed in relation to the small bowel (see p. 130), but here its relevance to the large bowel is considered. The vast majority (98%) of colon cancers are adenocarcinomas.

This disease occurs mostly in the older age population, with a peak between 60 and 70 years of age. Less than 20% of cases exist below the age of 50 years. Men suffer about 20% more cases than women, and the underlying lesion is thought to be, in the majority of cases, a pre-existing adenoma. The number of adenocarcinomas arising directly from normal mucosa has not been established, and is probably very low. The disease is very unequally distributed geographically, with high incidence in the 'developed' countries, notably Europe, Australia and North America, and low incidence in Africa, Asia and South America. The incidence correlates well with dietary factors, in particular the presence of meat in the diet. A high level of meat consumption is associated with higher incidence of the disease, and this may be due to the higher levels of saturated fatty acids that come with the meat. High levels of saturated fatty acids in the diet are linked to a greater output of bile acids in the faeces, and these can be converted to dangerous carcinogens by the intestinal flora (see p. 299). But this is not the only dietary consideration. Linked to this are other risk factors, such as a low level of vegetable fibre, low levels of protective micronutrients and high consumption levels of refined carbohydrates in the diet.

Low dietary fibre (fibre is found particularly in the green leafy vegetables) is thought to reduce the faecal bulk in the colon which in turn increases the transit time, i.e. how long faeces are held in the colon. Faeces that are held in the colon for a long time create a greater opportunity for the development of harmful carcinogens which are then exposed to the colonic mucosa for longer periods. Faeces must be transported to the rectum and eliminated in reasonable time to excrete the dangerous carcinogens from the bowel.

Low dietary micronutrients, such as vitamins A, C and E, reduce the antioxidants in the bowel, i.e. chemicals which neutralise the harmful effects of **free radicals** (i.e. dangerous reactive chemicals which damage cells, including DNA, and cause gene mutations) (see p. 38). Antioxidants protect the mucosa from the harm of free radicals, e.g. one vitamin E molecule can neutralise two free radicals. An absence of micronutrients increases the free radicals in the bowel and therefore the risk of genetic mutations.

High dietary refined carbohydrates, such as sugars, can lead to the formation of harmful toxic products by the intestinal flora, and these can damage mucosal cells, especially when the faecal transit time is increased due to low dietary fibre (i.e. the factors work together, not in isolation, to cause the disease)(see also Chapter 11, nutrition, p. 286) (Woolf 1998).

Genetic factors

Genetic factors also have a major role to play in the causation of this disease. The following section should be read in conjunction with the genetic basis of cancer in Chapter 2 (see p. 35). **Familial adenomatous polyposis coli** (**APC**), **Gardner's syndrome** and **Turcot's syndrome** are examples of genetically inherited disorders that include a distinct increase in the risk of colon cancers (Table 5.3).

The tumour suppressor gene involved in APC and Gardner's syndrome is found at 5q21 (see pp. 12–13 for an explanation of this chromosomal shorthand). APC occurs as multiple (more than 100, and sometimes as many as 5000) pre-malignant adenoma polyps in the colon of the affected individual. Sporadic (non-familial) cases of colon cancer often demonstrate a mutation in the APC gene at an early stage. Excision of the affected part of the bowel is the only preventative measure to stop further malignancy.

Other genetic errors in colorectal cancers include *ki-ras*, DCC and *Ki-ras* and *Tp53*. (see Chapter 2, p. 41) is found at 12p12. Mutations that result in the formation of this important oncogene are found in 50% of adenomas over 1 cm across, and in half of all colon cancers.

TABLE 5.3 The major syndromes involving increased risk of colorectal cancer

Syndrome	Notes
Familial adenomatous polyposis coli (APC)	Pre-malignant collection of multiple polyps of the colon and duodenum, carcinoid tumours of the ileum (see p. 130), papillary tumours of the thyroid and increased incidence of brain tumours. It has autosomal *dominant* inheritance resulting in loss of the tumour suppressor gene *APC* at 5q21. An association of APC with brain tumours is called Turcot's syndrome. The *APC* gene mutation is inherited in an autosomal *recessive* pattern (see p. 43)
Gardner's syndrome	Cysts of the epidermis, dermoids (cysts containing hair, hair follicles and sebaceous glands) and increased risk of colon cancer. Gene involved is also the tumour suppressor gene *APC* at 5q21, inherited in an autosomal *dominant* pattern (see p. 43)
Peutz-Jeghers syndrome	Gastrointestinal cancer with ovarian and testicular cancers. An autosomal *dominant* inheritance pattern results in a loss of the tumour suppressor gene *STK11* at 19p13.3
Hereditary non-polyposis colorectal cancer (HNPCC) (Lynch syndromes I and II)	Lynch syndrome type I: HNPCC involving cancer of the colon and rectum only. Lynch syndrome type II: HNPCC involving cancer of the colon and rectum with increased risk of cancer of the ovary, endometrium (see p. 198) and pancreas (see p. 131). An autosomal *dominant* inheritance of loss of any of several DNA repair genes at 2p16, 2p22, 2q31, 3p21 and 7p22

DCC (**deleted in colon cancer**) is a tumour suppressor gene at 18q21 (see p. 35) that is inactivated in over 70% of colon cancers and in 50% of large adenomas. The addition of this deletion to **carcinogenesis** (*carcino* = cancer, *genesis* = creation, i.e. the cause of cancer) gives a poorer prognosis, with a major drop in the 5-year survival rate. *Tp53* (see p. 40) at 17p is found to be mutated in 70 to 80% of colon cancers.

Large bowel cancers

About 50% of large bowel cancers occur in the rectum, i.e. within 15 cm of the anus, and in the sigmoid colon closest to the rectum (Woolf 1998)(Figure 5.10). From here, rectal tumours can spread through the rectal wall into the prostate in men or the vagina in women. Systemic and pulmonary metastases can occur from malignant cells getting into the **inferior vena cava** (the main vein returning blood to the heart from the lower parts of the body). Other sites for cancers within the bowel, and the frequencies at each site can be seen in Figure 5.11.

Staging of disease

Staging of colorectal cancers is important for two reasons: to make decisions with regards to the treatment and to give some idea as to the patient's prognosis. The **Duke classification** is as follows:

Duke stage A	The tumour remains within the bowel wall, i.e. no spread to lymph nodes.
Duke stage B	The tumour has spread locally through the bowel wall but has not involved lymph nodes.
Duke stage C	The tumour has involved lymph nodes.
Duke stage D	The tumour has spread to involve metastases in distal organs.

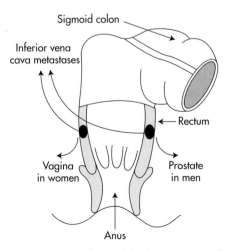

FIGURE 5.10 Rectal carcinomas (shown black) can spread into the vagina in women, into the prostate in men, and cause metastases in the inferior vena cava in both sexes.

137

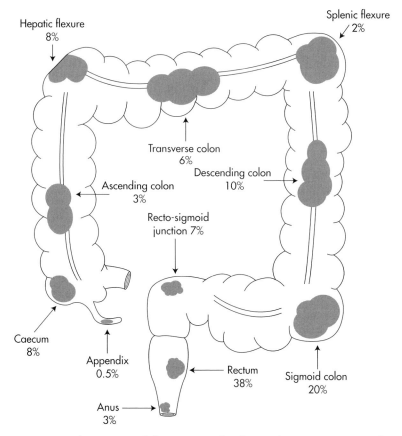

FIGURE 5.11 The sites and frequency of colorectal carcinomas. (Redrawn from Souhami and Tobias 2003.)

Another means of staging this disease is the **Astler–Coller** system:

A The cancer is limited to the mucosa.

B1 The cancer extends into the muscle wall, but no lymph nodes are involved.

B2 The cancer penetrates through the muscle wall but no lymph nodes are involved.

C1 The cancer extends onto the muscle wall and lymph nodes are involved.

C2 The cancer penetrates the muscle wall and lymph nodes are involved.

D There are distal organ metastases.

What is interesting is the predicted 5-year survival rate for each of the Astler-Coller system categories, as follows: **A,** 100% of patients will be alive after five years because surgical resection of the cancer is expected to be 100% curative; **B1,** 67% of patients alive at 5 years; **B2,** 54%; **C1,** 43%; **C2,** 23% and **D** has no rating (presumably very low).

Colorectal cancers may possibly be asymptomatic for years. When symptoms do arise these include fatigue, weakness, anaemia (due to bleeding), abdominal pain and discomfort, progressive bowel obstruction and **hepatomegaly** (enlarged liver due to metastases).

A third system is the **TNM** (**tumour, nodal, metastasis**) staging method. Here letters are used to indicate variations in the nature of the three main components, the tumour, nodal spread and metastases. It is as follows:

T, Primary tumour

TX The primary tumour cannot be assessed.
T0 No primary tumour found.
Tis Carcinoma *in situ* (see p. 27)
T1 Tumour has invaded the submucosa.
T2 Tumour has invaded the **muscularis propria** (a layer of muscle that separates the mucous membrane from the serosa in the colon wall, see Figure 5.12).

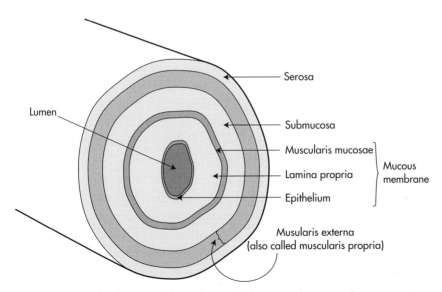

Serosa
Lumen
Submucosa
Muscularis mucosae
Lamina propria
Mucous membrane
Epithelium
Musularis externa (also called muscularis propria)

FIGURE 5.12 The layers of the colon wall showing the muscularis propria.

T3 Tumour has invaded through the muscularis propria or into tissues surrounding the colon or the rectum (without entering the peritoneum).

T4 Tumour has entered the peritoneum and invaded other organs.

N, Regional lymph nodes

NX The regional lymph nodes cannot be assessed.

N0 No regional lymph node metastases.

N1 Metastases in one to three lymph nodes around the colon or rectum.

N2 Metastases in four or more lymph nodes around the colon or rectum.

N3 Metastases in any lymph node along the course of a local blood vessel.

M, Distal metastases

M0 No distal metastases.

M1 Distal metastases found.

Symptoms of bowel cancer

Symptoms are dependent on the site of the cancer within the bowel. In the **ascending colon,** tumours are often large and bulky, they can bleed (causing dark red blood *mixed with* stools and anaemia). They can ulcerate, causing pain. A palpable mass can be felt in the right side of the abdomen. Spread is to the liver via the **portal vein** which runs from the gut to the liver.

Tumours in the **descending colon** start as small button-like elevated masses and eventually ulcerate centrally causing some pain. They can obstruct the lumen (they grow circumferentially, i.e. around the tube to form a ring that then closes across the lumen) and this causes vomiting and constipation. Abdominal distension can occur, and bleeding causes bright red blood *on* the stool surface. Spread is via the lymph nodes in the abdomen and pancreas, then to the liver via the **mesenteric veins** (part of the venous drainage of the abdomen).

Vomiting (or **emesis**) is a common symptom of most gastrointestinal disorders and is another management challenge for the nurse. Vomiting is a complex series of co-ordinated activities involving muscles of the digestive and respiratory systems, and the muscles of the abdominal wall. The **vomit centre** that controls these events is in the **medulla** of the brainstem, close to the **respiratory centre** (see p. 280) and the **cardiac centre**. Near the vomit centre also is the **chemoreceptor trigger zone** that is sensitive to chemical stimuli and the site where anti-emetic drugs act. Stimulation of the chemoreceptor trigger zone by emetic drugs (i.e. those that cause vomiting, e.g. morphine or cytotoxic agents), other chemicals (e.g. toxins in the blood), unusual movements (e.g. sea sickness), bad sight or unpleasant smells causes activation of the vomit centre and the person will vomit. Whilst a single bout of vomiting is not especially harmful (it is, after all, a normal protective mechanism against harm), persistent vomiting for hours or even days is not only unpleasant for the patient but can cause deterioration of health.

Long-term vomiting can lead to distress, **dehydration**, **hypokalaemia** (low blood potassium levels) and **hyponatraemia** (low blood sodium levels) (i.e. an electrolyte imbalance), **alkalosis** (a blood pH higher than the normal level of 7.4), **malnutrition** (see p. 305), reduced effectiveness of oral medication and a risk of inhalation of vomited matter. Drug treatment is often the only effective way of relieving vomiting (anti-emetic agents include **hyoscine**, **cyclizine**, **promethazine**, **metoclopramide** and **domperidone**). Nurses should remain with the vomiting patient and give privacy, support, a bowl and tissues, and a mouthwash for after. In prolonged vomiting, consideration must be given to the immediate management of dehydration and electrolyte imbalance (oral fluids are not likely to be tolerated, so an intravenous infusion may be required), and to the prevention of malnutrition.

Nursing skills: surgery and stomas

The treatment of colorectal cancers usually involves surgery, often **resection** (removal of the affected part of the bowel) and **anastomosis** (joining the cut ends of a tube, in this case the remaining bowel), with or without the formation of a **stoma** (*stoma* = hole or opening). Surgery is necessary, of course, to save lives and to improve the quality of that life. However, complications can occur, both physically and mentally (see the case history on p. 145). One postoperative complication of bowel surgery that nurses need to be aware of is **paralytic ileus**. This is where the bowel movements that drive the contents along stop (see **peristalsis** on p. 118), and this is caused by the handling of the bowel during surgery. Bowel handling by the surgeons is kept to a minimum in order to prevent this particular problem, but it can still occur. The effect of paralytic ileus is the cessation of all bowel movements and therefore bowel sounds, which are caused by bowel movements, stop. The content does not flow and therefore the patient is unable to eat or drink, they may feel nausea and may vomit, and they will become malnourished if this continues. Fortunately this problem normally corrects itself as the **autonomic nervous system**, which drives bowel movements, begins to function again. In the meanwhile the patient is usually kept *nil by mouth* until bowel sounds are heard again. Water is introduced by mouth in small quantities at first, and if this is tolerated the amount of water can be gradually increased until food is re-introduced back into the diet.

Colostomy and **ileostomy** are openings into the bowel (*colostomy* is an opening into the colon, *ileostomy* is an opening into the ileum) for the collection of faeces into a bag worn on the abdomen. Stomas are used either temporarily, as in inflammatory bowel disease (IBD) (see p. 133), or permanently, when bowel resection involves the rectum so there is no longer an option available for a normal anastomosis with the anus, as in the case of an **abdoperineal resection**. A colostomy can be sited anywhere along the colon (see Figure 5.13), so it is important to know if the patient has an **ascending**, **transverse**, **descending** or **sigmoid colostomy**. Owing to the water absorption function of the colon (see p. 122), the site of the colostomy will affect the nature of the faecal material eliminated from it. Ascending and early transverse colostomies are likely to eliminate more fluid faecal matter since the organ has had, at that point, little opportunity to absorb the water. Colostomies sited further along the organ will produce progressively more solid faecal matter, although all colostomies can, given enough time and the right diet, produce solid or at least semi-solid faecal matter. Ileostomies (see Figure 5.13) eliminate the contents into a bag before any colonic function occurs, so the stoma bag is likely to contain purely liquid drainage.

A stoma means that the patient is required to wear a bag permanently over the stoma opening to collect the faecal matter. At first faeces can be eliminated into the bag at any time, probably multiple times per day, but again with time the stoma can be managed in a way that it will empty once or just a few times per day. The choice of stoma bag appliance is very important since different appliances may affect the patient in different ways. One such complication, which

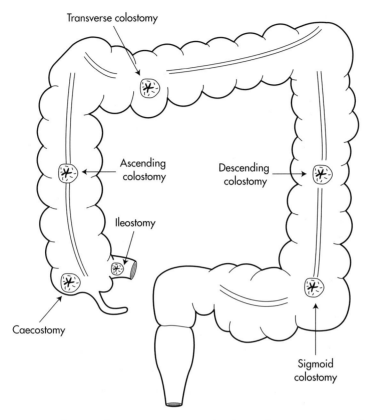

Transverse colostomy

Ascending colostomy

Descending colostomy

Ileostomy

Caecostomy

Sigmoid colostomy

FIGURE 5.13 The sites for various stomas. (Redrawn from LeMone and Burke 2004.)

should be avoided if possible, is soreness and breakdown of the skin around the stoma, and the wrong choice of appliance can cause this to happen by putting excessive pressure on the skin or causing irritation. Good skin care is vital, the skin around the stoma should be a normal colour (not red), it must be clean with no irritations, no rashes and no signs of inflammation or **excoriation** (the surface of the skin breaks down and is lost). The factors that lead to skin problems, and therefore should be avoided are:

1 A badly fitting or irritating stoma bag appliance.
2 Excessive pressure on the skin caused by an appliance that is too tight.
3 Stoma bag appliances that stick to the skin, because these remove skin cells each time they are peeled off, and the adhesive may irritate the skin and cause contact **dermatitis** (inflammation of the skin).

143

4 Changing the stoma bag too frequently.

5 A leaking stoma appliance that causes faecal contamination of the skin, since this is likely to have an effect similar to burning of the skin. This is particularly important with regard to ileostomies, where the bag content will have digestive enzymes and bile salts that can cause considerable skin destruction around the stoma site.

6 Excessive or rough cleaning of the skin can cause skin damage.

7 Infections of the stoma site and surrounding skin, notably fungal infections.

The stoma must be observed to ensure it is healthy, i.e. it has the necessary blood supply and is not infected, so it should be a red colour (not brown, black or pale) with no signs of inflammation (see p. 82) and no pus. It should not be **retracted** (re-entering the abdomen) or **prolapsing** (extending too far out from the abdomen).

Patients with colostomies need a lot of input from nursing care and considerable understanding of their situation, particularly at first. This operation is a major change of body image for the patient, and a big obstacle for the patient to overcome. It is so important to involve the **advanced nurse practitioner** (**ANP**) for stoma care (sometimes called the **stoma care nurse**) from a very early stage when the decision for creating a stoma is first made. This specialist nurse can get to know the patient and family and discuss the problems, solutions and appliances, and answer all their questions. Education is a key component for both the patient and family, and this is going to be a major learning curve for all concerned. The ANP in stoma care can do much to facilitate the patient's adjustment to their new life, teach them the daily management of their stoma, and be alert to the complications and problems, and have solutions readily available.

Nurses that do not have this expertise should be guided by the ANP in stoma care in the care of their client. The following passage (from LeMone and Burke 2004, p. 675) and the case history both highlight the importance of body image change and the need for professional guidance.

Clients undergoing ostomy [*stoma*] surgery for cancer may be more concerned about the effect of the cancer on their lives than the effect of the ostomy. Adaptation to a life-threatening disease and survival are more critical issues for the client and deserve higher priority for nursing care focus. As the threat of the cancer diagnosis is reduced [over *time*], strategies to improve and reintegrate body image will be more effective. Nurses need to acknowledge and accept the client's feelings and behaviour toward the ostomy [*stoma*] in the initial post-operative period. Progressive involvement in stoma care is important, as is preventing major leakage accidents. Education is a key strategy to promote body image; as the client acquires new skills, self concept is enhanced.

The case history concerns a middle-aged professional and very intelligent gentleman, who held a very good job and had a loving supportive family. He was generally fit and well and enjoyed life. He came into hospital with a bowel disorder, and went to the operating theatre where a colostomy was performed. Unfortunately the stoma functioned almost constantly, every few minutes, with liquid faeces. Each new bag needed changing very quickly, and the colostomy would also function whilst the bag was being changed causing faecal contamination of both him and his immediate environment. The nurses did everything necessary to keep him clean and protect him against unpleasant smells. However, no matter what he or the nurses did he quickly got the impression that he was constantly contaminated with liquid faeces, and he convinced himself that he was destined to be like this for life. He quickly began to lose the will to live. It was a disastrous change of body image that the patient could not cope with. This unpleasant situation continued and, despite all the help available, this gentleman became very depressed with his plight. Within a week or so of the surgery he was dead. Effectively, the colostomy, rather than improving his quality of life, had actually killed him. It is true to say that this is an exceptional case, and that most patients will not have such a bad experience. Thousands of patients all over the world live with and cope well with a colostomy, and many of their friends, colleagues and even family do not know they have a stoma. But this case does show that problems and complications of surgery can quickly destroy the patient's own view of themselves, and destroy the confidence they once had in themselves. It can cause them to view their body in a very negative way. The effects of changes in body image on the patient offer a powerful message to all nurses who care for patients with bowel problems.

Key points

Oral cancers

- Digestive cancers can all seriously impact on the patient's nutritional status, and therefore nurses must try to ensure optimum nutrition in their patients.
- Smoking and alcohol are often major contributors to oral cancers.
- About 95% of cases of mouth cancers are squamous cell carcinomas.

Oesophageal cancers

- Most oesophageal cancers are squamous cell carcinomas or adenocarcinomas.
- Oesophageal cancers can spread locally into the wall and beyond into the lower respiratory tract, the lung and the mediastinum.

Gastric carcinoma

- Gastric carcinoma occurs in two forms, the intestinal and the diffuse forms.
- The degree by which the cancer has infiltrated into the stomach wall is the important factor, i.e. the depth of invasion.
- Gastric carcinoma usually begins insidiously and may show vague, obscure symptoms, or may even be asymptomatic at first.
- The earliest symptoms are usually abdominal discomfort and weight loss.
- Dumping syndrome occurs after partial gastrectomy of the distal portion of the stomach and anastamosis with the jejunum or duodenum.
- Gastrectomy can cause pernicious anaemia due to the loss of intrinsic factor in the formation of vitamin B_{12}, and this is corrected by vitamin B_{12} injections.
- Weight loss is also a problem after gastrectomy because of reduced calorie intake, smaller meals eaten and malabsorption of nutrients.

Intestinal cancers

- Small bowel cancers, i.e. those of the duodenum and ileum, are 40 to 60 times less frequently seen than those of the colon.
- About 45% of small bowel cancers are adenocarcinomas, about 30% are carcinoid tumours, a further 10% are small bowel lymphomas and the rest are sarcomas.

Pancreatic cancer

- Pancreatic cancers are mostly adenocarcinomas.
- The two forms of pancreatic cancer are the ductal and non-ductal types.
- The ductal type accounts for most of the pancreatic tumours and two-thirds of them arise from the head of the gland.

Colorectal cancers

- Non-malignant (benign) and non-neoplastic (no malignant potential) polyps of the large bowel are growths arising from the mucosal or submucosal lining of the gut wall.
- Adenomas are neoplastic tumours (with malignant potential) derived from the glandular epithelial components of the mucous membrane lining of the bowel.
- Adenocarcinoma is the malignant growth of the bowel (i.e. cancer of the small or large bowel).

Stomas and surgical complications

- A colostomy and an ileostomy are openings into the bowel (*colostomy* is an opening into the colon, *ileostomy* is an opening into the ileum).
- Good skin care around the stoma is vital, the skin should be a normal colour (not red), clean, with no irritations, rashes or signs of inflammation or excoriation.
- Paralytic ileus is a postoperative complication of bowel surgery where the bowel movements that drive the contents along have stopped.
- Problems and complications of surgery can quickly destroy the patient's own view of themselves, and destroy the confidence they once had in themselves. It can cause them to view their body in a very negative way.

References

Anonymous (2004) CRP – tests predict risk of heart attack, *in* Bredenberg J. (ed.) *Medical Breakthroughs 2004*, Reader's Digest Association, London.

Blows W. T. (2001) *The Biological Basis of Nursing: Clinical Observations*, Routledge, London.

Cottrill R. B. (1996) *Helicobacter pylori*, *Professional Nurse*, 12 (1): 46–8.

Kumar V., Cotran R. S. and Robbins S. L. (1997) *Basic Pathology* (6th edn), W. B. Saunders Company, London.

LeMone P. and Burke K. (2004) *Medical-Surgical Nursing, Critical Thinking in Client Care* (3rd edn), Pearson Education International, Prentice Hall, New Jersey.

Souhami R. and Tobias J. (2003) *Cancer and its Management* (4th edn), Blackwell Science Publishing, Oxford.

Woolf N. (1998) *Pathology, Basic and Systemic*, W. B Saunders Company Ltd, London.

Chapter 6

Cancers of the respiratory and renal systems

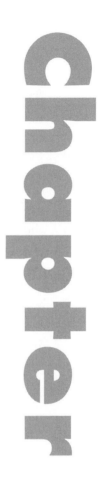

- Introduction
- Nursing skills: carbon dioxide and oxygen administration
- Laryngeal cancers
- Cancer of the bronchus and the lung
- The renal system
- Cancer of the kidney
- Bladder cancers
- Key points

Introduction

Breathing is taken for granted, but as soon as something goes wrong with the respiratory system, breathing becomes a major emergency. This illustrates the essential nature of respiration on a minute by minute, and even a second by second basis. When a person cannot breathe properly they panic, followed sooner or later by collapse and loss of consciousness. One of the hardest challenges for nurses is in assisting patients who are fighting for their breath. Cancer of the respiratory system makes this challenge faced by nurses on the wards even harder, because there is no easy answer to the management of the acutely breathless patient caused by a tumour blocking the airway. Lung cancer is clearly a case of prevention being far better than the cure.

The essential nature of the renal system, both as an excretory pathway for wastes and as a regulatory system for fluid, electrolyte and pH balances, is highlighted in this chapter. The respiratory and renal systems are linked both by their joint nature as excretory organs, and by their joint co-operative role in stabilising the blood chemistry.

The respiratory system is described in Blows (2001, Chapter 4) along with the respiratory observations that may prove useful when nursing patients with lung cancers. It would be of value, therefore, for students and nurses to read this current chapter in conjunction with Chapter 4 of Blows (2001).

Nursing skills: carbon dioxide and oxygen administration

If asked 'why do we breathe?', students and even many trained nurses would often answer 'because we need oxygen'. But this is only part of the story. In fact, it may be surprising to learn that the real reason we breathe at all is not so much to do with oxygen. Yes, we need oxygen (we will find out why in a moment), but this is not the main driving force that keeps us breathing. That main driving force is **carbon dioxide** (**CO_2**), i.e. the need to eliminate CO_2. The removal of CO_2 from the body puts the need for oxygen into second place, such that if all the CO_2 in a person's body were to be totally removed, breathing would almost certainly stop, irrespective of the need for oxygen. But that scenario is not possible in a living body since CO_2 is constantly being produced by the metabolism of the cells. To stop CO_2 production would require energy production to stop, and that is incompatible with life. So where does that put oxygen?

Oxygen (O) (notice the chemical symbol for oxygen is O, not O_2, since the chemical symbol for an element is the same as *one atom* of the substance, and the symbol O_2 represents *two* atoms together, i.e. a *molecule* of the element) is vital for life. But when asked 'what does oxygen actually do inside the cell?', students and many trained nurses do not know. And yet, oxygen is all around them in the clinical areas. It is piped to the bedside or delivered in cylinders, it can be found on the anaesthetic trolleys, on the resuscitation trolleys, on patient trolleys, or just on its own trolley. Try and find some carbon dioxide; there may be some on the anaesthetic trolley, but that is probably all. It seems that oxygen is so important, and just as soon as someone gets any breathing difficulty we dash for the oxygen. But consider for a moment the following: give just a little too much oxygen to a patient with breathing difficulties due to **chronic bronchitis** and his breathing will slow down, and it is possible that it could sometimes even stop.

So does giving oxygen help to relieve the difficulty experienced by the patient with **dyspnoea** (difficulty or great effort needed for breathing)? Well, clearly, not always. We have seen how oxygen is *not* the main respiratory drive, and that it can actually *reduce* respiration in chronic bronchitis. So the answer to this particular question is that any help that oxygen offers to the breathless patient is *not direct*, it is only *indirect*. What giving oxygen does is to improve the O_2 saturation of the haemoglobin in the blood. This *does not* help to relieve the dypsnoea *per se*, but it does make the transport of oxygen more efficient and therefore delivers more oxygen to the tissues. This extra oxygen better satisfies the tissues' need for oxygen, and therefore reduces the body's demand on the respiratory system to acquire more oxygen, and so the patient's breathing should become less laboured. So this puts oxygen into a more realistic perspective; it is not the cure for all respiratory ailments, and may actually make some worse (see chronic bronchitis above). We know, for example, that pure oxygen (100%) is positively dangerous, as with the case of any newborn baby given 100% oxygen, it may well cause them to go permanently blind, and would stop the chronic bronchitis patient from breathing altogether (a state of **apnoea**, i.e. absence of breathing).

But what about that question 'what does oxygen actually do in the body?' Any answer like 'it is essential for tissue metabolism' is too vague, and it is not getting to the heart of the answer. The real answer lies in the following statement: oxygen is essential for the *removal of wastes* from tissue metabolism.

Oxygen is the waste removal system, and as such it is essential for keeping the cell chemistry going (known as **metabolism**, see Figure 6.1). It is the 'dustman' of tissue metabolism. Without it the wastes rapidly build-up and the cell's chemistry cannot continue, and will grind to a halt. Given this is essentially energy production metabolism, grinding to a halt means all energy production stops and the cell will die if the oxygen supply is not restored. There are three steps in energy production, and oxygen removes waste from two of them (see Figure 6.1). In the **tricarboxylic cycle** (previously known as the **Krebs cycle**) there is a tendency to build up too much carbon waste. So for each carbon atom (C) that needs to be removed, two oxygen atoms (O_2) come in and these combine with the carbon to form carbon dioxide ($C + O_2 = CO_2$), the CO_2 then being taken away and eliminated through the lungs. In the final stage of energy production there arises a surplus of hydrogen (H) which, if allowed to accumulate, would cause acidic conditions to develop (known as **metabolic acidosis**, see p. 307). Instead, every time two excess hydrogens (2H) need removal, a single oxygen atom (O, but sometimes written as $\frac{1}{2}O_2$) comes in and combines with the hydrogen to form water ($2H + \frac{1}{2}O_2 = H_2O$), water ($H_2O$) being a harmless substance removed from the body by the kidneys (and to a lesser extent through the lungs). So, if you thought the lungs and the kidneys had

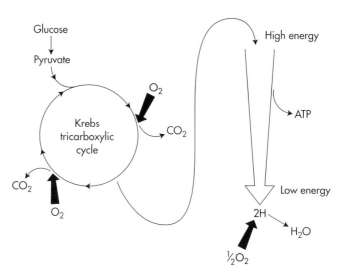

FIGURE 6.1 Oxygen is the waste removal system in tissue metabolism. In the Krebs tricarboxylic cycle oxygen collects unwanted carbon and removes it as carbon dioxide. Oxygen also collects unwanted hydrogen (as 2H) and removes it as water at the end of ATP production.

nothing in common, consider this. They both eliminate the oxygen-based waste products from tissue metabolism. An alternative title for this chapter could have been 'Cancers of the oxygen-based waste removal systems'. Water is, of course, also essential in the body (most of the body is water) but, just like CO_2 it is kept in strict balance because, again like CO_2, too much water is a dangerous thing.

The airway and gas diffusion

The respiratory system begins at the nose and mouth and ends as the microscopic air sacs in the lungs, called **alveoli** (see Figure 6.2). The passage from the mouth and nose to the alveoli is known as the **airway**. The tubing that makes up this airway has a **smooth muscle** wall (see p. 21) with **mucous membrane** (see p. 15) lining the inner surface. Some parts of the airway, i.e. the **larynx**, the **trachea** and the **bronchi** contain substantial amounts of tough cartilage, the purpose of which is to stop the airway from collapsing, which would, of course, prevent breathing.

The larynx is a cartilaginous hollow box with a mucous membrane lining from which the **vocal cords** are fashioned. The cartilages are hard tissue and cause the larynx to bulge out in the throat, particularly in men (the so-called **Adam's apple**). The vocal cords are stretched across the narrowest part of the airway inside the larynx, called the **glottis**. Above the glottis is a flap, the **epiglottis**, which closes the glottis during swallowing, like a door, to prevent food and water from entering the respiratory passages.

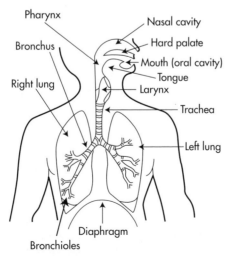

FIGURE 6.2 The respiratory system.

Below the larynx is the **trachea** (the 'wind-pipe'), which passes down through the neck into the **thorax**, or chest cavity. It has cartilaginous rings to prevent collapse and is lined with ciliated mucous membrane (see p. 15, and read also about the **muco-ciliary escalator** on p. 67). At the lower end the trachea divides into two **primary bronchi** (singular = **bronchus**), one for each lung, left and right. These also have cartilaginous rings and they subdivide into **secondary bronchi**, which supply air to the lobes of the lung, three lobes in the right lung and two lobes in the left lung. Within the lobes the airway further divides into many tiny branches that serve to bring air to the terminal air sacs, known as **alveoli**. Each of the lobes consists of millions of microscopic alveoli (there are 300,000,000 in the entire respiratory system), which are held together with **yellow elastic connective tissue** (see p. 17), plus the tiny air delivery tubes called **bronchioli**. Alveoli have very thin walls (only one cell thick) to allow exchange of the gases oxygen and carbon dioxide with the blood. The blood that passes through the lungs in the capillaries comes incredibly close to the airway (see Figure 6.3, and also Blows 2001, p. 69). This part of the circulation of blood, i.e. through the lungs, is called

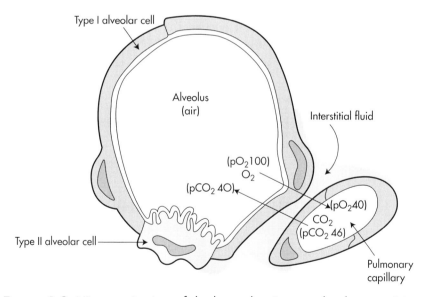

FIGURE 6.3 Microscopic view of the lung, showing an alveolus containing air, with the walls of type I and type II cells, a pulmonary capillary containing blood, and interstitial fluid between the capillary and the alveolus. The direction of gas movement and the pressures in mmHg for pO_2 and pCO_2 in the blood and air are shown. (Redrawn from Blows 2001, Figure 4.1.)

the **pulmonary circulation**. Oxygen leaves the alveoli and enters the blood by means of **diffusion** down a **concentration gradient**, i.e. moving from a high concentration (in the alveoli) into a low concentration (in the blood). Carbon dioxide moves in the opposing direction, again from a high concentration (in the blood) to a low concentration (in the alveoli)(see Figure 6.3, and Blows 2001, p. 79). Blood is the transport system for both oxygen to all parts of the body (mostly attached to the pigment molecule **haemoglobin**, see p. 21), and carbon dioxide back to the lungs (mostly in the plasma).

Laryngeal cancers

Only about 2% of all cancers in men are of the larynx, and only 0.4% in women. This disease occurs most frequently after the age of 40 years. The overwhelming factor in virtually all cases is tobacco smoking. This one factor alone is essentially responsible for this disease, which means that the prevention of laryngeal cancer is clearly available to everyone. Drinking alcohol may play a less significant role in the cause, but alcohol consumption combined with smoking carries the biggest risk. The vast majority of laryngeal cancers (95%) are **squamous cell carcinomas** with a very small amount of **adeno-carcinomas** seen. Both are derived from the mucosal lining of the larynx. The commonest site of tumour growth is the vocal cords within the glottis (see p. 153), and these are known as **glottic tumours**, accounting for up to 65% of laryngeal cancers. But cancers may arise from anywhere within the larynx (**intrinsic tumours**) or from outside (**extrinsic tumours**)(see Figure 6.4). Intrinsic tumours can develop from above the vocal cords (called **supraglottic**, about 35% of cases) or from below the glottis (called **subglottic**, less than 5% of cases). **Transglottic** tumours extend across the **laryngeal ventricle** (the space within the larynx). Spread from these locations usually follows these patterns:

1 Glottic tumours remain confined within the larynx for long periods of time giving the patient a better chance of a cure, and this improves the long-term prognosis. The reason for this is that the laryngeal cartilaginous wall surrounding the tumour contains the growth, with only a few lymphatic vessels available for spread.
2 Supraglottic tumours can spread into the local spaces within the larynx and to the **cervical** lymph nodes (those found in the neck

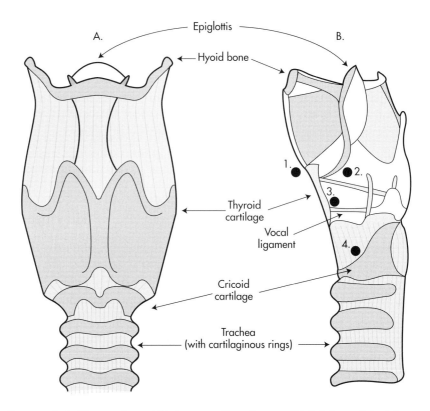

FIGURE 6.4 The trachea. (A) Anterior (front) view, (B) left lateral (side) view of cut section, with cancer sites shown as black spots: (1) extrinsic, (2) supra-glottic, (3) glottic, (4) subglottic (2, 3 and 4 are all intrinsic). (Redrawn from Martini 2004.)

area). The prognosis is reasonable with a 65% 5-year survival rate and many complete cures are possible.

3 Subglottic tumours most often involve the vocal cords as well as the structures below, and they frequently spread into the local tissues, especially the thyroid gland, the **cricoid cartilage** (see Figure 6.4) and the trachea (see p. 154). The survival rate at 5 years is about 40%.

4 Transglottic tumours are prone to spread more than the other types to the cervical lymph nodes and they require extensive excision of all affected tissues. The 5-year survival rate is about 50%.

Persistent hoarseness of the voice, beyond that expected from a sore throat, is a primary symptom. This is followed later by pain,

haemoptysis (coughing of blood) and **dysphagia** (pain or difficulty with swallowing).

The treatment for some of these tumours is surgical removal of the larynx, called a **laryngectomy**. Since the larynx is the 'voice box', surgical removal means that the postoperative patient will no longer be able to speak. Older techniques exist which allow the patient to 'fashion' a voice from air released from the stomach, and this method would have to be taught to the patient. However, modern technology allows for 'synthesised' voices to be generated by a computer, and this speaks for the patient.

Cancer of the bronchus and the lung

Bronchial cancers are one of the commonest causes of cancer deaths in both sexes, and the main cause, like laryngeal and mouth cancer (see p. 123), is smoking. Other factors play a role in the causation of this disease, like air pollution (urban deaths from this disease are twice as common as rural deaths), radiation, genetics and asbestos, but their effects are small compared with smoking. So again, like laryngeal and mouth cancer, individuals have a choice whether to run the risk and smoke, or not.

The disease usually starts in the bronchial mucosa close to the tracheal bifurcation (the point where the trachea ends and divides into the two main bronchi, left and right). From here it will spread into the lung, and metastases will spread to other parts of the body, commonly the cervical lymph nodes, the pleura, the liver, the adrenal glands, the brain and the bones (see Figure 6.5) (see also Chapter 9 for secondary growths of the brain, bone and liver). There are several different types of lung cancer, and Table 6.1 lists these in order of frequency.

Of these types, **squamous cell carcinoma** has the strongest link of all with smoking. This type accounts for an average of 30% of bronchogenic carcinomas (i.e. those arising in the bronchus). They metastasise late in the course of the disease but they are linked closely with two complications, **pneumonia** (an inflammatory fluid consolidation of the lung) and **atalectasis** (lung collapse). **Adenocarcinoma** is commonest in women and again it is closely associated with smoking. The early stages of the disease tend to be asymptomatic. **Small cell carcinoma** is the most malignant of all the lung cancers and carries the worst prognosis (less than 2% of patients are alive 2 years after diagnosis). There is a strong link with smoking.

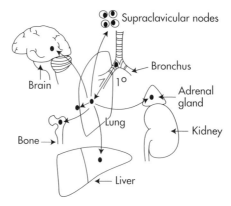

FIGURE 6.5 The spread of lung cancer. The primary site (1°) is usually at the division of the trachea into two bronchi. From here it can spread into the lung and pleura, to the bone, brain, liver, adrenal gland and the supraclavicular lymph nodes.

TABLE 6.1 Some of the types and frequencies of lung cancer

Cancer	Frequency (%)	Variant types
Adenocarcinoma	30 to 50	1. Acinar adenocarcinoma 2. Papillary adenocarcinoma 3. Bronchioloalveolar adenocarcinoma 4. Solid carcinoma with mucous formation
Squamous carcinoma	25 to 40	Spindle-celled squamous carcinoma
Small cell carcinoma	15 to 25	1. Oat cell carcinoma 2. Intermediate cell type 3. Combined oat cell carcinoma
Large cell carcinoma	10 to 20	1. Giant cell carcinoma 2. Clear cell carcinoma
Carcinoid tumour	1 to 2	1. 'Typical' 2. 'Atypical'
Bronchial gland carcinomas	Rare	1. Adenoid cystic carcinoma 2. Mucoepidermoid carcinoma

The cells are tiny with very little **cytoplasm** (see p. 4). It is also called **oat cell carcinoma** if the cells are compressed into ovoid shapes. **Large cell carcinoma** consists of giant or spindle-shaped cells with clear cytoplasm. They can grow in such a manner as to distort the trachea.

The patient with bronchogenic lung cancer is typically middle aged with a history of smoking. They mostly have a persistant cough, which later in the disease produces **sputum**. Sputum is a lung or bronchial substance secreted by the mucous lining of the respiratory tract and then coughed up. The mucous secretions usually contain microorganisms or cells, and these can be identified in the laboratory and may aid in the diagnosis. Sputum samples may be required from the patient for this purpose. **Haemoptysis** (coughing up blood from the respiratory tract) may occur at a late phase of the disease and suggests erosion of blood vessels by the tumour. The patient may be breathless, or have a wheeze and may have **dyspnoea** (pain or difficulty in breathing). Advanced stages of the disease can cause **air hunger**, where the patient is fighting for every breath. Such extreme difficulty may be eased by putting the patient in an upright position, leaning forward, and possibly by the use of oxygen (see p. 151), delivered in a low concentration, usually just a little above that found in normal air (the concentration of oxygen in normal air is about 20%). They may have chest pain and they find it very hard to eat properly (dyspnoea generally makes eating impossible), so they become malnourished and in time they will show evidence of **wasting** (loss of fat, and eventually muscle loss leading to weight loss, see p. 304). The overall prognosis is not good, only 13% of treated patients survive for 5 years, and if left untreated they are likely to be dead in nine months or so.

The treatment is surgery whenever possible to remove that part of the lung that contains the primary growth. A **lobectomy** is removal of one lobe of one lung, whilst the removal of one whole lung is a **pneumonectomy**. Patients in this latter category of treatment must rely on their one remaining lung for the rest of their lives. Whilst this is adequate for sustaining life it does curtail energetic exercise, where greater oxygenation of the blood is required. Radiotherapy and cytotoxic therapy (chemotherapy) will be required for the management of metastases and secondary growths.

Mesothelioma

Two layers of a single membrane, **the pleura**, which has a fluid-filled cavity between the layers, cover the lungs. **Mesothelioma** is a malignant tumour developing usually on the pleura, the covering of the lung. It tends to spread through the pleural double layers, and may involve the pericardium, the covering of the heart. Less often, the primary site may be the peritoneum. The vast majority of cases are caused by exposure to asbestos, i.e. the inhalation of fine asbestos fibres (less than 0.5 µm in diameter, 8 µm in length). The long delay between exposure and the start of the disease, some 20 to 40 years, means that despite the precautions now taken with asbestos, and its elimination where possible, the legacy of the past remains, and the disease is still on the increase. Males are affected more than females and it occurs mostly in the 50 to 70 years age range. The tumour grows along the membrane and covers the lung, making surgical removal possible in only a small number of cases where diagnosis is made early. There are epithelial and sarcomatous types and tumours of mixed types. Spread outside of the pleura (which occurs more often in the sarcomatous type) involves the local lymph nodes, the kidney, liver and the brain.

The features of the disease are chest pain, increasing to very severe, and **dyspnoea** (difficulty with breathing). The symptoms get worse as the tumour covers the lung, and causes considerable incapacitation, with reduced chest wall movements during breathing. **Pleural effusion** (fluid in the pleural space between the two layers) is common, adding to the dyspnoea. The prognosis is poor due to the limited ability to treat this condition satisfactorily. An early diagnosis is essential and this is rarely achieved. The hope for the future is that the precautions taken with asbestos now will result in a decline in the numbers of patients with this tumour.

The renal system

The renal system, like the respiratory system, is described in Blows (2001, Chapter 5) and this section should therefore be read in conjunction with it.

The kidneys provide the other major excretory pathway for the elimination of waste material from the body, not only unwanted water (see p. 164) but also **urea** (a waste from protein metabolism),

uric acid (waste from the nucleic acids RNA and DNA) and **creatinine** (waste resulting from muscle breakdown).

The kidneys

There are two kidneys, left and right, positioned on either side of the lumbar spinal column, and attached to the back wall of the abdomen. They each have about one million **nephrons**, the functional unit of the kidney, and these are in the **cortex**, the outer part of the kidney. A nephron (see Figure 6.6) consists of a microscopic tuft of **arterioles** (i.e. mini arteries) called the **glomerulus**. This is surrounded by the **Bowman's capsule**, the collecting 'cup' for what is called **filtrate**, the fluid product extracted from the blood though the glomerulus. Leading from this are two **convoluted tubules** (the first, or *proximal*,

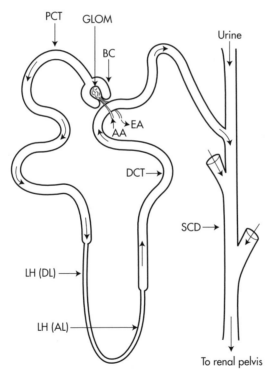

FIGURE 6.6 The renal nephron. AA = afferent arteriole, AL = ascending limb (of loop of Henle), BC = Bowman's capsule, DCT = distal convoluted tubule, DL = descending limb (of loop of Henle), EA = efferent arteriole, GLOM = glomerulus, LH = loop of Henle, PCT = proximal convoluted tubule, SCD = straight collecting duct. (From Blows 2001, Figure 5.1.)

and the second, or *distal*), and these are separated by a **loop of Henle**. Finally, the nephrons have **straight collecting ducts** that drain urine into the centre of the kidney (see Figure 6.6).

Central to the cortex is the **medulla**, which consists of the **pyramids**. These are made from numerous straight collecting ducts from one region of the cortex joined together and converged towards a point, and several of these pyramids drain urine from the entire cortical area. Urine from a pyramid first arrives in a cup-like structure called a **calyx**, then into the **renal pelvis**, the hollow core where urine collects. From here it drains down the ureter to the bladder (see Figure 6.7).

The kidneys each have three surface coverings, the innermost **renal capsule**, the middle layer of fat called the **adipose capsule** (which helps to attach the kidney to the posterior abdominal wall), and the outermost **renal fascia** made of dense fibrous tissue. This last structure is also important for anchorage of the kidney in place.

Urine formation

The formation of urine is complex. Blood is filtered by the two million glomeruli. The filtrate produced by the glomerulus is not urine

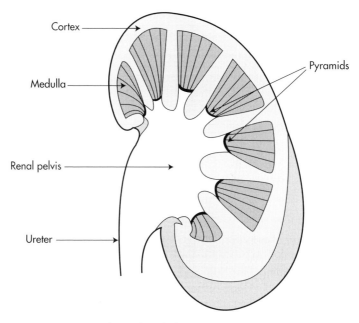

FIGURE 6.7 A section through a kidney.

yet as it must undergo many changes first. Urine formation falls into three main stages:

1 **Filtration** from the glomerulus into the Bowman's capsule.
2 **Re-absorption** of many substances in the filtrate that the body requires (occurs in the convoluted tubules).
3 **Tubular secretion** of specific substances (occurs in the straight collecting ducts).

Filtration from the glomerulus is the result of pressure from the blood in the glomeruli forcing fluid into the Bowman's capsule (see Figure 6.8, and see Blows 2001, p. 92). The blood supply to the kidney is critical to kidney function. Kidneys work on blood pressure like a vacuum cleaner works on electricity. Gradually reduce the electrical current and the vacuum cleaner becomes progressively less efficient, until a sufficiently low current will stop the cleaner altogether. So it is with the kidneys. If the blood pressure falls, kidney filtration becomes less efficient, until the **systolic pressure** falls below 50 mmHg, at which point the kidney is likely to stop filtration completely, a condition called **renal failure** (often referred to as **renal shutdown**). The systolic blood pressure is the maximum pressure of

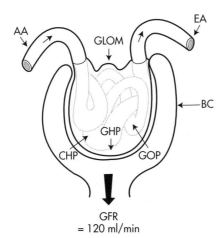

FIGURE 6.8 The glomerulus (GLOM) and Bowman's capsule (BC). Glomerular hydrostatic pressure (GHP) pushes filtrate out of the blood, which is shown as the afferent arteriole (AA) and efferent arteriole (EA). The forces opposing GHP, i.e. the capsular hydrostatic pressure (CHP) and the glomerular osmotic pressure (GOP) caused by blood proteins, return some filtrate back to the blood. The result of these forces is the glomerular filtration rate (GFR) of about 120 ml per minute. (From Blows 2001, Figure 5.2.)

blood at the time the heart is contracting. Blood pressure is measured in **mmHg**, i.e. **millimetres of mercury**, and low systemic blood pressure is termed **hypotension**. The blood supply to each of the kidneys is via the **renal arteries** (left and right), and these are branches of the **abdominal aorta**. Anything that interferes with the renal artery supply to the kidneys, e.g. tumours, may significantly disturb the kidney's ability to filter the blood, and can cause renal shutdown. Of course, if that happens it would, mostly likely, be in one kidney only, whereas a condition like shock, which causes systemic hypotension, would affect both kidneys simultaneously. The blood drainage from the kidneys is via the **renal veins**, which channels blood back to the **inferior vena cava**, the main vein returning blood to the heart from the lower parts of the body.

Once filtrate is produced by the glomerulus, and has entered the Bowman's capsule, it flows on into the first (proximal) convoluted tubule where essential substances, like glucose, are re-absorbed back into the blood. The loop of Henle, distal convoluted tubule and the straight collecting duct all have a role to play in maintaining correct fluid and electrolyte balance. The kidneys therefore, carry out the following vital functions:

1 Water balance in the body, excreting surplus water if there is too much, or conserving water if there is not enough (see Mr Wet and Mr Dry physiology in Blows 2001, pp. 98–9).
2 Electrolyte balance in the body, e.g. positively charged particles like sodium (Na^+) or negatively charged particles like chlorine (Cl^-).
3 pH balance (the maintenance of blood pH at close to 7.4 by the removal of H ions, H^+).
4 Excretion of wastes (see pp. 160–161).
5 The production of some hormones, notable **erythropoietin** (stimulates erythrocyte production, see p. 98) and other substances (e.g. modification of **vitamin D**, see p. 294).

The bladder

Once formed, urine flows into the **renal pelvis** of the kidney, then down the **ureter** into the **bladder** (see Figure 6.9). The ureter is a smooth muscle tube connecting the kidney to the bladder below. The bladder is also made from smooth muscle, lined with mucous membrane (made from **transitional epithelium**, see p. 16). Three

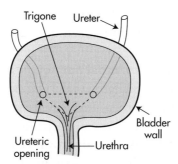

FIGURE 6.9 The bladder in section. Between the two ureteric openings and the urethra is the trigone (shown by a dotted triangle).

openings occur in the bladder, the two ureters, left and right, where urine enters from the kidneys, and the one **urethra** where urine leaves (see p. 218). The patch of bladder floor between the three openings is the lowest part of the bladder, and is called the **trigone** (see Figure 6.9). There is a ring of smooth muscle, called the **internal sphincter**, which guards the exit into the urethra, the tube to the outside world. Outside this internal sphincter is a second ring, the **external sphincter**, made from **skeletal voluntary muscle** (see p. 20). When urine is collecting in the bladder the sphincter muscles contract causing the sphincters to tighten up and close the exit. At the same time, the muscles of the bladder wall relax and stretch to allow the organ to fill with urine. At about 300 ml or so of urine, signals are sent via the nervous system to the brain which then co-ordinates emptying of the bladder, at a convenient moment of course. During the passage of urine (called **micturition**) both sphincter muscles relax and the sphincters open, the internal sphincter opens automatically, but the external sphincter remains closed until opened voluntarily, when the conditions are right. This allows urine to pass through the urethra to the outside world. Simultaneously, the bladder wall muscles help to push urine out by contracting.

Cancer of the kidney

The malignant tumours of the kidney are:

1 **Renal cell carcinoma**, i.e. those of the kidney substance seen in *adults*.
2 **Transitional cell carcinoma**, i.e. those of the kidney pelvis seen in *adults*.

3 **Wilms' tumour, rhadboid tumour** and **clear cell sarcoma**, i.e. those of the kidney substance seen in *children*.

Renal cell carcinoma (or **renal adenocarcinoma**) is the cause of 85% of all adult kidney malignancies. The age of onset is usually middle to later life rising to a peak incidence in the seventh and eighth decades of life. Men account for twice as many cases as women, and smoking doubles the risk for this disease. Renal cell carcinoma causes pain and a mass (or lump) in the loin, with haematuria (blood in the urine) as an important sign (seen in 60% of cases). Haematuria will require detection by testing the urine during the early stages of the disease, and if this is not done routinely the disease could be missed in its early stages (urine testing, specifically for blood, is discussed in Blows 2001, pp. 104–7). Invasion of the tumour at a later stage involves spread from the cortex into the medulla, extending into the renal pelvis. There is often spread along the **renal vein**, the vessel that drains blood from the kidney, and along the **inferior vena cava** (the main vein conveying blood returning to the heart). Variations of the tumour cell types include **papillary renal carcinoma** (papillary in nature, see p. 187) and **sarcomatoid renal cell carcinoma** (malignant spindle-shaped cells).

The **Robson method** of staging of renal cell carcinoma is as follows:

I   Entirely within the kidney.
II   Invasion through the renal capsule, but not through the renal fascia (see p. 162 for renal capsule and fascia).
III   Spread into the regional lymph nodes, renal vein or both without spread into the fat around the kidney.
IV   Distant metastases or invasion through the renal fascia into neighbouring structures.

Survival averages out at about 45% for this disease, with poor prognosis (10 to 15%) for those with metastases, but good prognosis (70%) for those without metastases.

Oncocytoma is a tumour with a particular cell type called an **oncocyte**. It is a malignant cell with a finely granular cytoplasm, the granules consisting of numerous abnormally large **mitochondria** (see p. 5). This tumour is three times more common in men than in women, and it has a benign growth pattern.

Wilms' tumour of the kidney (also called **nephroblastoma**) is the commonest of the child renal tumours, occurring mostly between 1 and 4 years of age. It may be associated with a range of other medical conditions, or appear alone. Some chromosome abnormalities are known in this disease, notably deletion of part of 11p (the short arm of the chromosome 11), which appears to result in the loss of a **tumour suppressor gene** (see p. 35). The tumour causes abdominal pain in the child, a palpable mass in the abdomen, abdominal distension and fever. Haematuria occurs in about 30% of patients.

The staging of Wilms' tumour identifies five points:

I   Tumour is confined to the kidney.
II Tumour extends beyond the kidney.
III Some tumour remains after surgical removal, lymph node involvement.
IV Distant blood-borne metastases.
V   The tumour is bilateral.

Prognosis has much improved with the introduction of surgery in combination with chemotherapy and radiotherapy (see Chapter 12).

Rhabdoid tumour is a rare disorder of early age onset (within the first year of life) in boys more often than girls. It is highly malignant and therefore is associated with a poor prognosis (only about 25% survival after two years). The abnormal cells have large amounts of cytoplasm containing twisted bundles of **cytoskeleton** filaments.

Clear cell sarcoma consists of abnormal cells containing small, round nuclei and multiple vacuoles within the cytoplasm (see p. 5 for vacuoles). The tumour spreads via the lymph and blood to many parts of the body, including bone metastases.

Bladder cancers

The vast majority of bladder neoplasms, some 95%, are both benign and malignant growths of the **transitional epithelium** (see p. 16), and the remaining 5% are of connective tissue origin. Of the malignant forms, about 90% are **transitional cell carcinomas** (**TCC**), 5% are **squamous carcinomas** and 5% are a mixture of the two. Bladder cancer affects men three times more than women, usually in middle to late age. The risk factors include smoking, industrial carcinogens (in particular those found in the cloth dyeing or rubber industries), drug abuse (especially of analgesic drugs, see p. 270) and

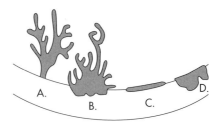

FIGURE 6.10 Bladder cancers: (A) papillary carcinoma, (B) invasive papillary carcinoma, (C) flat non-invasive carcinoma, (D) flat invasive carcinoma.

as a side effect of treatment with the drug **cyclophosphamide** (see p. 323).

There are four morphological (= shape) types of transitional cell carcinoma of the bladder (see Figure 6.10) where the invasive types are more advanced:

1 **Papillary carcinoma**.
2 **Invasive papillary carcinoma**.
3 **Flat, non-invasive carcinoma**.
4 **Flat, invasive carcinoma** (Kumar *et al.* 1997).

Grading of the tumours is important because, like other tumours, early staging is conducive to better survival rates than late staging. Several staging systems are in practice, and the following is a basic I, II, III staging system which can be applied to most TCCs:

I   Papillary tumours, non-invasive, tissue remains clearly transitional epithelium with some loss of orientation, and little mitosis is evident.

II   Tumours made from tissue that remains clearly transitional epithelium, greater degree of cell mitosis and growth than in grade I with more variation in the nucleus and greater disorientation of the tissue.

III A carcinoma, with loss of identity as transitional epithelium, loose cells washed off into the urine (**exfoliation**), later invasion of the bladder wall and metastases.

Other systems are the **TNM** and **P** systems (Souhami and Tobias 2003):

T_{is}	carcinoma *in situ.*
T_p	papillary non-invasive carcinoma.
T_0	No primary tumour found.
T_1 (P_1)	Tumour limited to the **lamina propria** (the bladder wall layer immediately below the transitional epithelium).
T_2 (P_2)	Tumour limited to the superficial muscle.
T_3 (P_3)	Invasion of bladder wall to the deep muscle layer.
T_{3a}	Invasion into the deep muscle layer.
T_{3b}	Invasion through the deep muscle layer.
T_4 (P_4)	Invasion of the local organs outside the bladder.
T_{4a}	Invasion of the prostate, uterus or vagina.
T_{4b}	Fixation of tumour to pelvis or abdominal wall.
N_0	Local lymph nodes involved.
N_1	A single lymph node group on same side as the cancer involved.
N_2	Lymph nodes on both or opposite sides are involved.
N_3	**Lymphadenopathy** (disease of the lymph glands) at a fixed distance from the tumour.
N_4	Lymph nodes in other regions of the body are involved.
M_0	No distant metastases involved.
M_1	Distant metastases are involved.

The benign papillomas (small, nipple-like growths on the inner surface of the bladder wall) of the bladder may well be the original source of any malignancy, so they should be removed when found. They can reoccur after removal, so regular (often annual) checks must be maintained. Checking consists of a **cystoscopy**, where the inner bladder wall is viewed using a **cystoscope** passed up the urethra under anaesthetic. Cystoscopy is often accompanied by **biopsy** (taking of a sample of the tissue) of any lesion found for **histological** examination. Taking a biopsy may cause some temporary bleeding to occur. Nurses should note, therefore, that while some post-procedural urinary bleeding is often encountered it should not persist. If bleeding continues after the patient has had three episodes of post-procedural micturition it should be reported to the surgeon (LeMone and Burke 2004).

The malignant transitional cell carcinomas may be nodular or flat, and these are commonly associated with mutations of the *Tp53* gene (see p. 12). There is a well-established association between the presence of extra DNA (called **ploidy**, see pp. 43–44 and 187), the depth of tumour invasion and the patient's response to various treatments.

TABLE 6.2 The genetic mutations found in bladder cancers

Chromosome	Mutation
1	Abnormalities may be of secondary importance
5	Short arm (i.e. 5p) changes found in 40% of cases
7	Trisomy 7 (see p. 43) in some cases. Mutation of the *c-erb* gene on this chromosome found in over 80% of invasive carcinoma cases
9	Monosomy 9 (see p. 44) seen in 50% of cases. 9q (long arm) deletions (see p. 38) seen in 67% of advanced bladder cases
11	11p (short arm) deletions (see p. 38) seen in 40% of cases
17	The *Tp53* gene mutations (see p. 12) found in 63% of cases

Also, expression of the mutant *ras* genes (see p. 41) is often associated with the higher graded tumours, and therefore a worse prognosis. Other genetic mutations found in bladder cancers are found in Table 6.2 (Woolf 1998).

Carcinoma *in situ* (CIS) (see p. 27) may occur adjacent to papillary lesions in the bladder wall, and 50% of CIS will become invasive carcinomas. These tumours at first cause a painless **haematuria** (blood in the urine)(Blows 2001, p. 106), frequency and urgency of micturition, or some obstruction to the flow of urine, with or without **dysuria** (difficulty or pain on passing urine).

Treatment depends on the stage of the disease. Surgical removal of the growth can eradicate the disease in the early stages, with repeated checks to look for possible future development of the tumour. More advanced disease with metastatic spread requires radical surgery (e.g. **cystectomy**, removal of the bladder). This will involve the cosmetic rearrangement of the urinary outflow (**ureteric diversion**) through an **ileal conduit**, the refashioning of a section of small bowel (ileum) into an artificial 'bladder' (or conduit) leading to a stoma (see p. 141). A stoma bag would then be worn on the abdomen over the stoma to collect the urine (see p. 142 for discussion of stomas). Additional to surgery, for metastatic spread, chemotherapy (see p. 322) and radiotherapy (see p. 334) are used.

Key points

Laryngeal cancer

- The overwhelming causative factor in virtually all cases of laryngeal cancer is tobacco smoking.

- The vast majority of laryngeal cancers (95%) are squamous cell carcinomas, the remainder includes some adenocarcinomas.
- The commonest sites of tumour growth are the vocal cords within the glottis.
- Persistent hoarseness of the voice, beyond that expected from a sore throat, is a primary symptom.
- The treatment for some of these tumours is surgical removal of the larynx, called a laryngectomy.

Bronchial carcinoma

- Bronchial carcinoma usually starts in the bronchial mucosa close to the tracheal bifurcation.
- All lung cancers have a causative link with smoking but squamous cell carcinoma has the strongest link.
- Small cell carcinoma (also called oat cell carcinoma) is the most malignant of all the lung cancers and carries the worst prognosis.
- Spread is into the lung, and metastases will spread to other parts of the body, commonly the cervical lymph nodes, pleura, liver, adrenal glands, brain and bone.
- The patient with bronchogenic lung cancer is typically middle aged with a history of smoking.
- The treatment is surgery, i.e. a lobectomy or a pneumonectomy, followed by chemotherapy and radiotherapy.

Renal system

- The kidneys provide water balance, electrolyte balance, pH balance, excretion of wastes and the production of some hormones.
- Blood pressure is the driving force for renal filtration.
- Urine formation occurs as three main stages: filtration, reabsorption and tubular secretion.
- Urine flows into the renal pelvis of the kidney, then down the ureter into the bladder.
- Micturition is the passage of urine down the urethra to the outside world.

Urinary system cancers

- The malignant tumours of the kidney are renal cell carcinoma and transitional cell carcinoma, both seen in *adults*, and Wilms' tumour, rhadboid tumour and clear cell sarcoma, all seen in *children*.

- Renal cell carcinoma, the commonest form of kidney tumour, causes pain and a mass in the loin, with haematuria as an important sign.
- The benign papillomas of the bladder may be the source of malignancy, so they should be removed when found.
- The malignant bladder cancers are 90% transitional cell carcinomas, 5% squamous carcinomas and 5% a mixture of the two.
- Initially these tumours cause a painless haematuria, frequency and urgency of micturition, with or without dysuria.

References

Blows W. T. (2001) *The Biological Basis of Nursing: Clinical Observations*, Routledge, London.

Kumar V., Cotran R. S. and Robbins S. L. (1997) *Basic Pathology* (6th edn), W. B. Saunders Company, Philadelphia.

LeMone P. and Burke K. (2004) *Medical-Surgical Nursing, Critical Thinking in Client Care* (3rd edn), Pearson Education International, Prentice Hall, New Jersey.

Martini F. H. (2004) *Fundamentals of Anatomy and Physiology* (6th edn), Benjamin Cummings, Pearson Education International, San Francisco.

Souhami R. and Tobias J. (2003) *Cancer and its Management* (4th edn), Blackwell Science, Oxford.

Woolf N. (1998) *Pathology, Basic and Systemic*, W. B. Saunders Company, London.

Chapter 7

Cancers in women

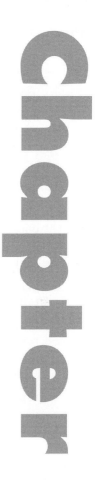

Introduction: the oestrogens

Cancers found specifically in women are often linked by one factor, a hormone group called **oestrogens**. In fact, there are three slightly different oestrogens found in women (and to a much lesser extent in men as well). These are **oestradiol (E2)**, **oestrone (E1)** and **oestriol (E3)**. They are produced originally from **cholesterol** (see Figure 7.1), and are, therefore, fat-based (or lipid-based) hormones known as **steroids**. Another female hormone, called **progesterone**, is also produced in the same sequence from cholesterol. In women the oestrogens are produced mostly in the **ovaries**, with smaller quantities being produced by the **adrenal cortex** (and that is why men also have small quantities of oestrogens, i.e. they also have adrenal glands, each with a cortex). Oestradiol (E2) is the most potent of the estrogens, and the one that has the greatest physiological effects. The potency of E2 is twelve times that of oestrone, and eighty times that of oestriol. This hormone promotes development of the female reproductive tract during the embryonic stages, and breast development during puberty. It continues to have a major influence throughout life, promoting cell division and maintaining health of the reproductive tissues. Oestrogen binds to **oestrogen receptors (ER)** within the cell (possibly inside the nucleus) and cells that have these

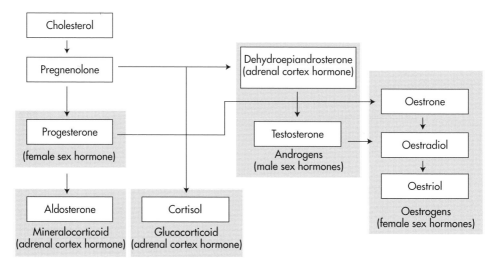

FIGURE 7.1 The oestrogens (oestradiol, oestrone and oestriol) and the androgens (testosterone and dehydroepiandrosterone) are produced from cholesterol. The diagram also shows that the hormones progesterone, aldosterone and cortisol are produced from the same pathway. (Blows 2003, Figure 4.4.)

receptors are said to be **ER positive (ER+)**. On binding to the receptor, E2 forms a complex with receptors, and this complex then binds to a **gene promoter** region on the DNA (see Figure 7.2). The binding of a second oestradiol-receptor complex to the same promoter site (two E2+ER complexes together is called a **dimer**) initiates **gene promotion**, i.e. it sets into motion the activation of the gene so that protein synthesis will commence (also known as **gene expression**). The genes that are switched on in this way are first, not surprisingly, a gene that replaces the original ER, otherwise the cell would use up all the ER and become ER negative (ER−), i.e. no longer able to respond to E2. But, other genes are activated, including those that code for **PgR** (the **progesterone receptor**), and various growth hormones (see p. 36 and Figure 7.2). The other oestrogens are less important. E1 (oestrone) is held in the body mostly in an inactive form bound to the protein **albumin** in the blood. It also stimulates breast cell growth but to a lesser extent than E2. It becomes a more important oestrogen in women after the menopause, when levels of E2 drop. E3 (oestriol) is the weakest of the oestrogens (as a comparison, E2 has a thousand times greater effect on breast tissue than E3). In fact, E3 may have a beneficial effect on the prevention of breast cancer by occupying ER instead of E2. E3 is the form in which much of the oestrogen is excreted from

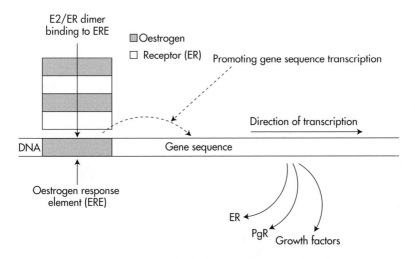

FIGURE 7.2 The oestrogen and oestrogen receptor complex binds with a second complex to form a dimer. The dimer binds to the oestrogen-response elements of DNA and begins transcription of the genes. The resulting proteins are more copies of the oestrogen receptor (ER), the progesterone receptor (PgR) and growth factors. (Redrawn from Blows 2003, Figure 4.2.)

the body. The importance of understanding the nature of the oestrogens becomes apparent in the subject of breast cancer.

The breasts and breast cancer

Breasts are modified sweat glands. This *does not* mean that breast milk is modified sweat, as suggested by one group of students. The two statements are very different, i.e. the first is true, but the second is quite definitely *not* true. The breast (see Figure 7.3) is constructed in the form of **lobes**. There are between 15 and 20 lobes set in a circular fashion, like spokes of a wheel, around a central point, the **nipple** (also called the **mammary papilla**). Each lobe is sectioned off from the neighbouring lobes by a wall of connective tissue. Lobes contain a tree-like system of ducts called a **lobule** (the milk-producing, or secretary portion of the breasts) (Marieb 2001). A lobule consists of one central duct with multiple branching ducts, each ending in a dilated segment (called an **acini**) the walls of which form terminal

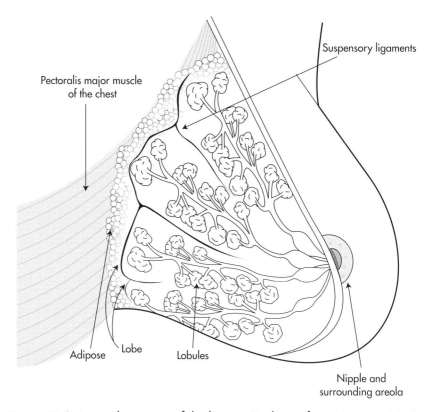

FIGURE 7.3 Internal structure of the breast. (Redrawn from Martini 2004.)

sac-like structures called **alveoli** (the same name as the sac-like structures of the lungs). The cells in the walls of the alveoli produce breast milk, when required, under hormonal control (called **lactation**). Special cells, called **myoepithelial cells**, have long thin extensions and these surround the alveoli in a network. Under hormonal control these cell extensions contract (like miniature muscles) and squeeze milk from the alveoli into the central duct. This is rather like a hand squeezing the rubber bulb when taking blood pressure to pump air into the cuff. The central duct in the lobule drains the milk towards the nipple (see Figure 7.3).

The nipple has a covering of pigmented and folded **epidermis**, which is rich in **sebaceous glands** producing **sebum**, an oily fluid that protects the skin surface during breastfeeding. Inside the nipple is **dense collagen** connective tissue with many elastic fibres. These fibres continue outward beneath the **areola**, a pigmented area of epidermis around the nipple which is also rich in sebaceous glands.

The breast is packed with a fibrous connective tissue called **stroma**, and this includes a number of supportive structures. The **adipose** tissue (i.e. fat) is present in variable amounts and has nothing to do with milk production. The volume of fat present determines the size of the breasts. There are loose connections between the breasts and the **deep pectoral fascia**, a connective tissue layer covering two main chest muscles, the **pectoralis major** and the **serratus anterior**. These muscle are sometime involved in advanced breast cancer.

Blood supply to the breast comes from branches of the **axillary artery** and the **internal thoracic artery**, plus some **intercostal arteries**. Venous drainage is via a **venous plexus** beneath the areola, then the **internal thoracic** and **intercostal veins**. The **lymphatic** drainage is important for the understanding of how breast cancers spread. Over 85% of lymph drains from the breast into the **axillary lymph nodes** (i.e. those of the armpit). There are 20 to 30 large lymph nodes (plus a number of smaller ones) clustered in the axilla, and these are grouped into five sets, the **anterior**, **posterior**, **lateral**, **central** and **apical** (or **infraclavicular**) sets. The anterior set are several large nodes with contacts within the tail of the breast that extend beneath the axilla (called the **tail of Spence**).

Two sets of lymphatic vessels drain the breast of lymph: (1) The **cutaneous lymphatic** plexus, which is within the skin (except the nipple and areola), and drains the skin surface; and (2) the **subareola plexus** (or **plexus of Sappey**), which drains lymph from the secretory

TABLE 7.1 The cells and tissues of the breast

Tissue type	Examples in the breast	Notes
Epithelial	Alveolar	Milk-producing cells; cuboidal in non-lactating phase, becoming columnar when lactating. These are ER+
Epithelial	Duct-lining	Cuboid or columnar. These are ER+
Epithelial	Myoepithelial	Long branching processes containing two contractile proteins, actin and myosin. Responds to the hormone oxytocin by contracting and squeezing the alveoli, pushing milk towards the nipple. These are ER+
Connective	Stroma	Connective tissue fibres containing fibroblasts, adipocytes, neutrophils, macrophages, lymphocytes (see pp. 95–96 for these cells)

tissues (the ductal system of the lobules) and the areola. The remaining 15% of the lymph drainage passes either into the **parasternal nodes** along the edge of the **sternum** (the breast bone) or crosses the midline via superficial lymphatic vessels from one breast to the other. Crossing between the breasts allows the chance of cancer to involve both breasts by this means. There are lymphatic connections between the breasts and the pectoralis major muscle, allowing for spread to the chest wall, and some lymphatic drainage through the diaphragm giving the potential for spread to the abdomen. Table 7.1 shows the tissues and cells present in the breast.

Breast cancer

Breast cancer is a huge and very important subject for two reasons: (1) it is still the cause of many needless deaths in women, and (2) because of the uncertainty surrounding the role of hormones (i.e. the contraceptive pill and hormone replacement therapy) in the cause of this disease. It is essential to point out that the debate over the hormones continues, and it is beyond the remit of this book to enter this debate.

The pathological types of breast cancer

The types of breast cancer can be classified into two groups (**non-invasive** and **invasive**), and are located as either **ductal** (inside or arising from the ducts) or **lobular** (within the lobes) (Kumar *et al.* 1997, Woolf 1998).

Non-invasive (carcinoma *in situ*)(see page 27)

Intraductal **ductal carcinoma** *in situ* (**A1a**)(also called **ductal carcinoma** *in situ*, or **DCIS**) causes 20 to 25% of all breast carcinomas, with malignant cells filling the ducts, but remaining within the basement membrane. They may be **non-Comedo** (differentiated with no central necrosis) or **Comedo** (poorly differentiated with central necrosis). Comedo can reach large size, 50% are over 2 cm across.

Ductal carcinoma *in situ* **with Paget's disease** (**A1b**) is seen mostly in older women. It is basically A1a (DCIS) with Paget's disease, which is described below (Table 7.2). The nipple is affected with symptoms similar to eczema, i.e. ulcerated and fissured, and oozing fluid. Table 7.2 describes two nipple disorders found in breast cancers.

Lobular carcinoma *in situ* (**LCIS**) (**A2**) is a distinct form of the disease that is found by tissue biopsy and examination. It can be multi-focal (many sites within the breast, accounting for 70% of patients) or bilateral (involving both breasts, about 30 to 40% of patients). Small, uniform cells occur within the smaller ducts or acini, and these become distended with central necrosis. Later invasion of surrounding tissues can occur in about 30% of patients.

Invasive

Invasive ductal carcinoma (**B1a**) is the most common form of breast cancer, between 70 and 85% of patients have this disease. It usually appears as a very hard nodule (the word **scirrhus** means very hard, like stone) making it easily detected by palpation. It is composed of dense fibrous stromal cells mixed with tumour cells, the surface of the tumour often infiltrates the surrounding tissues, including blood vessels. Microscopic variations of this type are seen, with different tumour cell types and abnormal tissue structures.

Invasive ductal carcinoma with Paget's disease (**B1b**) is type B1a with additional Paget's disease (see Table 7.2).

Invasive lobular carcinoma (**B2**) accounts for about 5 to 10% of all invasive breast tumours. One-fifth of these are bilateral (in both

TABLE 7.2 Two main nipple disorders in breast cancer

Nipple disease	Description
Paget's disease	Paget cells are large with abundant pale cytoplasm and large nuclei with a prominent nucleolus. They occur in surface epithelium of the nipple (i.e. epidermis) and are probably derived from glandular cells, i.e. ductal cells (therefore they are a type of adenocarcinoma). They originally cause simple reddening of the nipple and areolar with pruritis. This leads on to scaling (i.e. eczema-like changes) and eventually to erosion of the skin (ulceration).
	Often there is a painless palpable mass in the underlying breast tissue (in about 50% of cases). Up to 95% of patients have underlying carcinoma, frequently intraductal carcinoma, although it is not always palpable.
	Paget's disease of the nipple is generally unilateral, but can be bilateral
Nipple duct carcinoma (NDC)	This can be mistaken for Paget's disease. It is usually unilateral.
	Nipple discharge is commonly reported (in about 60–70% of cases).
	Then follows enlargement and induration of the nipple with ulceration. There is also pain, itching or burning. The margins of the lesion are well-delineated. Cystic dilation can occur in the underlying ducts.
	The pathology begins with a small number of ductules clustered around a major duct.
	The advanced lesion replaces part or all of the nipple stroma, causing enlargement and expansion of the nipple and erosion of the surface epithelium (ulceration)

breasts), and they tend to become multifocal. The cells are smaller and more uniform than in ductal carcinoma causing a poorly circumscribed mass (i.e. the edges are not easily defined).

Medullary carcinoma (B3) accounts for about 1% of all breast cancers. It forms a large mass (anything from 2 cm up to 10 cm diameter is possible) which is soft in nature with a well-defined edge. Growth causes the tumour to 'push' into the surrounding tissues rather than infiltrate. The large cells of the tumour grow in sheets with no stroma between them

Colloid (mucinous) carcinoma (B4) accounts for about 2 to 3% of breast cancers. Most are seen in women after menopause, and they carry a good prognosis, owing to very few nodal metastases. The tumour is a jelly-like bulky mass with a well-defined edge. It is largely **mucin** produced by the islands of tumour cells scattered throughout.

Tubular carcinoma (B5) accounts for about 2% of invasive carcinomas. The prognosis is better for this than for invasive ductal carcinoma. It consists of a small tumour (about 1 cm in diameter) with a poorly defined edge. The cells form tubes which can be oval or elongated and arranged randomly. There is a family history of the disease in about 40% of patients.

Adenoid (cystic) carcinoma (B6) is very rare, accounting for only about 0.1 to 0.2% of breast carcinomas. The tumour is about 1 to 5 cm in size and is painless. It arises from the nipple or areola area and has well-defined edges. It carries a good prognosis.

Apocrine carcinoma (B7) is a solid mass, about 2 cm in diameter, and may be ductal or lobular. **Apocrine metaplasia** is a premalignant change in the epithelial cells sometimes seen in otherwise normal breasts in women over 20 years of age. It consists of pink cells present during fibrocystic changes, increasing the risk of malignancy. Such a malignancy would be a solid mass, about 2 cm in diameter.

Invasive papillary carcinoma (B8) accounts for only about 1.5 to 2.5% of breast cancers. The highest incidence of this disease occurs in post-menopausal and non-Caucasian women. It is an intraductal palpable tumour in 90% of patients with this disease.

Generally, hard tumours cause inflammation at the interface between the tumour and surrounding tissues, and this results in **fibrosis** (involving cells called **fibrocytes**, derived from **fibroblasts**). This is not the case with soft tumours.

The risk factors for breast cancer

The risk factors involved in causing breast cancer are the following.

The disease increases with **age**, doubling the risk every 10 years until menopause, then the risk increase slows down. Also, **menarche** (the age at first period) before 11 years and late **menopause** (i.e. after 54 years) have higher risk (i.e. twice the risk of those women with later menarche and menopause at about 45 years). The reasons are not clear, but perhaps could be to do with the length of time the breasts are exposed to the oestrogens. Oestrogens are highest between menarche and menopause, and the more years this involves the greater the risk.

First pregnancy after the age of 30 years doubles the risk compared with those whose first pregnancy is before 20 years. **Breastfeeding** for a long term is protective against the disease. **The contraceptive pill** and **hormone replacement therapy** (**HRT**) as risk factors are inconclusive and under further research and discussion.

Family history of the disease increases the risk by three or more times that of the general population in all the female members of that family. Increased risk is seen in women who have a **first-degree relative** (mother, sister or daughter) with bilateral breast cancer, or unilateral breast cancer under 40 years of age, or have combined breast and ovary cancer (see p. 194). Also at higher risk are women who have two **first-** or **second-degree relatives** (granddaughter, grandmother, aunt or niece) with breast cancer diagnosed between 40 and 60 years of age, or three first- or second-degree relatives with breast and ovarian cancer on the same side of the family. Four or more family members with breast cancer (with or without ovarian cancer) within three generations put the other women in that family at a very high risk. Identifying who is at risk is important because

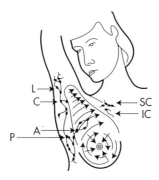

FIGURE 7.4 The breast is examined by palpation with the three middle fingers. It can be examined in different directions, either circular, or from the outside towards the nipple, as shown by the arrows. It is important to feel the entire surface, and to examine the tail of Spence under the arm. The lymph nodes are also shown: A = anterior, C = central, L = lateral, P = posterior, IC = inferior clavicular, SC = superior clavicular. (Redrawn from Kozier *et al.* 2000.)

these high-risk women should then be screened at very regular intervals by their doctor, as well as performing self-checks at home (see Figure 7.4), and they may be tested for the presence of specific genes.

Previous history of benign breast disease is important. Women with severe atypical epithelial hyperplasia (see p. 27) have four to five times greater risk of breast cancer. Women with benign breast changes like this and with a family history of breast cancer carry nine times higher risk.

Lifestyle factors, such as **diet, alcohol, smoking** and **night work** affect the risk. The risk is doubled with post-menopausal **obesity**, and eating high levels of meat and dairy products increases the risk. This is thought to be due to the consumption of higher levels of **IGF-1** (**insulin-like growth factor-1**, see Table 2.1, p. 36) associated with these foods. Post-menopausal women with higher than normal IGF-1 intake have three times the average risk of breast cancer. In women below the age of 50 years the risk was higher (up to seven times the average). Some studies show an increased risk by drinking excess **alcohol**. There is now a proven link between **smoking** and breast cancer. Smoking 20 cigarettes per day increases the risk by four times.

Women who work **night shifts** have been shown to increase their risk by 1.5 times. The reason is not clear, but may be due to working in artificial light conditions and with **melatonin** production. Melatonin is a hormone produced by the **pineal gland** in the brain, and whilst its functions are not fully understood, it is thought that this hormone has some influence over the sleep–wake cycle. The link between night duty and breast cancer is best explained by the following theory. Melatonin is produced mainly at night in dark conditions, but artificial light on night duty would suppress this natural cycle. Melatonin is also thought to suppress oestrogen levels, so oestrogen would be naturally lower at night. It is possible that women on regular night work have constantly low melatonin levels, which results in maintaining a high oestrogen level day and night. A persistently high level of oestrogen would promote breast cell replication and may therefore contribute towards breast cancer. Taking this theory further, blind women, because they never see any light and therefore are likely to have raised melatonin levels (and correspondingly lower oestrogen), have been shown to have 50% *less* risk of breast cancers.

Radiation increases the risk of breast cancer. The greatest risk is exposure to radiation at an early age, particularly between 10 and 14 years of age, when breast tissue is undergoing rapid development. Radiation-induced breast cancer comes on later in life, with a gap of at least 10 to 15 years after the exposure before symptoms arise. The effects of the radiation have been shown to last for 35 years, maybe longer.

The genetics of breast cancer

About 5% of breast cancers are caused by a **dominant** gene (see p. 43). This means that about 1 in 200 women in the Western world will develop a genetic predisposition for breast cancer.

The ***TP53* gene** at 17p13.1 (see p. 12 for a discussion of this gene) is an important **tumour suppressor gene**, and a factor in this disease. **Li-Fraumeni syndrome** is a rare **autosomal dominant** inherited disorder (see p. 43) involving the *TP53* gene, which causes the development of multiple cancers, including multifocal breast cancer early in life. Other inherited genes in breast cancer include the following.

hMLH1 and *hMSH2* are DNA repair genes (see p. 12), i.e. they code for proteins which repair mismatched bases on DNA (normally **adenosine** matches with **thymine**; **cytosine** matches with **guanine**) (see p. 6). They are linked to chromosomes 2p and 3p, and cause breast cancer in those families with **hereditary non-polyposis colorectal cancer** (**Lynch syndrome type II**)(see Table 5.3 on p. 136).

BRCA 1 (**BR**east **CA**ncer 1) gene is implicated as a causative factor in all hereditary breast with ovarian cancers. It is a large gene (18 million bases long) on chromosome 17 (17q21). The normal gene product may be involved in suppression of oestrogen-dependent breast cell proliferation, possibly by inhibiting ER production (see p. 174 for ER), and appears to have some control over the cell cycle by interacting with the protein products of the *Tp53* and *RB1* genes (see p. 12) (Passarge 2001). Women with mutations of the *BRCA 1* gene lose this function, and therefore have a 56 to 85% increased chance of developing the disease (different estimates of the importance of this gene vary). Five different mutations have been found for this gene, and during screening the entire gene must be examined for errors. With a gene this large screening is a huge undertaking that takes months.

BRCA 2 (**BR**east **CA**ncer 2) on chromosome 13 (13q12.3) is found in about one-third of all familial breast cancer patients. It appears to have a similar role in controlling the cell cycle as *BRCA 1* (Passarge 2001). Inheritance of *BRCA 1* and *2* is of the autosomal dominant mechanism (see p. 43). Less is known about *BRCA 3* (**BR**east **CA**ncer 3) gene than *BRCA 1* or *2*, but more research will produce further information.

Oncogenes (see p. 38) cause more sporadic cases of breast cancer.

The symptoms of breast cancer

The symptoms of breast cancer may be the presence of a solitary, painless lump in the breast, often found by the patient at self-examination. Lumps in the breast are *not* always cancer; the vast majority of lumps have benign causes, like **fibrocyctic** changes (non-malignant lesions of epithelial origin that come and go in relation to the ovarian cycle) (see p. 190). The involvement of axillary lymph nodes in those lumps that are malignant is a sign of advancement of the disease. The removal of the lump (often called a '**lumpectomy**') is a first step, and subsequent treatment depends on the histopathological result of the removed tissue (see p. 25).

Mammography, an X-ray procedure of the breast, can show shadows of dense tissue or **calcification** in the breast, although benign lesions can also calcify and show up on mammography. A valuable use of this examination is as an annual screening test for those women who carry a higher risk of the disease.

Breast pain is not commonly an early symptom, but may be a feature in advanced disease, i.e. 60 to 70% of patients with *advanced* breast cancer complain of pain. Those with metastatic disease usually have several different pain sites with probably different causes. Breast pain generally may be cyclic (occurs at specific points in relation to the menstrual cycle) or non-cyclic (unrelated to the menstrual cycle). Cyclic breast pain (**cyclic mastalgia**) is due to hormonal changes and is not caused by breast cancer. Non-cyclic pain is far less common and feels very different from cyclic pain. It does not vary over the menstrual cycle, it is often of unknown cause and usually in one spot or area ('**trigger zone pain**'), suggesting it is anatomical rather than hormonal in origin. Breast pain may sometimes be caused by trauma to the breast.

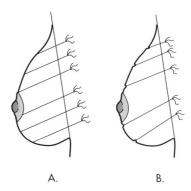

A.   B.

Figure 7.5 A schematic view of the cause of the peau d'orange effect. (A) Normal breast showing suspensory ligaments, (B) after the breast is swollen the suspensory ligaments hold parts of the breast back, causing a dimpling effect.

The spread of **metastases** from tumours is suggested by:

1 The tumour size being larger than 5 cm.
2 The formation of **oedema** (see pp. 305–306) of the skin around the tumour. Swelling causes dimpling of the skin where the ligaments attaching the breast tissue to the skin hold the skin in (called **peau d'orange**, or orange peel appearance) (see Figure 7.5).
3 Ulceration of the skin over the tumour.
4 Adhesion of the breast on the chest wall muscles preventing movement of the breast.
5 **Superclavicular** (i.e. above the collar bone) lymph nodes can be felt (i.e. palpable).
6 Large lymph nodes (e.g. walnut size) are found in the axilla.
7 The skin around the tumour mass is inflamed.

Important prognostic markers are:

1 **Lymph node metastasis**, i.e. the more nodes that are involved the worse is the prognosis.
2 **Tumour size**, the larger the tumour the worse the prognosis. Generally, tumours less than 1 cm have an excellent prognosis.
3 **Histological grade**, using cellular differentiation, nuclear pleomorphism and the number of mitotic figures present in the tumour. **Cellular differentiation**, i.e. *well differentiated*, means that the cells look normal, i.e. they look the same as the tissue of

origin, but *poorly differentiated* means that cells appear grossly abnormal. **Nuclear pleomorphism** concerns how abnormal the nucleus looks, (pleo = more; pleomorphism = more, or multiple shaped nucleus).

4 **Mitotic figures**, i.e. the number of cells in mitosis within the tissue (the more cells in mitosis the more aggressive is the tumour).

5 **Histological type**, i.e. what the abnormal cells are like, e.g. **tubular** are cells that appear like tubes; **medullary** are cells which have the colour of the brain (medulla); **mucinous** are tumour cells that produce mucus and **papillary** are cells that stick out in little finger-like projections (called **papules**).

6 **Hormone-receptor status** (also known as *biological markers*), e.g. cells that are **oestrogen receptor positive (ER+)** (see p. 174). ER+ tumours allow for treatment with anti-oestrogen drugs. About 60% of breast tumours are ER+. **Progesterone receptor positive (PgR+)** tumour cells exist mostly in relation with ER+, since the presence of PgR is dependent on an intact ER pathway. Their role in inducing breast cancer is not proven, and anti-progesterone therapy may only ease symptoms in advanced disease (see p. 189).

7 **Ploidy** is the measurement of the amount of DNA in the cell; i.e. **diploid** is the normal chromosome count (46) and carries a better prognosis if found in tumour cells than **aneuploid** (any abnormal chromosome count).

8 **Genetics**, the presence of mutations of the genes such as *erb-B2* (see p. 42) or *Tp53* (see p. 40).

Advanced breast disease is divided into local and metastatic. **Locally** advanced disease is characterised by the features of skin and chest wall infiltration, with or without axillary node involvement. *Skin features* include ulceration and the presence of satellite nodes, dermal infiltration, peau d'orange (see p. 186 and Figure 7.5) and erythema (redness) over the tumour site. *Chest wall features* include fixation of the tumour to the ribs, the intercostal muscles or the serratus anterior muscle (see p. 176). *Axillary node* features are where the nodes are fixed to each other or to other structures (i.e. they become matted together).

Metastatic disease may involve any site, but more often bone, lymph and chest wall (better prognosis), or lung, liver or brain (poorest prognosis)(see Chapter 9 for metastasis and secondary tumour growth).

Specific problems of advanced breast cancer

Lymphoedema is the collection of fluid on the tissues due to obstruction of the lymphatic drainage. In cancer, this is due either to blocking of lymph nodes with malignant cells, as in lymph metastases, or from treatment, e.g. surgical removal or irradiation of the lymph nodes (see also the causes of oedema, Table 11.3, p. 306). Upper limb lymphoedema is often caused by local recurrence of the disease within nodes of the axillary and supraclavicular regions. It is a cause of pain, discomfort and distress.

Hypercalcaemia (high blood calcium) can be caused by bone disease releasing calcium into the blood. The loss of calcium from the diseased bones makes them weaker and at risk of **pathological fractures**. Breathlessness can be caused by pulmonary (lung) disease, and **raised intercranial pressure** (**RICP**) may be caused by cerebral (brain) disease (see p. 245).

The treatment of breast cancer

Mastectomy is the surgical removal of the breast. This can be just the lump itself (a **lumpectomy**) or removing part or all of the breast (leaving all other structures) or can be *radical*, removing the breast and other structures like the chest wall muscles (see p. 176) and axillary lymph nodes (see p. 177). Total mastectomy, especially the radical procedure, is reserved for the management of more advanced disease since the surgery carries with it a considerable amount of disfigurement and alteration of body image. Lesser surgical techniques (e.g. lumpectomy) are available for the removal of smaller tumours where much or some of the breast can be preserved. Reconstructive surgery (called **mammoplasty**) is also available to re-establish, where possible, the normal contours of the breast. Women undergoing surgery to the breast should be under the care of the **advanced nurse practitioner** in breast care, who can support the patient and offer advice on restorative measures such as breast implants and prostheses.

Radiotherapy (see also p. 334, Chapter 12) is also used routinely to various degrees. Techniques change according to different units, and they also change in different patients according to the stage of the disease. In early disease, as a follow-up from simple surgery, two tangential fields of radiation are often used over the chest wall, one *lateral oblique* and the other *medial oblique* to arrest any remaining disease and prevent local spread. A radiation standard dose of between 4000 and 5000 centigray (cGy) is divided into 15 to 25 daily doses. It is important to avoid irradiating the lungs as this may cause post-radiation complications. For advanced disease with lymphatic spread, a wider field of irradiation to include lymph nodes and chest wall muscles could be used.

Cytotoxic therapy (or **chemotherapy**) is also used to destroy metastatic disease, and is discussed in Chapter 12 (p. 322). The cytotoxic drugs used in breast cancer particularly are: **cyclophos-phamide** (an **alkylating agent**), **methotrexate** and **5-fluorouracil** (**5-FU**) (both **antimetabolites**), **doxorubicin** and **epirubicin** (both **anthracyclins**), **taxol** and **taxotere** (both **mitotic inhibitors**), and **vinblastine, vindesine** and **vincristine** (all **vinca alkaloids**). The nature and function of these drugs are discussed in Chapter 12 (see p. 322). Nurses should be aware of the possibility of these drugs affecting the ovaries and therefore causing infertility. For younger patients particularly this could be a major problem, and nurses must be able to support and advise their patients about this.

Hormonal therapy is the use of drugs to block the hormones (notably oestradiol) that otherwise would promote breast cancer growth. Anti-oestrogens work by binding to the oestrogen receptors (ER) in breast cells that are ER positive (ER+)(see also pp. 175, 178), and this prevents the oestrogens from binding, and therefore elimi-nates the growth these hormones would promote. The difficulty is that in breast cancers not all the malignant cells are ER+. Many cells may be ER− (i.e. without ER), and therefore would not respond to this type of treatment. Some tumours are a mix of ER+ with ER− cells, and since only the ER+ cells respond to this treat-ment the tumour would regress but not respond completely. The anti-oestrogens include **Nolvadex (tamoxifen)** and **fareston**. They are often used in prophylaxis (i.e. prevention) to block further malig-nant growth after the tumour and any spread of the disease has been eradicated. Traditionally a drug like tamoxifen has been given for up to five years following completion of the initial treatment to prevent reoccurrence. **Aromatase inhibitors** are drugs that block the func-tion of **aromatase**, an enzyme that converts the androgens to oestro-gens (see Figure 7.6). This reduces significantly the amount of oestrogen produced. These drugs are **anastrozole** and **formestane**. Progesterone therapy is used to relieve symptoms in women with advanced breast disease involving metastatic spread that is not responding to other treatments. Progesterone cannot be given

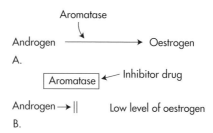

FIGURE 7.6 Aromatase inhibitors reduce the oestrogen levels by blocking the enzyme aromatase that converts androgens to oestrogens (see also Figure 7.9).

directly by mouth, but is given orally as a precursor called a **progestogen** (the drug is known as **megestrol**). Given the fact that not all breast cancers will respond to this form of treatment, hormonal therapy is considered as an adjunct (or additional) therapy alongside other treatments.

The ovaries and ovarian cancer

The two ovaries are situated low in the pelvic extension of the abdominal cavity, one each side of the uterus. They have a close association with the **uterine** (or **fallopian**) **tubes**, which carry the **ova** (the 'egg' cells) that have been discharged from both ovaries into the uterus. The function of the ovary is to produce the ovum (normally one each side per cycle) and to produce the hormone **oestradiol** (see p. 174).

The ovarian cycle

This section should be read in conjunction with Figure 7.7 and with the uterine cycle (see p. 197). This account is an illustration of the ovarian cycle based on the standard 28 days, although there is considerable variation in the timing of the cycle in different women. The **ovarian cycle** is controlled by two hormones from the **anterior pituitary gland** at the base of the brain, i.e. **follicle-stimulating hormone (FSH)** and **luteinising hormone (LH)**. These are together called the **gonadotropic hormones** (*tropic* means to influence, i.e. they influence the **gonads**, a collective term for the ovaries and testes). In women, ova develop up to the **antrum stage** (see Figure 7.8) without FSH, but FSH is required to stimulate the development of ova from the antrum stage on to full maturity (**follicular maturation**). At first, several ova develop, but then only one goes on to full

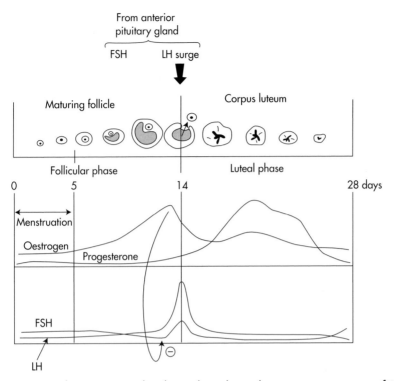

FIGURE 7.7 The ovarian cycle. The cycle is shown here over an average of 28 days although a variety of different time spans are seen. The first 14 days is the follicular phase, the second 14 days is the luteal phase, with ovulation occurring about day 14 due to a surge in LH (luteinising hormone). The maturing follicle in the first half releases more and more oestrogen as it gets bigger. This rise in oestrogen has a negative feedback on FSH (follicle-stimulating hormone) which then falls (see arrow). Progesterone is released from the corpus luteum in the second half, and rises to a peak before falling again as the corpus luteum disappears. Progesterone sustains the endometrium of the uterus, and due to the decline in progesterone towards the end of the cycle this lining is then shed over days 1 to 5 of the next cycle, a process called menstruation.

maturity. They are maturing inside a tiny ball of cells in the ovary called a **follicle**. This occurs during the first 14 days of the cycle, and this period is therefore called the **follicular phase** (days 0 to 14). The maturing follicle produces increasing amounts of oestradiol, so the level of this hormone increases in the blood over the follicular phase. At or about day 14 (mid-cycle) the high oestradiol level causes a surge in the release of LH from the pituitary gland, which in turn causes the mature follicle to rupture and release the ovum. The ovum is captured by the **fallopian tube** to begin its journey to the uterus, and it may or may not become fertilised in this tube.

The remains of the follicle in the ovary condense down to form a **corpus luteum**, so the second half of the cycle, after ovulation, is known as the **luteal phase**. During this phase the condensing corpus luteum produces the hormone **progesterone** that sustains the uterine lining until the fertilised ovum (if indeed it is fertilised) can become embedded in this lining. The decline in progesterone towards day 28, the end of the cycle, due to the disappearing corpus luteum, causes shedding of the uterine lining (called **menstruation**, or a **menstrual 'period'**) over the first five days of the *next* cycle (days 1 to 5), in those cycles where fertilisation did *not* occur. If fer-

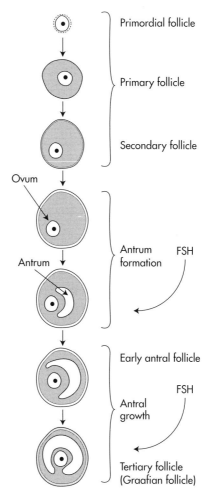

FIGURE 7.8 The developing follicle and ovum (days 1 to 14 of the ovarian cycle). The stimulus for development during the early stages is not known, but from antrum (or cavity) formation onwards the stimulus is FSH (follicle-stimulating hormone).

tilisation does occur, the ovum (which has now developed into a cluster of cells) becomes embedded in the uterine lining and establishes a connection with the maternal blood circulation through the developing **placenta**. Part of the embedding cell cluster (called a **blastocyst**) produces a hormone called **human chorionic gonadotrophin (HCG)**, which enters the mother's blood and causes retention of the luteal phase. Keeping the corpus luteum means that the progesterone production does not diminish, thus preventing the loss of the uterine lining, and retaining the pregnancy, so that the menstrual period will be missed because the next cycle will not start. HCG levels rise over the first two months of pregnancy, then fall to a low level by the fourth month, and remain at this lower level for the remainder of the pregnancy (Marieb 2001). Excretion of HCG in the urine forms the basis of pregnancy tests since it can only be present as a product of a blastocyst, i.e. a pregnancy.

Two particular cell types are important in the ovary; the **theca** cells and the **granulosa** cells. The theca cells are stimulated by LH, and they produce **androgens** (mostly **androstenedione**) from **cholesterol** (see Figures 7.1 and 7.9). The granulosa cells are stimulated mostly by FSH (but also some LH) and they produce oestradiol from the androgen (see Figure 7.9). One effect of oestradiol is to suppress the release of FSH (as a negative feedback system). As the follicle reaches full maturity so the oestradiol reaches the greatest output. This peak of oestradiol blocks FSH release (since FSH will no longer be required for follicular maturation) and the oestradiol also triggers

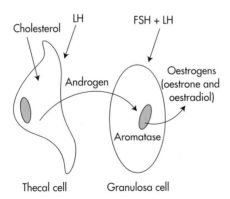

FIGURE 7.9 Two cell types in the ovary. The first, the thecal cell, converts cholesterol to androgens (male hormones), and the second, the granulosa cell, converts the androgen to oestrogen using the enzyme aromatase. The thecal cell responds to LH (luteinising hormone) and the granulosa cell responds to LH and FSH (follicle-stimulating hormone).

the LH surge that causes ovulation. So oestradiol is a major hormone in the control of the ovarian cycle.

Ovarian cancer

Cancer of the ovary is the cause of more deaths per year than all the other malignancies of the female reproductive tract put together. As such, like breast cancer, it is another very important female neoplastic disorder. The highest risk seems to be related to a Western lifestyle, with higher risks seen in women who have never had children, or have never been pregnant, or those who are smokers or exposed to asbestos. Three categories of malignant potential occur in these tumours, *benign, borderline (low malignant potential)* and *overtly malignant.* Many are associated with **cysts**, which are fluid-filled cavities within the tissues. Neoplasms of the ovary are a wide assortment of diseases which can be broadly placed into the following two main groups (according to the cell of origin) (Kumar *et al.* 1997).

TABLE 7.3 The types of surface epithelial ovarian tumours

Tumour type	Notes
Serous (cystadenomas, cystadenocarcinomas)	Most frequent type, presents at 30 to 40 years of age. Solid tumour often with cysts; 60% are benign, 15% borderline and 25% malignant
Mucinous	Very similar to serous, derived from mucin-secreting epithelium. Less likely to be malignant than serous (only 20% are borderline or malignant)
Endometrioid	Usually malignant form derived from the walls of cysts. They take on a microscopic appearance similar to endometrial cells; 30% are bilateral, and 15 to 30% are associated with endometrial cancer (see p. 198)
Clear cell (mesonephroid)	A spongy, partly cystic tumour of cells with clear cytoplasm. Most are malignant
Brenner	Rare, solid tumour of transitional epithelium (see p. 16) set in stromal cells (see p. 178). Mostly benign
Cystadenofibroma	Similar to serous cystadenoma, malignancy is rare

1 Tumours of **surface epithelial** origin make up the largest proportion of ovarian cancers seen. The malignant forms of the disease account for about 90% of all malignant ovarian cancers. The
   group as a whole includes benign and malignant, and there are
   different types (see Table 7.3).
2 Tumours of **germ cell** origin (germ cells are the ova and its
   surrounding follicular tissues) account for about 3 to 5% of all
   malignant ovarian tumours. Like surface epithelial tumours,
   there are a number of different types (see Table 7.4).

TABLE 7.4 The types of germ cell ovarian tumours

Tumour type	Notes
Teratoma	About 15 to 20% of all ovarian tumours. They appear at an early age. *Mature* and *immature* forms occur. Mature are rarely malignant (99% are benign) but immature have a greater tendency to become malignant (see also teratoma of testes, p. 216)
Dysgerminoma	These appear around 20 to 30 years of age. They are solid malignant tumours, about one-third spread to other sites
Endodermal sinus tumour (yolk sac tumour)	Appears in the young (average age is 19 years). It is highly malignant. The tumour secretes a protein called α-fetoprotein (AFP) which can be monitored to assess the progress of the disease
Choriocarcinoma	Appear in those under 30 years of age. They are malignant and metastasise early. They often have areas of necrosis and haemorrhage
Sex-cord tumours	Sex cords are primitive germ cells that migrate into the ovary during embryonic development. They can retain the ability to differentiate in the adult gonads, and give rise to tumours. This category includes granulosa-theca cell tumours (see p. 193 for granulosa and thecal cells) that account for about 1.5% of all ovarian tumours and which may produce oestrogens, thecomas (usually benign tumours of thecal cells seen mostly in post-menopausal women) and Sertoli–Leydig tumours (see p. 210 for Sertoli and Leydig cells), which are very rare in the ovary (0.2% of ovarian cancers)

Ovarian cancers are often symptom free at first, which gives the tumour time to spread unless found on routine examination. When symptoms arise they are often pain in the abdomen, swelling of the abdomen and sometimes **ascites** (oedema collecting in the abdomen) (see p. 306 for oedema). In advanced disease the patient can suffer from nausea and vomiting, bowel changes and vaginal bleeding from local spread into the vagina.

Staging for ovarian cancer uses four major grades, **I** to **IV** with divisions **A**, **B** and **C** (Woolf 1998):

IA   One ovary involved, capsule intact, no ascites.

IB   Both ovaries involved, capsules intact, no ascites.

IC   Capsule involved and malignant cells present in peritoneal fluid.

IIA   Extension of the tumour to the uterus or fallopian tubes (see p. 197).

IIB   Extension of the tumour to other pelvic organs.

IIC   Pelvic extension and malignant cells present in peritoneal fluid.

IIIA   Microscopic metastases outside of the pelvis.

IIIB   Metastases smaller in size than 2 cm.

IIIC   Metastases greater in size than 2 cm.

IV   Distant organs involved.

Oophorectomy is the surgical removal of an ovary. Removal of both ovaries is a big change in body image (despite the fact that they are internal organs), and as such the surgery is potentially a major problem, especially for younger women. With both ovaries removed the patient is immediately rendered infertile, and she will go directly into menopause (due to the loss of the oestrogen production). In older women who are already in menopause and who do not want any further children the effects of the surgery are much less of a problem. For younger women having bilateral oophorectomy the infertility problem must be discussed with them and their partners, and the patients should be supported in their decisions. The issue of immediate menopause in younger patients can be overcome to some extent by the administration of oral hormone.

The female reproductive tract

The **uterus** (commonly known as the **womb**)(see Figure 7.10) is the main organ low in the female pelvis where development of first the embryo and later the foetus takes place. It is a hollow organ with a smooth-muscle wall (the **myometrium**) lined internally by a layer of glandular cells set in stromal connective tissue (the **endometrium**). This inner layer has a rich blood supply and is shed regularly as part of the **uterine cycle**. This cycle is linked to the ovarian cycle, and the following account of the uterine cycle should be read in conjunction with the ovarian cycle on p. 190. Over the first 5 days or so of the ovarian cycle a large amount of the endometrial lining is lost through the vagina in a flow known as **menstruation**. It then begins to thicken over the remaining follicular phase up to day 14, but becomes thicker still under the influence of progesterone during the luteal phase (day 15 onwards). Towards the end of the 28-day cycle the progesterone production (which has sustained the endometrium) released by the corpus luteum declines and the endometrium can no longer survive. By day 1 of the next cycle the endometrium is shed and a new menstruation starts (see Figure 7.7) (see p. 193 for the events that change this in early pregnancy).

Linking the uterus to the ovaries are the **fallopian** (or **ovarian**) **tubes**, one each side, and these capture and pass the released ova

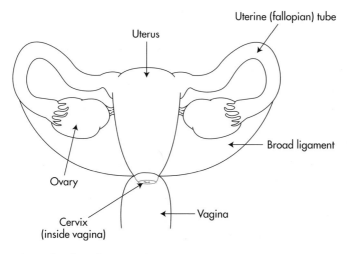

FIGURE 7.10 The female reproductive tract. The ovaries are suspended on the broad ligament. Ova shed from the ovaries are captured by the fimbriae (finger-like projections from the fallopian tubes). The cervix is the opening of the uterus into the vagina. (Redrawn from Martini 2004.)

from the follicle of the ovary to the uterine body (Marieb 2001). If fertilisation has taken place in the fallopian tube (the commonest site for fertilisation of the ova by sperm) then the developing cells of the **blastocyst** (see p. 193) will attach to the endometrium and become buried in it (a process called **implantation**). The lower portion of the uterus is the **cervix** (meaning *neck-like*), a narrow opening into the **vagina**. This is a collapsible tube extending from the cervix to the outside world, and is the organ of **coitus** (sexual intercourse) for the female. It is also the *birth canal*, i.e. the route for the natural birth of a foetus, and the route for menstrual flow. It is made of smooth muscle with a mucous membrane lining.

The **external genitalia** in females, i.e. the **vulva**, consists of the: (1) **mons veneris** (the skin covered pad of fat over the symphysis pubis bearing pubic hair); (2) **labia majora** (folds of skin-covered fat on each side of a space called the **vestibule**); (3) **labia minora** (inside the labia majora), these smaller folds of modified skin enclose the vestibule; (4) **clitoris** (an erectile organ, the tip of which is positioned at the anterior union of the two labia minora); (5) **urethral opening** (for the passage of urine), just anterior to the **vaginal opening**, both openings are in the vestibule; and (6) **Bartholin's glands** and **Skene's glands** which secrete lubricating fluid and mucus, respectively, into the vestibule.

Uterine and cervical cancer

Endometrial carcinomas

The tumours of the uterus are usually **endometrial carcinomas** (Woolf 1998). They are quite rare under 40 years of age, but are often seen in women aged 55 to 65 years. Risks factors of the disease are the presence of obesity, diabetes, hypertension and infertility, and some of these, like obesity, are linked to raised levels of oestrogen in circulation. The origin of the disease often lies in the occurrence of **endometrial hyperplasia** (see p. 26), and post-menopausal women who develop endometrial hyperplasia whilst on hormone replacement therapy (HRT) are at particular risk. This disease is often associated with breast cancer. Uterine cancers erode into the muscle wall of the uterus and also fill the uterine cavity. They are mostly **adenocarcinomas** (derived from, and looking like, the glandular cells of the endometrium), and some may also contain well-differentiated squamous-like cells (the tumour is then called an **adenocarcinoma**

with squamous metaplasia). Squamous cells that become overtly malignant within an adenocarcinoma produce a tumour called an **adenosquamous carcinoma**.

An early sign of an endometrial carcinoma is irregular vaginal bleeding, which in a post-menopausal woman is indicative that something is wrong. Bleeding is from erosion of the endometrial surface. In time the uterus may become enlarged and palpable. Spread beyond the uterus can cause fixation of the uterus against surrounding structures. The grading of these tumours follows the lines of whether the growth of the mass is **solid** or **acinar** (i.e. having sac-like cavities) (Woolf 1998):

I   About 5%, or less, of the tumour is of the solid type of growth (about 50% of endometrial carcinomas; 90% of patients show a 5-year survival rate with treatment).

II   Between 5 and 50% of the tumour is of the solid type of growth (35% of endometrial carcinomas; 30 to 50% of patients show a 5-year survival rate with treatment).

III   More than 50% of the tumour is of the solid type of growth (15% of endometrial carcinomas; less than 20% of patients show a 5-year survival rate with treatment).

Grades I and II may be raised a grade if the tumour shows predominant signs of atypical cells. (see p. 27).

Cancers of the myometrium

The smooth muscle lining of the uterine wall is the site of origin for the **leiomyosarcoma**, a moderately rare neoplasm affecting older post-menopausal women (50 years old or more). The prognosis is not good, with about 20 to 30% surviving for 5 years. A poorer prognosis is associated with a younger (pre-menopausal) onset and a high frequency of mitosis seen in tissues under examination. Spread can be into the pelvic organs, and also via the blood to involve the lungs.

Cancer of the cervix

Cancer of the cervix is, worldwide, the second most common female malignancy after breast cancer. The link between cervical cancer and the woman's sexual history relates to the age at first intercourse (i.e. before 18 years of age increases the risk by 2.5 times), and the number of sexual partners (the more partners the greater the risk). This suggests a viral agent may be a major causative factor, and the **human papillomavirus** (**HPV**) (see p. 47) is a good candidate. There are over 50 different varieties of HPV, and HPV types 16 and 18 are oncogenic (see p. 48). HPV is sexually transmitted, and it appears to infect the cells of the cervix, which then produce proteins that interfere with the function of the **RB1 gene** (see p. 41). Other causative factors include smoking (both **nicotine** and its breakdown product, called **cotinine**, are found in the cervical cells of smokers).

A pre-malignant phase occurs where the squamous epithelial cells of the cervical mucosa show increasing degrees of abnormal change (see dysplasia, p. 27) (Woolf 1998). Indentifying these pre-malignant changes is the goal for **cervical cytology**, where screening by cervical smears can allow early intervention to save lives and improve the prognosis. **Cervical intraepithelial neoplasia** (**CIN**) is the termed used to describe the degree of these dysplastic changes. **CIN I** means one-third or less of the cells show dysplasia (i.e. mild), **CIN II** means that one- to two-thirds of the cells show dysplasia (i.e. moderate), and **CIN III** means that more than two-thirds of the cells show dysplasia (i.e. severe, or **carcinoma *in situ***). Evidence for the inclusion of HPV is strong for CIN I and II, but rarer for CIN III where full integration of the HPV genome into the host cell makes the virus invisible.

About 70% of invasive cancers of the cervix are **squamous carcinomas** (Kumar *et al.* 1997). Spread from the site of origin can occur directly to the uterus (above), the vagina (below) or into the bladder or rectum. Lymph node involvement and blood-borne metastases also occur, leading to secondaries in the lungs, liver and bone at a late stage. Survival rates at 5 years stand overall at about 55%.

Removal of the uterus is a **hysterectomy**, although not all cancers are treated by total removal of the organ. Cervical cancers, especially in the early stages of the disease, may be treated by removal of the affected tissues only, resulting in various degrees of cervical **resection** (see p. 141). Loss of the whole uterus is another major challenge to body image. Since the organ is the site for pregnancy, total hysterectomy renders the patient unable to bear children. For the older lady, who is not expecting any further children, this may not be a problem. For the younger woman, the effects of this surgery must be discussed with her and her partner, and support should be given to their decisions.

Vaginal and vulval cancer

The majority of vaginal cancers are those spread from the cervix (see p. 199) (Woolf 1998). Malignancies primarily occurring in the vagina are rare (about 1% of all cancers of the female reproductive tract). Most are **invasive squamous carcinomas** occurring in the upper parts of the vagina in elderly women, but some **adenocarcinomas** occur. Spread is into the bladder, the rectum and the local lymph nodes, and in the later stages secondaries in the lungs and bone can be seen. Several variations of adenocarcinoma of the vagina occur, and one of these, called **clear cell adenocarcinoma**, is a rare but important disease as it causes cancer in *young* women of about 17 years of age (it is rare before 12 years and after 30 years). This there-fore affects women, in most cases, *before* child-bearing has occurred.

The staging of vaginal cancers is (Woolf 1998):

I   Tumour limited to the vaginal wall.
II   Tumour involves local tissues but not the pelvic wall.
III Tumour has reached the pelvic wall.
IV   Tumour has extended beyond the pelvis or involves the bladder or rectum.

Stage I carries a very good prognosis (80% of patients will have a 5-year survival) but for stages III and IV the survival rate is poor.

Visual examination of the vagina and the cervix (called **col-poscopy**) is done using an instrument called a **colposcope**. This is often carried out in specialised colposcopy units as an outpatient procedure. Surgery on the vagina may be required as a first step in the management of this disease. If this means removal of part or the entire vagina it is going to have a massive impact on the woman's body image and sexual life. This is the case at any age, although younger women will also be faced with the prospect of not being able to deliver a child normally, therefore pregnancy may no longer be an option. Reconstruction surgery to create a new vaginal open-ing (a **vaginoplasty** or **colpoplasty**) is available in most cases, and is essential in menstruating women.

Neoplasms of the **vulva** fall into **Paget's disease** of the vulva and **invasive carcinoma** of the vulva. Paget's disease is the presence of Paget's cells (see p. 180, Table 7.2), the origin of which is controver-sial. These cells invade the epidermis of the vulva (about 70% of patients) or the local glands (about 30% of patients). Invasive carcinomas are mostly squamous in origin (about 90% of cases). The majority of patients are women in their sixties with a history of smoking and sexually transmitted diseases. It affects the **labia majora** in most patients, with the **clitoris** being the second commonest site. Itching or irritation of the vulva (**pruritis vulvae**) is a common sign, with the formation of a mass or ulceration of the tissues, bleeding and local discharge. Spread into the lymph nodes on both sides of the vulva can happen, and surgical removal of the tumour usually involves dissection of lymph nodes on both sides. Staging (Woolf 1998) consists of:

I   Confined to vulva, tumour is 2 cm or less.

II   Confined to vulva, tumour is more than 2 cm.

III   Tumour extends beyond the vulva, no nodes involved, or tumour of any size with unilateral nodes involved.

IVa   Spread involves the bladder, rectum, upper urethra or the pelvic bones, with or without bilateral node involvement.

IVb   Distant metastases with pelvic nodes involved.

Patients with early stage disease have a good prognosis, up to 90% with 5-year survival rates. Only 25% survival rates occur in women with pelvic node involvement.

Surgical removal of the vulva (a **vulvectomy**) is often a radical means of eliminating the tumour, and can involve removing the labia, the clitoris, much of the surrounding skin and subcutaneous tissues and the regional lymph nodes (LeMone and Burke 2004). This seems to be a dramatic step to take, but it is important to remember that this is life-saving surgery. But, even so, this surgery will have a massive impact on a woman's body image and sexuality. Apart from the disfigurement it causes it may mean that this lady cannot undertake normal sexual relations again. Age may make a difference to the patient's response, with the younger woman suffering the consequences more than the older woman, but it is going to be tough for any woman to endure this surgery at any age. They will need great support from everyone involved, particularly their partner, family and the doctors and nurses during this period.

Key points

Hormones

- Three oestrogens are found in women: oestradiol (E2), oestrone (E1) and oestriol (E3).
- In women the oestrogens are produced mostly in the ovaries.
- Oestrogen binds to oestrogen receptors (ER) within the cell and cells that have these receptors are said to be ER positive (ER+).
- Oestradiol (E2) is the most potent of the oestrogens.
- Another female hormone, called progesterone is produced by the corpus luteum in the ovaries.

The breasts

- Epithelial cells make up the alveolar (milk producing), ductal and myoepithelial cells.
- The breast is packed with a fibrous connective tissue called stroma.
- The adipose (fat) tissue is present in variable amounts.
- Over 85% of lymph drains from the breast into the axillary (armpit) lymph nodes.
- Breast cancers can be classified into non-invasive and invasive, and are located as either ductal or lobular.
- Invasive ductal carcinoma is the most common form of breast cancer.

The ovaries

- The two ovaries are the glands for the maturation of ova, and the production of the hormones oestrogen and progesterone.
- The control of the ovarian cycle is by the pituitary hormones: follicle-stimulating hormone (FSH) and luteinising hormone (LH).
- The ovarian cycle is linked to the uterine cycle.
- Tumours of surface epithelial origin make up the largest proportion of ovarian cancers.
- Ovarian cancers are often symptom free at first.

The uterus

- The uterus has a smooth-muscle wall (the myometrium) lined by a layer of glandular cells in stroma (the endometrium).
- The tumours of the uterus are usually endometrial carcinomas.

- An early sign of an endometrial carcinoma is irregular vaginal bleeding, which in a post-menopausal woman is indicative that something is wrong.

The cervix

- Cancer of the cervix is, worldwide, the second most common female malignancy after breast cancer.
- The human papillomavirus (HPV) is a potential cause of this disease.
- About 70% of invasive cancers of the cervix are squamous carcinomas.
- A pre-malignant phase occurs where the epithelial cells of the cervical mucosa show abnormal changes and this is the reason why screening by cervical smears is so important.

The vagina

- The majority of vaginal cancers are those spread from the cervix.
- Most are invasive squamous carcinomas.
- Clear cell adenocarcinoma occurs in women of around 17 years of age, i.e. *before* child-bearing has occurred in most cases.

The vulva

- Neoplasms of the vulva are Paget's disease and invasive carcinoma.
- Itching or irritation of the vulva is a common sign, with ulceration of the tissues, bleeding and local discharge.

References

Blows W. T. (2003) *The Biological Basis of Nursing: Mental Health*, Routledge, London.

Kozier B., Erb G., Berman A. J. and Burke K. (2000) *Fundamentals of Nursing* (6th edn), Prentice Hall Health, New Jersey.

Kumar V., Cotran R. S. and Robbins S. L. (1997) *Basic Pathology* (6th edn), W. B. Saunders Company, Philadelphia.

LeMone P. and Burke K. (2004) *Medical-Surgical Nursing, Critical Thinking in Client Care*, Pearson Education Inc., Prentice Hall, New Jersey.

Marieb E. (2001) *Human Anatomy and Physiology* (5th edn), Benjamin Cummings, San Franscico.

Martini F. H. (2004) *Fundamentals of Anatomy and Physiology* (6th edn), Benjamin Cummings, Pearson Education International, San Francisco.

Passarge E. (2001) *Color Atlas of Genetics* (2nd edn), Thieme, Stuttgart.

Woolf N. (1998) *Pathology, Basic and Systemic*. W. B. Saunders Company, London.

Chapter 8

Male cancers

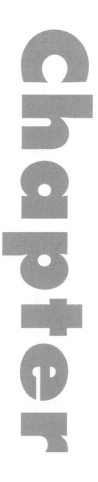

- Introduction: the androgens
- The male reproductive system
- Prostate cancer
- Testicular cancer
- Penile cancer
- Nursing skills: catheterisation
- Key points

Introduction: the androgens

The male hormones are **androgens**, of which, like oestrogens, there are three: **testosterone** (the most potent), **dehydroepiandrosterone** (**DHEA**) and **androstenedione** (both weaker forms). The cortex of the **adrenal gland** is the site for the production of these hormones in small quantities in both sexes, but the main source in males is the **testes**. Androgens have masculinisation effects on a number of tissues. For example, they build muscle and bone by inducing cell and tissue growth, and so are sometimes abused by athletes and body builders (they are sometimes known as **anabolic steroids**) (Marieb 2001). These effects are seen during male puberty, when testosterone levels rise and growth accelerates. It is this cellular growth effect that is a problem in a number of male tumours that respond to androgens. Testosterone and the other hormones bind to **androgen receptors** (**AR**) in cells that are androgen receptor positive (AR+, similar to ER+ in women, see p. 174). Any male tumour that is AR+ will grow faster with androgen stimulation, and treatment with an oestrogen causes the tumour to regress.

The male reproductive system

The organs of the male reproductive system are the testes and its associated ducts, the prostate gland and the penis (Figure 8.1). The distal urethra is important as the common duct conveying both urine and sperm to the outside world.

Testes

The testes (singular = testis)(Figure 8.2) are the organs that produce both sperm (a process called **spermatogenesis**) and the hormone testosterone. They begin by developing within the abdomen and must descend through a canal in the groin region (the **inguinal canal**) to a position within the **scrotum** (a sac of skin behind the penis) prior to birth. The reason is because the core temperature of 37°C within the abdomen is too high for the testis to function correctly. Babies born with undescended testes (called **cryptorchidism**) must have the problem corrected or risk infertility and testicular cancer later in life.

Internally, the testis is divided into sections (called **lobules**) by **septa** (singular = **septum**, a wall or partition) (see Figure 8.2). Each lobule contains a convoluted and twisted tube called the **seminifer-**

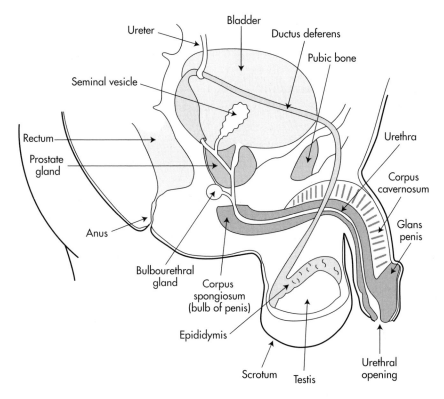

FIGURE 8.1 Section through the male reproductive system. (Redrawn from Marieb 2001.)

ous tubule where spermatogenesis takes place (*seminiferous* means 'sperm carrying'). The septa are internal extensions of the outer coat of the testis, called the **tunica albuginea**. Outside this layer is the double membrane of the **tunica vaginalis** with a fluid-filled cavity between the membranes.

The seminiferous tubules from the lobules unite in a network of tubes called the **rete testis**, and this in turn opens into the head of the **epididymis**. This structure is positioned close to the outside of the testis and has a head end (connected to the rete testis) and a tail end. It contains a single tightly coiled tube which, when uncoiled, would be six metres (20 feet) in length. It takes about 20 days for sperm to move through this duct, and it is the site for the storage of sperm for up to several weeks.

During ejaculation, sperm are pushed by smooth muscle contractions from the tail of the epididymis into the next duct (the **ductus deferens**, or **vas deferens**). This is a much straighter tube that doubles back on itself and joins the **spermatic cord**.

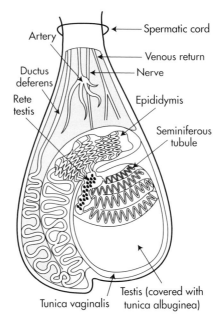

FIGURE 8.2 Section through the scrotum and testis showing the spermatic cord. (Redrawn from Marieb 2001.)

The testis is suspended on the spermatic cord, which is positioned between the scrotum below and the abdomen above, extending through the inguinal canal. In this respect, it is possible to see the similarity between the testis suspended on its spermatic cord and a puppet on a string.

The spermatic cord and the pathway for sperm

The spermatic cord is a sheath forming a tube, and passing through this tube are the following structures (Figure 8.2): the ductus deferens, the arterial blood supply to the testis, the venous drainage from the testis and the nerve supply to the testis.

The two ductus deferens, one from each testis, extend into the abdomen, over the urinary bladder and down the posterior wall of the bladder where they join the duct from the **seminal vesicles** on each side (Figure 8.1). The seminal vesicles produce a fluid which makes up about 60% of the **semen** (the fluid containing sperm that is ejaculated). This alkaline fluid contains sugar and vitamin C for nutrition of the sperm. The ductus deferens and the duct from the seminal vesicles join to form a single duct, the **ejaculatory duct**, on each side. The left and right ejaculatory ducts extend into the

prostate gland on both sides and both join with the **urethra** inside the prostate.

The prostate gland

This gland lies immediately below the urinary bladder (at the 'neck' of the bladder) and is made up of three main compartments (or zones)(see Figures 8.1 and 8.3). The **central zone** surrounds the ejaculatory duct as far as its junction with the urethra. The **transitional zone**, the smallest region, encompasses the *proximal* (upper) portion of the urethra (i.e. *before* its junction with the ejaculatory ducts). The largest region, the **peripheral zone**, surrounds the previous two zones on most sides, and encompasses the *distal* (lower) portion of the urethra (i.e. *after* its junction with the ejaculatory duct) (Kumar *et al.* 1997).

The function of the prostate gland is to produce fluid (about 30% of the fluid component of semen), and to produce other nutrients for sperm (Marieb 2001). The 'gland' is in fact about 25 smaller glands set in a connective tissue called **stroma** (see p. 178) surrounded by a fibrous outer cover.

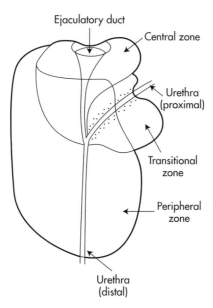

FIGURE 8.3 The prostate gland showing three zones and the junction of the ejaculatory duct with the urethra. (Redrawn from Kumar *et al.* 1997.)

The urethra and the penis

The distal urethra leaves the prostate and extends through the **penis** and opens on the tip of the **glans penis** (Figure 8.1). This portion of the urethra acts as both a duct for urine and for sperm. The penis is the male erectile organ of sexual intercourse. The body of the organ contains two types of cavity filled with spongy tissue; the **corpora cavernosa** and the **corpus spongiosum** (*corpus* = body). These extend along the full length of the penis. The corpora cavernosa are a pair of cavities touching along the midline and positioned within the dorsal (upper) region of the penis. The single corpus spongiosum is positioned more ventrally (i.e. below the corpora cavernosa), and it contains the urethra. It is this cavity that expands at the end of the penis to form the **glans penis**, which is covered by a fold of skin, the **prepuce**. Erection of the penis can occur as a result of filling these cavities with blood, and emptying of blood restores the flaccid state.

Spermatogenesis

Sperm are produced in the seminiferous tubules from **germ cells** called **spermatogonia**. The germ cells entered the testes during embryonic development from their site of production in part of the embryo called the **yolk sac**. In the healthy adult male, sperm are produced at the rate of *200 to 400 million per day* (compare that with the production of ova in women at the rate of *one from each ovary per month*). Sperm production requires a good supply of concentrated testosterone, and specialised cells in the testis, called **Leydig cells**, produce testosterone (Figure 8.4). Leydig cells are under the control of the male version of **luteinising hormone** called **interstitial cell stimulating hormone** (**ICSH**) from the **anterior pituitary gland** (Figure 8.4). Other specialised cells, called **Sertoli cells**, within the lining of the seminiferous tubules, are under **follicle-stimulating hormone** (**FSH**) control from the anterior pituitary gland (see p. 190 and Figures 8.4 and 8.5). FSH and testosterone between them stimulate sperm production. The Sertoli cells regulate the process of spermatogenesis and provide nutrition to the germ cells. They also form a barrier, the **blood–testis barrier**, between the outer surface of the tubule (the **basal compartment**) and the inner lumen of the seminiferous tubule (the **adluminal compartment**)(Figure 8.5). The fluid derived from blood in the basal compartment is different from the adluminal compartment fluid, which has the correct constituents needed for developing sperm. The purpose of the blood–testis bar-

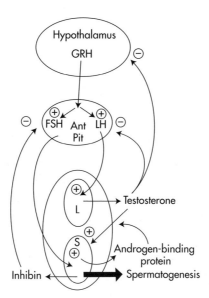

FIGURE 8.4 Control of the testis by the hypothalamus. Gonadotrophin-releasing hormone (GRH) causes release of follicle-stimulating hormone (FSH) and luteinising hormone (LH) from the anterior pituitary (Ant Pit) gland. FSH acts on Sertoli cells (S) to promote spermatogenesis, and the release of two substances, androgen-binding protein and inhibin. Androgen-binding protein binds testosterone and ensures its concentration needed for sperm production in the Sertoli cells. Inhibin provides a negative feedback system to the anterior pituitary gland reducing FSH release. LH acts on the Leydig cells (L), promoting the release of testosterone. Testosterone has a double negative feedback, on the anterior pituitary (reducing LH release) and on the hypothalamus (reducing GRH production).

rier is to maintain this difference. The Sertoli cells also produce the hormone **inhibin** and a protein called the **androgen-binding protein** (Figure 8.4). The hormone inhibin provides a negative feedback mechanism to the anterior pituitary regulating the release of FSH, because increasing levels of inhibin will switch off FSH release. The androgen-binding protein binds testosterone and this ensures the correct concentration of testosterone needed for sperm production (see Figure 8.4).

Prostate cancer

Before looking at prostatic cancer, it would be useful to identify some facts about a *very common benign* form of prostatic enlargement which the patient may think is cancer. **Benign nodular prostatic hyperplasia** is a problem experienced by a relatively large number of men in late middle or old age (50% of males show evidence of the problem by

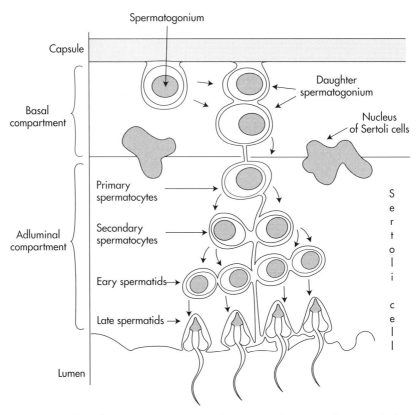

FIGURE 8.5 Sertoli cells nurture sperm production in the seminiferous tubules of the testis. Spermatogonia in the basal compartment divide to form daughter cells. One goes on into the adluminal compartment to further divide into four early spermatids. These will become sperm which break free in the lumen of the tubule. (Redrawn from Marieb 2001.)

50 years of age, and 75% of men by 80+ years). This is an increase in the size of the prostate due to an overgrowth of the cells forming nodules in the periurethral transitional zone (see p. 209, and Figure 8.3) which encroaches on the urethra. It is generally benign but a number of cases may go on to malignancy. There is much evidence now to show that the hyperplasia is due to the conversion of testosterone to another hormone called **dihydrotestosterone** by the enzyme **5α-reductase** (see Figure 8.6). Dihydrotestosterone binds to androgen receptors in cells within the transitional zone of the prostate and promotes cell growth there. The symptoms are those of urinary obstruction, i.e. **hesitancy** (a delay between starting urination and the actual flow of urine, which can be a considerable time delay), incomplete emptying (retaining some urine after micturition),

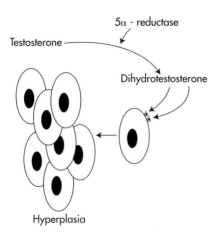

FIGURE 8.6 The conversion of testosterone to dihydrotestosterone by the enzyme 5α-reductase is thought to be a factor in prostate gland cells going into hyperplasia.

urgency (the need to pass urine urgently), **frequency** (passing urine more that seven times per day) and **nocturia** (passing urine at regular intervals throughout the night). There is a need to exclude prostatic cancer as the cause of the symptoms, even though the majority of men with benign hyperplasia do not develop malignancy. Surgical removal of the gland (a **prostatectomy**), or re-establishment of the urethral passage through the prostate (a **transurethral resection of prostate**, or **TURP**) are some options for treatment.

Cancer of the prostate is unfortunately also relatively common, ranking high in the list of cancer deaths in males over 50 years of age (Woolf 1998). Again, like prostatic hyperplasia, there is evidence to show that the action of androgens on the gland has a role to play in the causation of the disease. The majority of tumours (about 70%) develop from the peripheral zone of the gland (see p. 209), with only 25% within the transitional zone, and 5% within the central zone (Figure 8.3). It is interesting that most hyperplasias arise within the transitional zone, but most cancers are within the peripheral zone, and this highlights the absence of any link between the two disorders. Peripheral zone tumours cause less urinary obstruction symptoms than nodular hyperplasia, and they are more susceptible to palpation via rectal examination of the prostate. Two tumour markers are useful diagnostic tools, particularly the **prostate-specific antigen (PSA)**. This is a glycoprotein normally found in the **endoplasmic reticulum (ER)** (see p. 5) of prostatic cells, but released into the blood serum in large quantities in disease of the gland. The normal PSA in serum is 4 ng/ml (nanograms per millilitre), but can be raised in up to 60% of patients with prostate cancers and up to 40% of those with benign nodular hyperplasia. **Prostate-specific acid phosphatase** is another marker found in the lysosomes of prostate cells and released into the blood in disease of the gland (some 60% of patients with cancer and 80% of those with bone metastases show raised levels of prostate-specific acid phosphatase).

Prostate cancers are mostly **adenocarcinomas** (derived from glandular tissue) and they fall into a wide range of behaviour patterns, from those that show no signs of their presence (and may only be found at post-mortem) to those that are very aggressive and spread widely, often causing the death of the patient. The prognosis in each case can be assessed from the grading of the tumour. Those that are graded as poorly differentiated tumours tend to grow and spread quickly, whilst those that are well-differentiated tumours progress more slowly. Staging of these tumours uses either the **Tumour Node Metastasis** (**TNM**) system (see p. 168) or a clinical staging system shown here:

A   Not found on clinical examination.
A1 Focal, within the gland.
A2 Diffuse.
B   Palpable by rectal examination.
B1 Focal.
B2 Diffuse.
C   Local spread beyond the prostate.
C1 Seminal vesicles are not involved.
C2a Seminal vesicles are involved.
C2b Fixation to the pelvic wall.
D   Spread by metastases.

Testicular cancer

More than 90% of all testicular cancers arise from the **germ cells** within the lining of the seminiferous tubules (see p. 210). Leukaemia and lymphoma aside, testicular cancers are the commonest malignant disease in men aged between 15 and 34 years (the time of highest testosterone levels), and most of these cancers have the potential to cause metastases if not found early. Self-examination of the testes is an important step forward in the early detection of cancer (Figure 8.7).

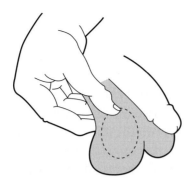

FIGURE 8.7 Self-examination of the testis. The testis should be felt by rolling the fingers over its entire surface to check for enlargement or lumps. Comparison with the other side will help to establish what is normal or not. If in doubt seek advice from a doctor. (Redrawn from LeMone and Burke 2004.)

The staging used for testicular cancers may be as follows:

I   Tumour confined to the testis.
II   Metastases spread only to the lymph glands below the diaphragm.
II   Spread to the lymph nodes above and below the diaphragm.
IV   Spread to other organs.

Tumours of the testes are not easy to classify because of the variation of tissue types and mixtures that occur, but they fall broadly into four main categories:

A   Germ cell tumours (about 90% of all testicular cancers).
B   Sex cord–stromal tumours (about 2% of all testicular cancers).
C   Mixed germ cell and sex cord–stromal tumours.
D   Others, including **secondaries** (metastases from primary tumours at other sites).

Germ cell tumours

Male germ cells (known as **spermatogonia**) (see p. 210) are the cells from which the sperm originate within the seminiferous tubules. It should not be surprising that tumours develop from these cells since they are naturally rapidly reproducing cells, and are therefore vulnerable to the effects of radiation. These tumours can be divided into **seminomas** (about 30 to 40% of all germ cell tumours), **teratomas** (about 10% of all germ cell tumours) (see also teratomas in

Chapter 7, p. 195) and others (e.g. **malignant lymphoma** and **adenomatoid tumour**).

Seminomas (or **germinomas**) are the male equivalent of the female ovarian dysgerminomas (see p. 195) and are sometimes subdivided into (1) **classical** (or **typical**) which account for more than 90% of seminomas and arise mostly in men between the ages of 30 and 50 years; and (2) **spermatocytic** which account for about 5% of seminomas and arise in men around 55 years of age. Classical (typical) seminomas consist of sheets of primitive-looking germ cells forming a well-defined mass. Spermatocytic seminomas are very large lesions containing sheets of cells of mixed sizes.

Teratomas are tumours that are composed of tissue types not usually found at that site, and the cells can differentiate into other cell types. They occur most frequently in female ovaries (see Table 7.4, p. 195) and in testes of young men. The risk of teratoma of the testes is higher in men with a history of undescended testes (see p. 206). Teratomas often produce markers such as alpha-fetoprotein (see p. 195) or human chorionic gonadotrophin (see p. 193), which can be monitored to assess the extent of the tumour and progress of the treatment.

Germ cell tumours usually begin as a painless swelling of one testis (rarely both are involved). The spread of germ cell tumours is first into the retroperitoneal lymph nodes (i.e. behind the peritoneum) around the abdominal aorta and iliac regions, then to the supradiaphragmatic lymph nodes (i.e. those above the diaphragm) in an **ipsilateral** manner (i.e. on the same side as the tumour). Spread can then be into the blood to the liver, bone and lung.

Treatment of germ cell tumours begins with surgical removal of the tumour. The prognosis has been improved considerably by the use of the cytotoxic drug **cisplatin** (see cytotoxic drugs, Chapter 12, p. 325), and a cure is now possible in many cases.

Sex cord–stromal tumours

These are rare, only 2% of testicular cancers, and although they can occur at any age, about 40% are found in children. **Sex cords** are the name given to the original embryonic cords of cells that in the adult form the tissues that house the ova and sperm cells; in females these are the follicles, and in males they are the seminiferous tubules. These tumours are a mix of sex cord cells with stromal (connective tissue) cells (see also stromal cells of the breast, p. 178). The tumour can cause **gynaecomastia** (i.e. male breast development) in children below puberty or in men over 50 years of age, and 40% of these tumours can be aggressively malignant.

Mixed germ cell

The **gonadoblastoma** is a mix of germ cell tumour elements with sex cord cancer components within separate compartments of the tumour. It occurs mostly in men below the age of 20 years who may also have a mix of other male developmental and gender problems.

Others

Leydig cell tumours comprise 1 to 3% of testicular cancers. They happen at any age and cause an initial testicular swelling and gynaecomastia in 30% of patients. The mass is composed of Leydig cells (see p. 210) in sheet form or mesh. **Malignant lymphoma** is the commonest testicular cancer in men over 55 years of age. They are mostly non-Hodgkin's lymphomas (see p. 107). There is testicular enlargement, about 60% in one testis, 40% in both. The tumour will infiltrate into the testis. **Adenomatoid tumours** occur mostly in the epididymis of men aged 30 to 40 years. The first sign is a small lump of 1 to 2 cm, just above the testis. They tend to be benign.

Surgical removal of the diseased testis (**orchidectomy**) is a vital first step in the treatment, particularly since the testes are, in surgical terms, relatively easy to get to. Chemotherapy as a follow-up treatment for any spread of the disease is the usual course. Orchidectomy has body image implications, and replacement of the removed testis with a prosthesis may be important, especially for younger men. If both testes are removed the patient will become infertile with low testosterone levels.

Penile cancer

Squamous carcinomas account for the majority of invasive tumours, which are rare in the Western world, but more common in parts of Asia, Africa and Latin America. The disease is closely associated with uncircumcised males; circumcision reduces the risk dramatically, especially if circumcision is carried out at an early age. **Phymosis**, the inability to retract the foreskin, increases the risk further. Also associated with an increased risk of penile cancer is the sexually transmitted **human papillomavirus** (**HVP**) infection (see p. 47 for the HPV organism). The tumour may develop as a mass extending from the **glans penis** or the **prepuce** (see p. 210 and Figure 8.1), or as an ulcerating lesion infiltrating into the penis. Excision of the lesion means the loss of part, or all, of the penis. Clearly this operation has body image and sexual implications, and the full outcome of the surgery needs to be discussed with the patient and, with their consent, their partner.

Nursing skills: catheterisation

In many **urogenital disorders** (diseases of the urinary and genital systems), difficulty with passing urine (**dysuria**) may lead to a complete failure to pass urine (**urinary retention**). Acute urinary retention is relatively rare, but when it happens it is a clinical emergency. The way to manage this initially is to pass a sterile tube, a **catheter**, up the urethra into the bladder and drain off the urine, a procedure called urinary **catheterisation**. Catheters are also essential to retain urinary drainage during, and following, surgical techniques that cause gross disturbance of the normal anatomy of the urinary system, as may be the case in the removal of a urogenital tumour. Catheterisation of a patient has a number of implications, some of which are related to the gender of the patient. Catheterisation requires the passage of the tube through the bladder sphincters, and this may be a problem in a few patients of either sex. In most patients this is not generally a problem. However, male catheterisation is a significantly more difficult procedure than female catheterisation for other reasons of anatomy. The differences between the male and female urethra are shown in Table 8.1, and Figure 8.8.

Of the criteria used in Table 8.1, the length, the numbers of bends and the prostate gland affect catheterisation. Being longer, the male urethra offers the greater challenge to the passage of a catheter,

TABLE 8.1 The differences between the male and the female urethra

	The male urethra	*The female urethra*
Length	Long; variable length, averaging about 20 cm	Short; about 2 to 3 cm
Bends	Two	None
Prostate	Present; enlargement causes resistance to the passage of a catheter	Absent
Function	Carries urine and sperm	Carries urine only

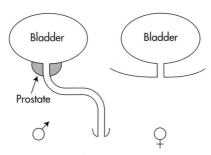

FIGURE 8.8 The differences between a male (left) and a female (right) ure-thra. The female is easier to catheterise because the male urethra is much longer, has two bends in it, and has a prostate gland at the entrance to the bladder.

simply because the catheter has further to go to reach the bladder, and it becomes more difficult to instil the entire urethra with local anaesthetic. The two bends will also need negotiation with the catheter. Whilst the nurse can reduce the outer bend by straightening out the penis, the inner bend remains. But it is the prostate that can cause the biggest problems. The presence of any prostatic enlargement (see p. 211) makes the passage of a catheter harder, and if the enlargement of the gland is considerable, the catheter may not pass at all. If this is the case, the relief of acute urinary retention requires a different approach, i.e. the insertion of a **suprapubic catheter**. This is a surgical procedure where a catheter is passed through an incision above the pubic bone (in the lower abdomen) and through the bladder wall. The catheter remains in place and drains urine continually until the prostate problem is resolved.

Catheters are often kept in the bladder semi-permanently (called **indwelling**), i.e. they remain in place using an inflatable balloon at the tip, inside the bladder, the balloon being inflated with sterile water. The catheter then stays throughout the duration of the disorder until normal micturition can be restored. But normal micturition is not always achievable, and after discharge into the community, some patients may be required to catheterise themselves each time they wish to pass urine.

Biologically, it is important to remember that each catheter insertion opens the bladder to the risk of infection. So patients with long-term indwelling catheters, or who are subject to multiple repeated catheterisations each day, are at a high risk of **urinary tract infections** (**UTI**). Not only the passing of catheters, but the changing of catheter bags, the collection of urine samples from a catheter and the washing out of the bladder through a catheter all carry a risk of infection for the patient. These procedures must be sterile and carried out using an **aseptic technique** (i.e. under strict sterile conditions). Aseptic technique involves more that just sterile equipment, it means the careful washing of hands, the use of sterile gloves, and the careful disposal of unwanted items afterwards. Urine samples should be monitored for signs of infection and other problems. Urine testing is routine, along with recording fluid balance, and the testing of urine in the laboratory for infection (i.e. *culture and sensitivity*) is carried out when the urine is cloudy, or smells foul or contains protein or blood (for urine testing see Blows 2001, Chapter 5).

When it comes to aseptic techniques, here is a personal observation. The practice of carrying stethoscopes slung around the neck is problematic. When the owner is bending forward, particularly whilst doing an aseptic technique, and the stethoscope is dangling in the sterile field, or worse still, the patient's wound, the stethoscope becomes a dangerous menace. Each nurse should consider carefully carrying their equipment in their pockets where it will not dangle. Dangling hair is not normally acceptable in the clinical area, so why are dangling stethoscopes accepted?

Infection can also gain entry to the bladder by ascending the urethra around the outside of the catheter, and indwelling catheters must be kept clean, particularly around the urethral opening. Sterility is not easily achieved in the community, especially during self-catheterisation by the patient. The ever-growing problem of the hospital so-called *superbugs* makes the issue of sterility absolutely essential in this procedure. 'Superbugs', like **methicilline-resistant *Staphylococcus aureus* (MRSA)** are bacterial organisms which are resistant to many, if not virtually all, the known antibiotics and are therefore very difficult to treat. There is a current increase in MRSA and similar organisms in the hospital environment, with a corresponding increase in patient deaths from these infections. A UTI caused by MRSA would be the worse case scenario for urogenital patients, and can be caused directly by poor catheterisation technique; in other words, it could be **iatrogenic** (i.e. caused, or spread, by the doctors or nurses). Consultation with the nurse experts in this field can prevent many problems and even save lives. The **advanced nurse practitioner (ANP)** in **urogenital nursing** will advise the patient, relatives and nurses on catheterisation techniques and problems, and the advice of the ANP in **infection control** should be sought if there are fears concerning infections, especially with MRSA.

Key points

Hormones

- The male hormones are androgens: testosterone (the most potent), dehydroepiandrosterone (DHEA) and androstenedione.
- Testosterone binds to androgen receptors (AR) in AR positive cells.
- Any male tumour that is AR+ will grow faster with androgen stimulation.

The reproductive system

- The testes produce both sperm (spermatogenesis) and testosterone.
- The testis is divided into lobules, each lobule contains a seminiferous tubule where spermatogenesis happens.
- Testes must descend through the inguinal canal to a position within the scrotum prior to birth.
- Undescended testes increase the risk of testicular cancer in later life.
- The prostate lies immediately below the urinary bladder and is made up of the central zone, the transitional zone and the peripheral zone.
- Sperm are produced in the seminiferous tubules from germ cells called spermatogonia.
- Leydig cells produce testosterone. They are controlled from the anterior pituitary gland by luteinising hormone, also called interstitial cell stimulating hormone (ICSH) in males.
- Sertoli cells line the seminiferous tubules and are under follicle-stimulating hormone (FSH) control from the anterior pituitary gland.
- The Sertoli cells regulate spermatogenesis and provide nutrition to the germ cells. They also form the blood–testis barrier.
- The Sertoli cells produce inhibin that provides a negative feedback mechanism to the anterior pituitary regulating the release of FSH.
- Sertoli cells also produce androgen-binding protein that binds testosterone, essential for spermatogenesis.

Prostatic hyperplasia

- Benign nodular prostatic hyperplasia occurs in late middle or old age in men.
- This is an enlargement of the prostate due to excess cells forming nodules in the periurethral transitional zone, which then encroaches on the urethra.

Prostatic cancer

- Prostate cancers are mostly adenocarcinomas.
- About 70% of cancers develop in the peripheral zone of the gland.
- Two tumour markers are useful diagnostic tools, prostate-specific antigen (PSA) and prostate-specific acid phosphatase.
- The normal PSA in serum is 4 ng/ml, but can be raised in up to 60% of patients with prostate cancers and up to 40% of those with benign nodular hyperplasia.

Testicular cancer

- More than 90% of all testicular cancers arise from the germ cells.
- Testicular cancers are the commonest malignant disease in men aged 15 to 34 years.
- Self-examination of the testes is an important step forward in the early detection of this cancer.
- Four main categories are germ cell tumours, sex cord–stromal tumours, mixed germ cell and sex cord–stromal tumours and others, including secondaries.
- Germ cell tumours are divided into seminomas and teratomas.
- Orchidectomy has body image implications, and replacement of testes with a prosthesis is important.
- If both testes are removed the patient will become infertile with low testosterone levels.

Penile cancers

- Squamous carcinomas account for the majority of invasive tumours of the penis.
- The uncircumcised penis, and particularly phymosis, carries a higher risk of penile cancer.
- A higher risk occurs with a human papillomavirus (HVP) infection.

Catheterisation

- The length of the urethra, the number of bends and the presence of the prostate gland make male catheterisation more difficult than female, especially in prostatic disease.
- Catheterisation must be a sterile technique.

References

Blows W. T. (2001) *The Biological Basis of Nursing: Clinical Observations*, Routledge, London.

Kumar V., Cotran R. S. and Robbins S. L. (1997) *Basic Pathology* (6th edn), W. B. Saunders Company, Philadelphia.

LeMone P. and Burke K. (2004) *Medical-Surgical Nursing, Critical Thinking in Client Care*, Pearson Education Inc., Prentice Hall, New Jersey.

Marieb E. (2001) *Human Anatomy and Physiology* (5th edn), Benjamin Cummings, San Franscisco.

Chapter 9

Metastases

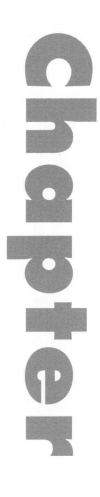

- Introduction: cell attachment
- Metastases
- The liver
- Liver cancer
- Lung secondary tumours
- Bone cancer
- The brain
- Brain and intracranial cancer
- Malignant melanoma
- Key points

Introduction: cell attachment

The study of the way cancers free themselves from the constraints of body needs, and of the way they spread, has shed much light on the natural history of this disease. Cells normally exist attached to each other and to the extracellular matrix (see tissues in Chapter 1, p. 15). Blood cells (p. 21), especially white blood cells, are an exception to this rule. Red blood cells (RBCs) are loose but are confined to circulation. They must be free in order that the tissue we call blood behaves as a fluid. White blood cells (WBCs) are completely free to pass through capillary walls into the tissues, and they need this ability in order to fight infection. Inflammation (p. 82) is all about facilitating this freedom of movement for WBCs in and out of tissues during infection.

But other cells must remain locked in their correct position within the tissues. We are what we are because of this principle. It would make no sense to have skin cells inside our bones or brain cells inside our lungs. So cells must stay where they are put, and to achieve this they are anchored down.

Cells have an internal structure which provides shape and support, and in some cells, movement. This is the **cytoskeleton**, a protein framework consisting of three elements: (1) the **microfilaments** (5 nm in diameter) made from the protein **actin**; (2) the **intermediate** filaments (10 nm in diameter) made from six different proteins; and (3) the **microtubules** (25 nm in diameter) made from two strands of a tubular protein called **tubulin**.

The attachment of cells to external surfaces and other cells is by a combination of four different groups of receptors called **cell adhesion molecules** (**CAM**s) (King 2000). Being receptors means that they bind to a particular molecule, called a **ligand**. CAMs are *transmembranous glycoproteins* (transmembranous means the molecular structure extends right through the cell membrane, and a glycoprotein is simply a protein with one or more sugars attached). By binding to an extracellular ligand, e.g. part of the matrix surrounding the cell, CAMs form links between the elements inside the cell and those of the external matrix, or to other cells.

The CAM receptor groups are (see Figure 9.1): integrins, cadherins, selectins and immunoglobulin-like proteins.

Integrins are a group of surface receptors which are made from various combinations of alpha (α) and beta (β) protein elements. The binding of the ligand promotes further integrin clustering and bind-

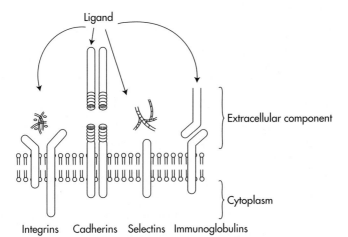

Ligand

Extracellular component

Cytoplasm

Integrins   Cadherins   Selectins   Immunoglobulins

FIGURE 9.1 Cell adhesion molecules (CAMs). What they bind to is called the ligand. Integrins bind to extracellular matrix, cadherins bind to cadherins of the next cell, selectins bind to extracellular polysaccharides and immunoglobulins bind to immunoglobulins of the next cell. (Redrawn from King 2000.)

ing which then strengthens the cell's adhesion to the extracellular matrix. They promote the assembly of elements of the **cytoskeleton** (see p. 226) internally in response to binding to a range of components of the extracellular matrix, such as **collagen** (see p. 17). Some integrins are involved in cellular migration rather than adhesion. Binding of the migratory integrins to extracellular ligands facilitates greater movement within the extracellular matrix. In cancer cells, generally, integrins involved in adhesion are reduced whilst those involved in migration are not, and they may even be increased. This is a process that promotes the chance of cancer cells moving, a prerequisite for invasion and metastases.

Cadherins (Figure 9.1) are receptor molecules that provide cell-to-cell adhesion, like intracellular 'glue' (see also **desmosomes** below). They often have the letter associated with the tissue that produces them, e.g. E-cadherin from epithelial tissue. On *extracellular* binding between cadherins, the *intracellular* components of the cadherins interact with a protein (called **β-catenin**) from the cell cytoplasm by affecting the available pools of this protein within the cell. There are two pools of β-catenin in the cell, one attached to the microtubules and actin microfilaments (see p. 226) and the other unattached and able to influence gene expression. Changes in these pools of β-catenin by binding cadherins lead to changes that control the cell cytoskeleton and gene expression. Which genes are involved is not fully understood in humans. In cancers, the loss of cadherins releases cells from cell-to-cell adhesion and causes a loss of control over the expression of certain genes.

Selectins are receptors that bind carbohydrate side-chain mole-cules (the ligand) found in the extracellular matrix. They are limited to vascular cells (i.e. cells of the blood vessels) and may play a role in stopping cancer cells that have got into the blood. Their intracellular activity when bound to the ligand is not clear.

Immunoglobulin-like proteins are a large family of single-stranded proteins that provide cell-to-cell adhesion, the ligand being integrins or other immunoglobulin-like proteins on other cells. Their intracellular activity when bound to the ligand is not clear.

In addition to CAMs, other mechanisms of cell attachment exist. **CD44** is an important receptor that binds some proteins within the extracellular matrix (see p. 79 for CD). A wide range of normal cells produce CD44 and its variants, but this process is down-regulated (reduced) in metastatic cancers of the colon, prostate and ovary. Some variants of CD44, however, are overexpressed (up-regulated) in other metastatic cancers, such as melanomas, so the picture of what is happening among the variants of CD44 is complex. **Syndecans** are transmembranous glycoproteins that bind to other protein compo-nents of the extracellular matrix and act as a co-receptor with integrins and cadherins.

The matrix around the cells contains **cell adhesion proteins**, and these provide a means by which connective tissue cells can bind to the structures around them. Cell adhesion proteins include **laminin**, **fibronectin** and **proteoglycans** (all glycoproteins). They form a kind of *glue*, i.e. they keep structures in place, and provide anchor-age binding points for the integrin CAMs.

Cell junctions, the point where epithelial cells touch, are tight junctions, gap junctions and desmosomes (see Figure 9.2).

Tight junctions are where nothing can pass between the cells. These are formed by the fusion of proteins in one cell membrane with the proteins in the neighbouring cell membrane. An example of this junction is found between cells lining the digestive tract.

Gap junctions are where the membrane of one cell is very close to the neighbouring cell membrane, but there is enough space to allow the passage of some substances between the cells. Openings (called **connexons**) between the two cells across the junction occur to allow movement of substances between the cells. Gap junctions occur in cardiac and smooth muscle (see p. 21).

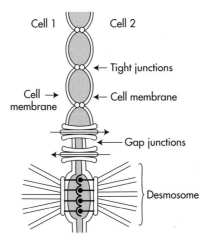

FIGURE 9.2 Cells are normally joined together by tight junctions, gap junctions and desmosomes. Gap junctions form channels between the two cells to allow passage from one to the other.

Desmosomes are junctions that actually anchor one cell to the next. At specific sites across the two facing cell membranes, proteins called **cadherins** (see above) extend out across the extracellular space between the membranes and lock onto each other, without the membranes actually touching. These junctions are also attached to the intermediate filaments of the cytoskeleton (see p. 226) on the inside of each cell. So, effectively, this locks one cell cytoskeleton to the next, and give great strength to cellular adhesion. They are found in tissues subjected to mechanical stress, like the skin and heart muscle (Marieb 2001).

Metastases

Malignant tumours can spread by (see Figure 9.3):

1 *Direct invasion* of tissues neighbouring the tumour, requiring the ability of tumour cells to establish an adequate blood supply for their needs (the creation of new blood vessels is called **angiogenesis**) and to produce enzymes that dissolve the body tissues (see discussion below).
2 *Via the lymphatic system* (see discussion below).
3 *Via the blood* (see discussion below).
4 *Transcoelomic*, i.e. malignant cells moving through a body cavity after they have invaded through the wall of the organ that contains the primary and broken free.

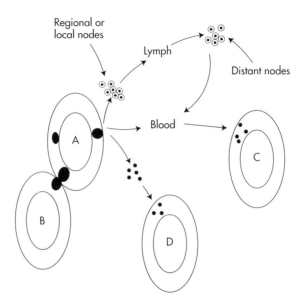

FIGURE 9.3 Spread of tumours. The tumour in organ A can undergo direct spread locally and infiltrate into part or all of the wall, and into the next organ (B). Metastases can move into the local (regional) lymph nodes, then on to distant lymph nodes. From there they can pass into the blood. Direct metastatic spread into circulation can lead to secondary growths in distant organs (C). Metastases from the primary tumour can sometimes spread across a body cavity (transcoelomic) to distant organs within that cavity (D).

Most of the cells of the body must remain anchored in place in order to survive. For epithelial cells this means resting on a **basement membrane**, which is made from glycoproteins like **collagen**, **laminin**, **fibronectin** and **proteoglycans** (see above, p. 228). For connective tissue cells this means binding to **extracellular stroma**, a mixture of proteoglycans and other glycoproteins (see also stromal cells on p. 178). Epithelial and connective tissue cells are therefore *anchorage dependent*. Any cell that breaks free from anchorage stops growing and may die, the cell triggers apoptosis.

Metastases are malignant cells that have broken free from anchorage and have survived, and they can continue to grow (i.e. they are *anchorage independent*). Malignant metastases have overcome the apoptosis trigger to ensure their survival. They have broken away from the original tumour, called a **primary**, by reducing the normal cell-to-cell adhesion (see p. 226), and they may cause another tumour, a **secondary**, to arise elsewhere in the body. One class of CAMs called **E-cadherin** (see p. 227) is important in the breaking free mechanism. The invasiveness of a malignant cell appears to be related to the amount of E-cadherin produced. To invade other tissues successfully malignant cells must have *very low* E-cadherin levels (i.e. E-cadherin is down-regulated, meaning that the gene that codes for E-cadherin is 'switched off'). Malignant cells also reduce the amount of **fibronectin** (also found in basement membranes, see p. 228) from their cell surface. Normally this acts like a cell-to-cell glue, so this loss again helps to free the cell.

The change to metastatic cells at a cancer primary site marks a bad development, from carcinoma *in situ* to invasive carcinoma (see p. 27). Invasive carcinoma is the generation of metastatic cells that have penetrated the basement membrane. Penetration of the basement membrane requires that the malignant cell binds to the **laminin** component of the membrane (see Figure 9.4, and p. 228), so the malignant cell must express laminin receptors. In order to cross the basement membrane the cancer cells must produce a collection of enzymes called **metalloproteinases**. These are **proteolytic enzymes**, i.e. enzymes that break down proteins, as found in the

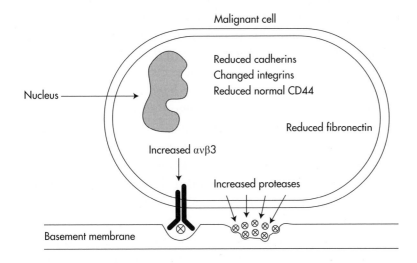

⊗ Metalloproteinases

FIGURE 9.4 Changes in a malignant cell to become a metastatic cell. To become free the cancer cell reduces the level of cadherins (that would normally bind it to the next cell), fibronectin (cell to cell 'glue') and CD44. The pattern of integrins changes from those keeping the cell in place to those promoting movement. One integrin, called αvβ3, is particularly important since it binds proteases (called metalloproteinases) which help to dissolve away the basement membrane. Extra metalloproteinases are produced for this purpose.

basement membrane. There are three main groups of these enzymes in the metalloproteinase family, the **collagenases** (that break down collagen), the **gelatinases** (that break down a range of different proteins) and the **stromelysins** (that break down stromal elements). The activity of the gelatinases appears to be particularly important as invasiveness is directly proportional to the amount of gelatinases produced by the cell. These enzymes allows the cancer cells to enter the blood, but entry into the lymphatic system is easier since there is a difference in the basement membrane (no collagen or laminin to get through) (Woolf 1998; King 2000). Carcinomas have a greater tendency to invade the lymphatic system, whilst sarcomas have a greater affinity for invading the bloodstream.

The blood is not a good place for cancer cells. They are washed along by the blood flow with no control over their destiny. Estimates put cancer cell destruction in circulation as high as 99%, and that less than 1 malignant cell in 10,000 will become a secondary tumour elsewhere. The reason is because malignant cells are removed and destroyed by the body's immune cells (see Chapter 3), and because they are destroyed by **proteolytic enzymes** or by mechanical stresses. Cancer cells in the blood become coated with **platelets** (see p. 97), and this makes them larger and stickier. They are then more likely to become jammed in the next capillary bed. It is possible that platelets may allow cancer cells to survive by secreting growth factors. The question arises: how do cancer cells in circulation know when to leave the blood vessel and invade the tissues? This is not fully understood, particularly when malignant cells produce most secondaries in lung and liver tissues, with high incidences also in bone. How do they know when they are passing through these structures? The possibility is that certain malignant cells recognise differences in the surface of blood vessels that are inside the structure, e.g. bone, and only there do they stick to the blood vessel wall and invade. It could be to do with certain CAMs (see p. 226) on the blood vessel epithelium surface that 'capture' malignant cells from the blood at specific sites. A similar question arises as to why some tissues, like cartilage, actually resist malignant cells, making secondaries there very rare indeed. Perhaps the relevant CAMs are missing from those sites. Clearly much is still to be learnt.

Lymph metastases may adhere to the lymphatic wall and grow along the lymphatic vessels. Indeed, malignant cells in the lymph have a slightly easier time than in the blood until they arrive in a lymph node. Here they accumulate and are attacked by activated **lymphocytes** (see Chapter 3). Lymph nodes containing malignant metastases are sometimes called *seeded*, and the node may become overwhelmed by cancer cells where they form a focus for malignant growth. Naturally, the nearest lymph nodes to the tumour are the first to be affected, particularly if they directly drain lymph from the tissues containing the tumour. They need to be inspected and any nodes suspected to contain malignant cells must be removed. Lymph nodes that are more distant from the primary site can also become seeded over time. Ultimately, the lymph will drain into the blood (see Figure 4.5, p. 106), and malignant cells may enter the circulation via this route.

The liver

The liver is a complex but fascinating organ. Excluding the skin, it is the largest organ inside the body. Liver cells (called **hepatocytes**) are packed in communities called **lobules** (see Figure 9.5), with numerous lobules occurring throughout the gland. A single liver lobule consists of a central blood vessel, which is a branch of the **hepatic vein**, and from this extend out tiny vessels called **sinusoids**, radiating like the spokes of a wheel from a central hub (see Figure 9.5). The hepatocytes are lined up along each side of the sinusoid like houses along a street. From the outside of the lobule blood is supplied to the sinusoids from branches of both the **hepatic artery** and the **hepatic portal vein**. The hepatic artery branch has arrived from a main branch of the **abdominal aorta**. *But the hepatic portal vein is something special.* The questions are *what is a portal vein* and *what makes it different to any other vein?* Also, another question could be *how many portal veins have we got?* These questions are answered later, for now it just needs to be said that the hepatic portal vein conveys blood rich in the nutrient products of digestion from the bowel (from the lower oesophagus to the rectum) on to the liver. So the sinusoid is getting a rich mix of arterial blood (containing oxygen) and hepatic portal blood (containing nutrients). The hepatocytes can carry on their function using these materials delivered to them until the blood drains into the central hepatic vein and leaves the liver. The hepatocytes also produce **bile** which drains from the liver via the small **biliary ducts** into the larger **common bile duct** outside the liver (see Figure 5.4 on p. 122). The function of hepatocytes (and therefore the functions of the liver) are:

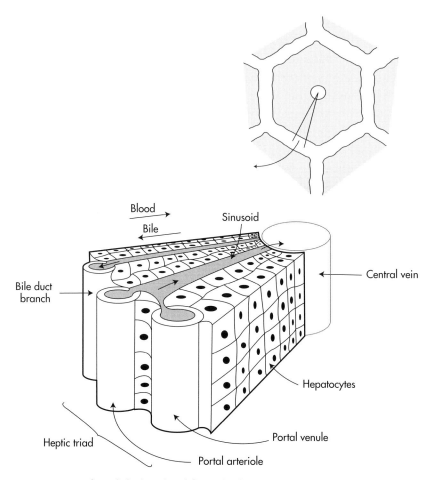

FIGURE 9.5 A liver lobule. Blood from the hepatic triad (arteriole and venule) mixes and flows down the sinusoid towards the central vein. Bile drains the other way towards the branch of the bile duct in the triad.

1 **Deamination** of excess amino acids from the diet (see p. 287 for amino acids). Deamination is the splitting off of an amine group, containing the **nitrogen**, from the amino acid, leaving the non-nitrogenous component, which can be converted to glucose (the creation of new glucose from a non-carbohydrate source like protein is called **gluconeogenesis**). The amine group is further converted by the liver first to **ammonia** (NH_3) then to **urea** (see liver failure, p. 239) for excretion.

2 Conversion of amino acids from one form (of which there is plenty) to another form (which is in short supply).

3 The formation of most blood proteins, like **albumin**, and the clotting proteins like **prothrombin** and **fibrinogen**, **lipo-**

proteins, and transport proteins like **transferrin** (transporting iron), or **transcobalamin** (transporting **vitamin B$_{12}$**).

4 Storage of glucose in the form of **glycogen**.

5 Conversion of **fructose** and **galactose** to glucose (see p. 123).

6 Preparation of fats for use as an energy source when glucose (the main energy source) is in short supply.

7 Conversion of fats into a form used for **adipose** (fat storage form called **triglycerides**, see p. 290).

8 Usage of fats for lipoproteins and for **phospholipids**, the formed fats are used in cell membranes (see p. 86).

9 Production of bile.

10 Metabolism of drugs in two phases; a **phase I reaction** and a **phase II reaction** (**conjugation**, meaning joining drugs to other substances, for excretion).

11 Storage of iron, vitamins A, B$_{12}$ and D, and folic acid (see p. 328).

But what about those questions asked earlier, i.e. *what is a portal vein* and *what makes it different to any other vein?* There are two types of veins in the body, *systemic veins* and *portal veins*. A portal vein conveys blood containing something special from one organ to another. The hepatic portal vein conveys blood with nutrients from the gut to the liver. The difference between the two types of vein is:

1 *Systemic veins* have capillaries at one end and the heart at the other, so all the blood is returned to the heart.

2 *Portal veins* have capillaries at both ends, so blood in a portal vein is not going to the heart.

Also, the other question, *how many portal veins have we got ?* The answer is two. The hepatic portal vein is one, the other is tiny and extends from the hypothalamus (at the base of the brain) into the anterior pituitary gland. And here is another question.

Whilst systemic veins get their blood from arteries (via capillaries), *where do portal veins get their blood from?* The answer is from systemic veins. There are junctions (called **anastamoses**) between the two types of veins. For the hepatic portal system these junctions occur at the base of the oesophagus and at the rectum (the two extremes of the gut that the portal veins collect from). And when bleeding occurs from the portal veins, due to **portal hypertension** (see Figure 9.6), the sites of these junctions become swollen veins and

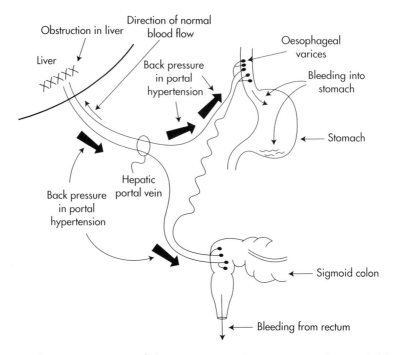

FIGURE 9.6 Hepatic portal hypertension. The passage of portal blood through the liver is obstructed. The pressure of the blood builds up in the portal vein, putting increasing pressure on the vein's capillary bed that spans almost the entire digestive tract from the lower oesophagus to the rectum. The capillaries swell with blood, especially at the lower oesophagus (varices) and rectum. Bleeding is sometimes a feature at these sites.

can bleed (they are called **oesophageal varices** in the lower end of the oesophagus).

Liver cancer

There are various types of liver cancer (Woolf 1998):

1 **Hepatocellular carcinoma (HCC)**, the commonest form of liver tumour.
2 **Fibrolamellar carcinoma**, a variant of HCC.
3 **Cholangiocarcinoma**, an **adenocarcinoma**.
4 **Hepatoblastoma**, an **embryonic carcinoma**.
5 **Angiosarcoma** of connective tissue origin.
6 Others (including secondary metastases).

Hepatocellular carcinoma (HCC)

This is a relatively common primary tumour worldwide, although the disease is less common in the Western world, and more common in South-East Asia. Some of the causative factors include: (1) infection with **hepatitis B virus** (**HBV**, see p. 47), even if it is mild with no symptoms; (2) the presence of **cirrhosis** (a disease of the liver where hepatocytes are replaced by fibrosis and abnormal nodule formation), often caused by chronic alcohol abuse; (3) metabolic disorders (e.g. **haemochromatosis**, a disease where excessive iron is

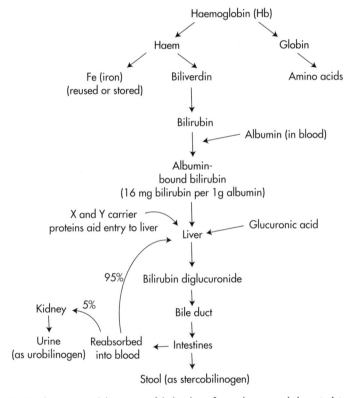

FIGURE 9.7 The natural history of bilirubin from haemoglobin (Hb). When released from old red cells, Hb splits into the haem component and the globin component. Globin can be broken down to recover the amino acids. From the haem component the iron can be recycled, but the biliverdin must be removed. It is first converted to bilirubin and then bound to albumin. This enters the liver with the assistance of carrier proteins X and Y. In the liver bilirubin is bound to glucuronic acid and enters the bile duct as a component of bile. Bile reaches the intestines and is partly reabsorbed. Most of it goes back to the liver, the rest is excreted in the urine as urobilinogen. What is not absorbed from the bowel is excreted in the stools as stercobilinogen.

absorbed and stored, damaging a number of organs); and (4) some drugs (e.g. chronic alcohol abuse) and toxins (e.g. from smoking).

The commonest features are **hepatomegaly** (enlargement of the liver) and abdominal pain with discomfort, but other symptoms include a loss of appetite (called **anorexia**), jaundice, weight loss and fever. Swelling, pain and discomfort in the abdomen are an indication of developing **ascites** (a collection of lymphatic fluid within the abdomen). It is a lymphatic oedema (see p. 306) due to obstructive lymphatic drainage within the liver. A sudden worsening of these symptoms is suggestive of a developing tumour. **Jaundice** is a yellow colour of various tissues, notably the skin, due to deposits of **bilirubin** in the extracellular (tissue fluid) space (the bilirubin is either *free* or *conjugated*, see Figure 9.7). Bilirubin is normally a bile pigment derived originally from **haemoglobin** (**Hb**) and excreted through the urine and faeces (see Figure 9.7). The normal level of bilirubin in the blood plasma is about 0.5 mg/dl (milligrams per decilitre of blood plasma) and this is mostly *free* bilirubin. In jaundice it can rise to 40 mg/dl, mostly of the *conjugated* type. The three main causes of jaundice are (1) **haemolytic jaundice**, excessive **haemolysis** (breakdown of red blood cells) releasing too much Hb; (2) liver disease (e.g. liver failure due to cirrhosis or cancer of the liver); and (3) **obstructive jaundice**, where the bile drainage is blocked, often by bile stones but this can also be by cancer (especially cancer of the head of the pancreas, see Figures 5.3 and 5.4, pp. 120 and 122).

Variations occur in the pathology of hepatocellular carcinoma. It may be a large single mass, it may be infiltrative or multifocal. It can spread through the branches of the portal vein and hepatic artery, although distal metastases usually occur only late in the course of the disease. Other variations of the histology include **minute carcinoma**, tiny patches of carcinoma sometimes set against a widespread cirrhosis of the liver (often seen in Japan), and less common are the **pedunculated tumours** (see p. 132) which protrude from the liver surface.

HCC tumour cells produce a marker which can be a useful diagnostic tool: **alpha** (α) **-fetoprotein** (**AFP**). This is not normally found in circulation after birth, and blood serum levels consistently above 500 µg/l are highly suggestive of a liver cancer. However, the minute carcinoma, pedunculated tumours and fibrolamellar carcinoma are exceptions since they produce only low levels of AFP (Woolf 1998).

HCC has rather a poor prognosis generally, death being caused by **cachexia** (see p. 305), bleeding into the digestive tract, **liver failure** (with hepatic coma) and more rarely liver rupture. Liver failure means that the functions of the liver (listed on p. 234) fail, and this condition is recognised by the presence of:

1 Jaundice (see above).
2 Low blood albumin levels (**hypoalbuminaemia**) leading to tissue oedema (see p. 306).
3 High blood ammonia levels (**hyperammonaemia**), which, along with other metabolic disturbances, lead ultimately to coma.
4 The presence of a characteristic musty body odour (called **fetor hepaticus**).
5 Impairment of the blood clotting mechanism (a **coagulopathy**) which leads to bleeding (notably into the digestive tract), due also to the back pressure of blood along the portal vein, called **portal hypertension**, from the obstructed liver (see p. 235).
6 Various skin manifestations, such as **spider angiomas** (small spider-like collections of blood vessels seen in the skin) or **palmar erythema** (local vasodilation and redness), both caused by abnormal oestrogen metabolism.
7 Failure of other body organs (called **multi-organ failure**), in particular the kidneys.

Other liver cancer variations

Fibrolamellar carcinoma is a variant usually seen in female patients below 25 years of age. About 65% arise in the left lobe of the liver. It consists of islands of tumour cells with collagen bands running between them. This tumour carries a better prognosis than other forms of HCC because it can normally be totally excised.

Cholangiocarcinoma is an **adenocarcinoma** arising from the bile ducts within the liver. The tumour cells secrete mucin, and spread to distant organs is more common in this tumour type than for HCC.

Hepatoblastoma is an **embryonic carcinoma**, which means the tumour contains cell types normally seen in the developing embryo. It arises in children (mostly boys) up to 3 years of age. Primitive foetal liver cells make up the **epithelioid** type, and in the **mixed** type primitive stromal cells separate foetal from embryonic liver cells. The children suffer anorexia, nausea and vomiting, and abdominal pain. The liver is usually enlarged and they have a raised serum AFP (see p. 238).

Angiosarcoma is a rare tumour of connective tissue origin. This is found mostly in adult males, often with a background of cirrhosis or exposure to industrial chemicals such as **arsenic** or **vinyl chloride**. The liver is very enlarged and spread of metastases is usually rapid. The tumour carries a very poor prognosis with patient survival usually being little more than 1 year from presentation.

Liver secondary tumours

The liver is the site for most metastases, and the majority of liver tumours are caused by metastastic spread from a primary elsewhere. Approximately 40% of cancer patients are likely to have liver metastases. Most of these secondaries will have come from a primary tumour in the stomach, pancreas, gall bladder and bile ducts, large bowel, lung, breast, kidney, or from a **malignant melanoma** (see p. 247) (Figure 9.8). The tumours that arise from the metastases develop as nodules mostly on the liver surface, but some occur deeper in the organ. A rise in the serum level of **alkaline phosphatase** (an enzyme involved in phosphate metabolism, as in the chemistry of glucose, cell membrane phospholipids and DNA, and in the calcification of bone) is an early warning that liver secondaries are likely to be present. This is followed later by the development of jaundice. Untreated, the prognosis following the discovery of liver metastases is poor, with patients surviving a matter of months. Resection of these tumours

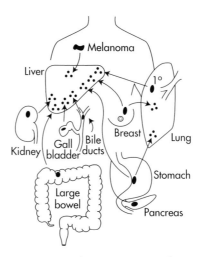

FIGURE 9.8 Liver metastases. The main sites for primary tumours are melanomas, lung, kidney, gall bladder, bile ducts, breast, large bowel, pancreas and stomach.

should improve the prognosis, with 40% of patients surviving 3 years or more (Woolf 1998).

Lung secondary tumours

The primary tumours of the lung are considered in Chapter 6 (see p. 157). After the liver, the lungs provide the second largest amount of metastatic spread. The commonest primary sites contributing to lung secondaries are breast and stomach carcinomas, and various sarcomas (Figure 9.8). The tumours that develop may be singular or multiple, and they tend to form round masses in the lung tissue.

Bone cancer

Bone is discussed in Chapter 1 (see p. 19). Primary bone tumours fall into two main groups (Woolf 1998): (1) **cartilaginous differentiation**, i.e. those where the neoplastic cells show a tendency to form cartilage; about 40% of this group are malignant, and these are the various forms of **chondrosarcoma**; and (2) **bone forming**, i.e. those where the neoplastic cells show a tendency to form bone; about 87% of this group are malignant **osteosarcomas**.

Chondrosarcomas form abnormal cartilage on bone, and they are the second commonest bone tumour (see osteosarcoma). The tumour forms lobules and is made largely of cartilage, sometimes with necrotic areas, and causes bone destruction. The causes of the tumour are not fully understood. Most (75%) occur in the skeleton of the trunk (ribs and pelvis) in principally the middle to elderly population.

Osteosarcomas are the commonest form of malignant bone tumour. The diagnosis is based on the fact that the malignant cells produce **osteoid** (an unmineralised matrix of **mucopolysaccharides** and **collagen**) which is the base upon which the bone minerals are deposited. Three main types of osteosarcoma are recognised depending on how much osteoid is present in the tumour: (1) **osteoblastic**, where osteoid and bone formation is the key feature; (2) **chondroblastic**, where the cells are mostly neoplastic cartilage, with some osteoid present; and (3) **fibroblastic**, where there is some osteoid present but cells produce large amounts of collagen.

The commonest site for osteosarcoma is around the knee (the lower **femur** and upper **tibia**), but other sites include the upper part of the **humerus** (the upper arm bone) and the **ilium** (the upper bone of the pelvis). Males develop this disease more often than females and are typically between 10 and 25 years of age. Some gene mutations play an important role in the cause of this disease, notably *Tp53* and *RB* gene mutations (see p. 40).

Osteosarcoma usually begins with a fracture at the site (called a **pathological fracture**, i.e. caused by disease weakening the bone), and on physical and X-ray examination the bone is enlarged by a mass. The tumour destroys the **cortex** (the outer layer) of the bone and extends both outward into surrounding soft tissues and inwards into the intramedullary canal. Tumours tend to metastasise via the blood early in the course of the disease, with most secondary tumours occurring in the lungs. The prognosis was originally poor, but has improved with advances in treatment, even for those with spread of the disease outside the bone.

Patients over 40 years of age are likely to have developed osteosarcoma as a complication of **Paget's disease** of the bone. Sir James Paget described several diseases in the 1800s that now carry his name (see also Paget's disease on p. 180). Paget's disease of the bone is a disorder of bone reabsorption and formation, and is not in itself a neoplastic disorder, but an osteosarcoma is sometimes seen as a complication of this disease.

Bone secondary tumours

Bone is the third most frequent site for metastatic spread. Common sites for primary tumours that cause bone secondary deposits are the thyroid, kidney, breast, prostate and lung (Figure 9.9). These tumours may destroy bone (**osteolytic tumours**) or produce extra bone (**osteoblastic tumours**). This latter category of tumour causes a very hard mass as a result of the new bone formation, and this may appear on X-ray screening. The bone formation also raises the blood level of **alkaline phophatase** (see p. 240). Osteolytic tumours cause thinning of the bone on X-ray examination (i.e. increased **radiolucency**). Pain is a common feature of these tumours, and the patient will be at risk of pathological fractures (see above), particularly as a result of osteolytic tumour activity. Bones become so weak they break very easily, with little pressure involved. How osteolytic tumours can cause such bone destruction is not fully understood. There is evidence to suggest that tumour-released enzymes, like **collagenase** (an enzyme for breaking down **collagen**, see pp. 17 and 232), may help to break down the protein component of the bone.

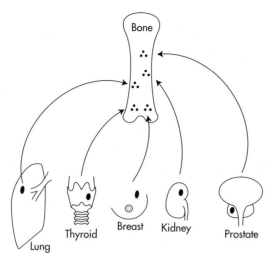

FIGURE 9.9 Bone metastases. The main sites for primary tumours are lung, kidney, breast, thyroid and prostate.

There is a possibility also that some prostaglandins (see p. 86) could be involved (Woolf 1998).

The brain

The brain is a complex organ and is not fully understood. It is beyond the scope of this book to discuss the brain in detail, the interested reader can find an overview in Blows (2003, Chapter 1). The functional cell of the brain is the **neuron** (see p. 23 and also Figure 1.13). The supportive tissue of the brain is the **neuroglia**, or **glial cells**, of which **astrocytes** are by far the most numerous. Table 9.1 lists the different types of glial cells.

Between the brain and the skull are three coverings called the **meninges**, the inner being the **pia mater**, the middle membrane is the **arachnoid mater**, and the outer, lining the skull, is the **dura mater**. Between the pia and the arachnoid is the **subarachnoid space** filled with **cerebrospinal fluid** (**CSF**)(Blows 2003, Figure 1.2). CSF originates from blood plasma inside the brain cavities (called **ventricles**) and returns to the blood via the arachnoid mater. So it has its own circulation, and malignant cells getting into this system can be washed to many parts of the **central nervous system** (**CNS**) (the CNS is the brain and spinal cord).

Between the blood and the brain is the **blood–brain barrier**, a system of tight junctions (see p. 228) between cells of the blood

TABLE 9.1 The cells forming the neuroglia

Glial cell	Notes
Astrocyte	Stabilises the tissue environment of the brain; provides nutrition to neurons; processes some neurotransmitters
Oligodendrocyte	Myelination of CNS neurons
Schwann cell	Myelination of PNS neurons
Ependymal cell	Lines the ventricles and ducts of the brain; assists in the formation and flow of CSF
Microglia	Phagocytic cells of the brain
Satellite cell	Not fully understood

vessel epithelium. These cells select what can and what cannot pass through and enter the brain (they are the least permeable of all the body capillaries) (Marieb 2001). This barrier may form a tough challenge for the entry of malignant metastases, and may partly account for the reason that most metastatic intracranial tumours do not occur inside the brain.

Brain and intracranial cancers

The types of primary brain tumours are gliomas, astrocytomas, oligodendrogliomas and ependymomas (Woolf 1998).

Gliomas (about 40 to 45% of tumours) are derived from **glial cells** (see p. 24). Various types occur based on the glial cell of origin.

Astrocytomas (derived from **astrocytes**, see Table 9.1) are probably the commonest form of tumour in the **central nervous system (CNS)**. They can be graded anything from slow growing (they are well differentiated and often just called *astrocytoma*), through to intermediate grade (called *anaplastic astrocytoma*) to aggressively infiltrative tumours (called *glioblastoma multiforme*).

Oligodendrogliomas are derived from **oligodendrocytes** (see Table 9.1). These are more common in childhood, and they often calcify, which means they may show up on X-ray examination (a valuable diagnostic point).

Ependymomas, derived from ependymal cells, can happen at any age but are commonest in the first 20 years of life. Most develop within one ventricle of the brain. They can interere with CSF flow and in smaller children could be a cause of **hydrocephalus** (fluid accumulation of the brain causing the head to swell). Spread of these tumours often involves entry into the subarachnoid space (see CSF, p. 243).

Medulloblastoma, is a tumour of the **cerebellum** derived from primitive cells during childhood. The cerebellum is the centre for many motor functions (Blows 2003), and the children will present with movement difficulties, like unsteady gait (**ataxia**). The tumour also spreads into the CSF and, like ependymoma, may cause obstruction to CSF flow. Such obstruction is likely to cause **raised intracranial pressure** (**RICP**)(see below).

Meningiomas (between 10 and 15% of tumours) are derived from the meninges (see p. 243) and therefore they are classified as *intracranial* (meaning *inside the skull*) tumours, not *brain* tumours (Figure 9.10). They are most often associated with the **arachnoid mater** in adults, predominately females, and can arise from this layer within

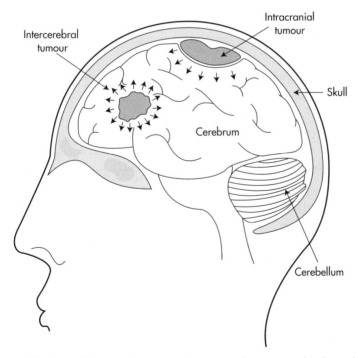

Figure 9.10 The difference between intracranial (extracerebral) and intra-cerebral tumours. The former occurs between the brain and the skull, putting pressure on the brain downwards. The latter occurs within the brain itself, putting pressure on the brain in all directions and disrupting the neurological structure of the brain.

the spine as well as inside the skull. They are often well-demarcated solid tumours that can invade the skull or the brain beneath. Most should be accessible by surgeons, and if this is the case, excision of the tumour improves the prognosis significantly.

A wide range of other tumour types occur based on different tissues of origin, some benign and others malignant, and there is some controversy regarding their classification due the range of variables possible and the confusing similarity between certain types.

Brain and other intracranial tumours cause their symptoms by a combination of:

1 Expansile growth putting pressure on surrounding tissues. The tumour creates what is called a **space-occupying lesion** (**SOL**), demanding space from brain tissues which are then pushed over. This raises the pressure (RICP) inside the skull (which cannot expand in adults).
2 Obstruction of CSF or blood flow through or around the brain. CSF obstruction leads to an accumulation of the fluid adding to the RICP.
3 Oedema formation around the tumour adding to the SOL and the RICP.
4 Irritation of neurons which then fail to function properly. Fits are one product of cerebral irritation.

The main symptoms of intracranial tumours are:

1 Those associated with RICP, which are headache, nausea and vomiting, altered state of consciousness, blurred vision, **diplopia** (double vision) pupillary changes, fits, disturbance to the pulse and blood pressure, **nystagmus** (involuntary rapid eye movements) and respiratory irregularities. The subject of RICP is discussed in more detail in Blows (2001, on p. 159). In the same reference there is a discussion of eye and pupillary changes (on p. 168), and of consciousness (on p. 138).
2 Those associated with the loss of neuronal function (called **neurological deficits**), such as **motor** (movement) weakness (movement is discussed in Blows 2001, page 190), sensory losses and speech disturbance.
3 Those associated with the brain's psychological functions, such as disturbance of behaviour, changes in personality, anxiety or depression.

Brain secondary tumours

The lung is one of the commonest sites for a primary tumour that gives rise to secondary brain metastases. Other primary sites are the breast and malignant melanomas (Figure 9.11). Most brain metastases are seen in the elderly population. The lesions are usually well-demarcated masses, either singular or multiple, and may occur in the meninges as well as the brain itself. Early signs of brain involvement include developing neurological deficits (e.g. limb weakness, speech difficulties) or psychiatric disturbance (e.g. personality changes, fits or depression) or physical symptoms associated with RICP.

Malignant melanoma

There are about 5,700 new cases of melanoma in the UK each year. It affects people mostly between the ages of 40 to 60 years. Under the age of 35 years it is the third most common cancer in women and the fifth in men.

Melanoma is a cancer of the pigment-producing cells, the **melanocytes**, mostly in the epidermis of the skin. Melanocytes normally produce the pigment **melanin** which gives colour to skin, hair and the eyes. The amount of colour present depends on the activity of the cell in producing melanin, not the number of cells present. Melanin is thought to be protective against the harmful effects of ultraviolet light (see p. 57). People with low levels of melanin production, i.e. the white population, are at greater risk of melanoma, especially those with a pale complexion, red hair or freckles. The risk factor is the amount of exposure to sunlight, and the health message

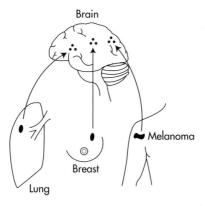

FIGURE 9.11 Brain metastases. The main sites for primary tumours are lung, breast and melanomas.

for some time has been to stay out of the sun during the times that the sun is hottest and brightest, cover-up exposed skin where possible and use sun-screen protection correctly. Sun bathing may be popular, but it just isn't healthy. It causes not only increased risk of skin cancer (the majority of melanomas occur on sun-exposed areas of the body) but also premature ageing of the skin and the risk of sunburn.

More than half of melanomas develop from a pre-existing skin lesion, like a **naevus** (a birthmark formed from malformed blood vessels in the skin, like a **strawberry naevus** or **port-wine stain**). The average white person is said to have about 12 pigmented naevi, any of which could become malignant.

There are two ways in which melanomas grow: (1) *radially*, called **radial growth phase** (**RGP**), i.e. growth is outwards in all directions from the central point; and (2) *vertically*, called **vertical growth phase** (**VGP**), i.e. growth extends deep into the lower half of the dermis. These two distinctions in growth are accompanied by differences in the type and behaviour of the malignant cells.

There are four main types of melanoma, accounting for nearly 90% of these cancers.

Lentigo maligna (**Hutchinson's melanotic freckle**) accounts for about 10% of all cases, occurring mostly in sun-exposed areas of skin in the elderly. It forms a flat, pigmented area in the epidermis which expands slowly. RGP is present. Surgical excision at the early stages is usually curative.

Superficial spreading melanoma (about 67% of cases) is generally larger than lentigo maligna (i.e. 2–3 cm in diameter), and occurs in middle age. The edge is irregular and after a few years the lesion begins to itch and ulcerate. RGP is present.

Acral lentiginous melanoma (about 4% of cases), mostly occurs in the feet, sometimes associated with the toe nail. It is commonest in dark-skinned races and carries a good prognosis if diagnosed early. RGP is present.

Nodular melanoma is a rapidly developing lesion which has nearly always reached deep dermal invasion by the time a diagnosis is made. A raised nodule forms which, if left, ulcerates within 2 to 3 months. RGP is absent, being totally VGP.

Staging of the tumour (i.e. the degree of invasion) and the vertical thickness of the tumour are the most important clinical aspects of this disease. There are a number of staging systems in use. The following is a good example of grading the level of invasion:

I   Confined to local site, less than 1.5 mm in depth.
II   Confined to local site, more than 1.5 mm in depth.
III Regional lymph node metastases.
IV   Lymph node metastases next to the region involved.
V   Distant metastases.

This is the 'Clark levels' of invasion and are shown in Figure 9.12.

The deletion of a tumour suppressor gene (see p. 35) has been identified in more than 50% of melanomas. A deletion of *CDKN2A* at 9p13 (see p. 41) causes a loss of p16 (see Figure 1.7, p. 14 for details).

Because metastases from a melanoma are a major problem, wide surgical excision of the primary lesion at as early a stage as possible is the most important treatment in most cases. The surgery will probably involve the regional lymph nodes in most cases, followed by chemotherapy and radiotherapy as appropriate.

Advances in the future management of melanoma

A new test, a new treatment and a new vaccine for melanoma are all possible within the next year or so. Trials of all these have proven successful (Anon. 2003, Anon. 2004). The new test will involve the identification of a protein that is expressed by cancer cells from a very early stage, making early diagnosis simpler (Anon. 2003). The new treatments include a modified **anthrax toxin**. Normally the deadly anthrax toxin links to a cellular enzyme called **furin**. It's this combination that turns anthrax into a killer. The modified anthrax toxin links only with another enzyme, **plasmogen**, which only cancer cells produce. Not linking to furin makes the toxin harmless to the body, but linking with plasmogen makes the toxin lethal to cancer cells (Anon. 2004). The other treatment is to take some immune

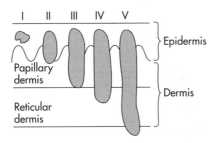

FIGURE 9.12 The Clark levels of invasion of melanomas. See text for details. (Redrawn from Woolf 1998.)

T-cells (see p. 70) from the patient, to boost their cancer killing properties artificially and to grow them in vast quantities. These T-cells are then given back to the patient (about 70 billion T-cells in 20 minutes) to increase greatly their immunity against the cancer (Anon. 2004). At least two vaccines are under development for melanoma (see Chapter 12, p. 341 for cancer vaccines).

Key points

Cell attachment

- Most cells remain locked in their correct position within the tissues.
- The cytoskeleton is a protein framework of the cell consisting of microfilaments, intermediate filaments and microtubules.
- Cells have tight junctions, gap junctions and desmosomes between them.

Metastases

- The change to metastatic cells in a cancer is a bad development, i.e. from carcinoma *in situ* to invasive carcinoma.
- Malignant tumours can spread by direct invasion, via the lymph or blood, and via transcoelomic spread.
- Malignant cells can become free from anchorage, i.e. they become anchorage independent.
- Cell adhesion molecules (CAMs) are transmembranous glycoprotein receptors, and they provide anchorage between cells (e.g. E-cadherin).
- To invade other tissues successfully malignant cells must have very low E-cadherin levels and must produce gelatinase (a metalloproteinase enzyme).

The liver

- Liver cells (called hepatocytes) are packed in lobules.
- The hepatic portal vein conveys blood rich in digestive nutrients from the bowel to the liver.
- The hepatocytes produce bile which drains from the liver via the small biliary ducts into the larger common bile duct.
- Other functions of the liver relate to protein, glucose and fat metabolism, the storage of certain nutrients and the metabolism of drugs.

Liver cancer

- There are various types of liver cancer, the commonest being hepatocellular carcinoma (HCC).
- Common features are hepatomegaly (enlarged liver) and abdominal pain.
- HCC tumour cells produce the marker alpha (α) -fetoprotein (AFP).
- Jaundice is a yellow colour of various tissues, notably the skin, due to deposits of bilirubin in the extracellular (tissue fluid) space.
- Liver failure involves bleeding caused by impairment of the blood clotting mechanism (a coagulopathy) and by portal hypertension from the obstructed liver.
- The liver is the site for most metastases, and the majority of liver tumours are caused by metastatic spread from a primary elsewhere.

Lung cancers

- After the liver, the lungs are the site of the second largest amount of metastatic spread.

Bone cancer

- Primary bone tumours fall into two main groups, cartilaginous differentiation (the neoplastic cells show a tendency to form cartilage, the chondrosarcomas), and bone forming (the neoplastic cells show a tendency to form bone, the osteosarcomas).
- Osteosarcoma begins with a pathological fracture at the site (often the knee), and an enlarged mass in the bone is seen on physical and X-ray examination.
- Bone is the third most frequent site for metastatic spread.
- These tumours may destroy bone (osteolytic tumours) or produce extra bone (osteoblastic tumours).

The brain

- The functional cell of the brain is the neuron.
- The supportive tissue of the brain is the neuroglia, or glial cells, of which astrocytes are by far the most numerous.
- Between the brain and the skull are coverings called the meninges.

- The inner covering is the pia mater, the middle covering is the arachnoid mater, and the outer is the dura mater.
- Between the pia and the arachnoid is the subarachnoid space filled with cerebrospinal fluid (CSF).
- CSF originates from blood plasma inside the brain ventricles and returns to the blood via the arachnoid mater.
- Between the blood and the brain is the blood–brain barrier, a system of tight junctions between cells of the blood vessel epithelium.

Brain cancer

- Gliomas account for 40 to 45% of brain tumours.
- They are derived from glial cells, including astrocytomas formed from astrocytes.
- Brain and other intracranial tumours cause their symptoms by expansile growth creating a space-occupying lesion (SOL).
- This causes raised intracranial pressure (RICP).
- Obstruction of CSF around the brain leads to an accumulation of the fluid adding to the RICP.
- Oedema formation around the tumour adds to the SOL and the RICP.
- Irritation of neurons may cause fits.
- The symptoms of intracranial tumours are those of RICP, neurological deficits and those associated with psychological functions.
- The lung is one of the commonest sites for a primary tumour that gives rise to secondary brain metastases.

Melanoma

- Melanoma is a cancer of the pigment-producing cells, the melanocytes, mostly in the epidermis of the skin.
- The risk factor is the amount of exposure to sunlight.
- More than half of melanomas develop from a pre-existing skin lesion, e.g. a naevus.
- Melanomas grow radially (radial growth phase, RGP), and vertically (vertical growth phase, VGP).
- Staging and the vertical thickness of a tumour are the most important clinical aspects of this disease.
- Because metastases from a melanoma are a major problem, wide surgical excision of the primary lesion is the most important treatment.

References

Anonymous (2003) *Medical Breakthroughs 2003*, The Reader's Digest Association, London.

Anonymous (2004) *Medical Breakthroughs 2004*, The Reader's Digest Association, London.

Blows W. T. (2001) *The Biological Basis of Nursing: Clinical Observations*, Routledge, London.

Blows W. T. (2003) *The Biological Basis of Nursing: Mental Health*, Routledge, London.

King R. J. B. (2000) *Cancer Biology* (2nd edn), Prentice Hall, London.

Marieb E. (2001) *Human Anatomy and Physiology* (5th edn), Benjamin Cummings, San Francisco.

Woolf N. (1998) *Pathology, Basic and Systematic*, W. B. Saunders Company Ltd., London and Philadelphia.

Chapter 10

Pain and analgesia

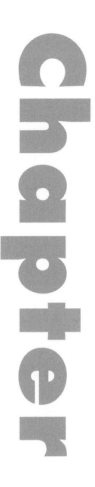

Introduction

Pain and death are perhaps the two most frightening aspects of cancer to any patient. And not just pain from the cancer, but also the pain associated with the medical investigations and treatments of various kinds is also a major source of concern. Many people who had previous family members or friends with cancer will often remember the pain they suffered from the surgery or other therapies. This colours their view of the illness, i.e. they conceive that cancer and its treatment cause pain, therefore the cancer patient is bound to suffer. But time and research have moved on, and the picture now is that with our greater understanding of the causes and effects of pain, the mechanisms of drug action, and of how to manage pain more effectively, prolonged suffering is no longer an inevitable consequence of cancer. A major part of that process is the understanding and commitment of the nurses, and doctors, in ensuring their patient is pain free and comfortable.

The neurophysiology of pain

There are several types of pain. **Acute pain** tends to be of sudden and relatively short duration. It serves a purpose in one sense, i.e. it alerts the individual that something is wrong and needs attention, or it protects the individual against further tissue injury. **Chronic pain** has a longer duration than acute, often lasting for weeks, months or even years. Some definitions put chronic pain as existing for longer than three months (Wood 2002) or longer than six months (Jacques 1994). **Intractable pain** is chronic pain unrelated to any detectable pathology. As such it is very difficult to treat and offers a major challenge to health-care professionals. Although there are some theories, there is no known cause of intractable pain.

Localised pain is often caused by **inflammation** of the tissues involved. Inflammation is in turn caused by local trauma or irritation of the tissues, as seen in infections, mechanical injury or tumour formation. Inflammation is a natural mechanism through which the **immune system** functions. We dislike inflammation because of the discomfort it causes, but the immune system could not function adequately without it. Inflammation causes an increase in capillary wall permeability, thus allowing increased amounts of water to leak into the tissues from blood plasma. And not just water, capillaries also allow the leakage of proteins from the blood, and allow larger numbers of white blood cells to leave the blood and enter the tissues. The protein leakage makes the tissue fluid protein rich, and this attracts more water from the capillaries. The result is a build-up of tissue fluid in the inflamed area; i.e. a local **oedema** (see p. 306). The pain is generated almost as a side effect. **Pain mediators** (i.e. chemicals causing pain) are released at the site; notably **histamine**, **prostaglandins** and **bradykinins** (Figure 10.1). These mediators bind to receptors on **nociceptors**, which are pain nerve endings (the word **nociception** is often used as another word for pain). There are two types of nociceptors: **mechanoreceptors** and **polymodal**. Mechanoreceptors are pain receptors that respond to mechanical injury, whilst polymodal receptors respond with pain caused by many types of tissue insult. Nerve impulses generated by nociceptors are recognised as pain by the brain only after certain criteria are reached. First, sufficient chemical mediator must bind to the nociceptors to raise the level of stimulation to **pain threshold** point or beyond. Threshold means the amount of chemical stimulation necessary to generate strong enough impulses from the nociceptors that are recognised as pain by the brain. With less chemical binding, i.e.

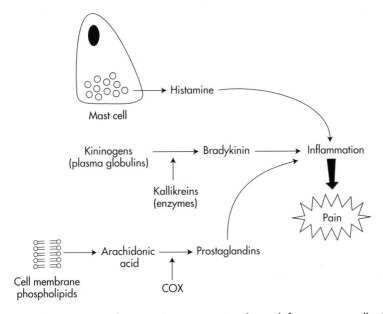

FIGURE 10.1 Pain mediators. Histamine is released from mast cells (see Figures 3.4 and 3.10), bradykinins are derived from the plasma globulins kininogens, and prostaglandins are formed from arachidonic acid (see Figure 3.11).

below threshold level, impulses can still be generated from the nociceptor, but these are weaker, and are recognised by the brain as **irritation**, rather than pain. **Itching** is one form of irritation caused by
mediators binding to nociceptors in concentrations below that
needed to activate the pain threshold level (Figure 10.2). Second,
even if the threshold is exceeded, the nature, severity and duration of
pain conceived by the brain is dependent on the intensity of neuronal
firing from the nociceptor. If the nociceptor firing is weak (i.e. just
above threshold level), the pain conceived by the brain will be significantly less than if the firing intensity is increased. It is a simple
relationship; the greater the intensity of impulses generated, the
greater is the perceived pain (Guyton 1981).

Pain impulses pass to the brain via the peripheral **sensory nervous system**. Two types of nerve pathways, '**A**' **fibres** and '**C**' **fibres**,
carry impulses destined to register as pain in the brain. 'A' fibres are
further divided into various subtypes of which the Aδ **fibre** carries
pain. Aδ fibres are fast, i.e. they convey impulses very quickly to the
brain, whilst 'C' fibres are slower. The difference is the thickness of
the fibres and the degree of **myelination** the fibre has. Myelin is the
fatty covering along the axon of neurons that is involved in impulse
conduction. The better the myelination (as in 'A' fibres) the faster the
impulse will travel, i.e. up to 25 metres per second in 'A' fibres. 'C'
fibres are unmyelinated and transmit impulses at speeds considered
as 'slow' in comparison, i.e. up to 2 metres per second. They are
important, however, since 'C' fibres carry about 80% of pain

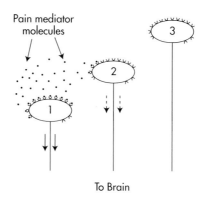

To Brain

FIGURE 10.2 Pain mediator molecules bind to nociceptors ('A', 'B' and 'C').
'A' has bound a lot of molecules and sends rapid impulses to the brain, and
pain is experienced, 'B' has fewer bound molecules and sends a slower rate
of impulses which the brain interprets as itching, 'C' has no molecules bound
and sends no impulses to the brain.

impulses to the brain, and they are widely distributed throughout the body. Nociceptors at the end of the Aδ fibres are found in the skin and mucous membranes where they are in the 'front line' for warning the brain against sudden, sharp pain due to trauma. Compare that to nociceptors of 'C' fibres which are also in the skin but are found in most other body tissues as well.

The pathway from the periphery to the brain is a three-neuronal system, i.e. the impulse must pass through three **sensory neurons** to get from the nociceptor to the brain (Figure 10.3):

1　*Neuron 1* passes from the nociceptor into the posterior part of the **spinal cord**. It is a specialised neuron having the cell body on a branch just outside the cord. This cell body is called the **posterior root ganglion (PRG)**.
2　*Neuron 2* synapses with the first neuron in the cord, the axon first crossing the midline before passing up the cord to part of the

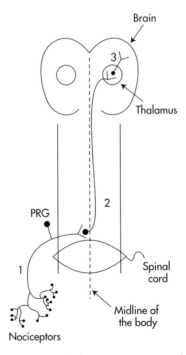

FIGURE 10.3 All sensations, including pain, use a three neuronal system from periphery to the brain. Neuron 1 extends from the nociceptors in the periphery to the cord (PRG = posterior root ganglion, the cell body of neuron 1). Neuron 2 crosses the midline in the cord and extends to the thalamus. Neuron 3 relays the impulses from the thalamus to the cerebral cortex of the brain.

brain called the **thalamus**. The crossover (called a **decussation**) means that impulses from the left of the body will continue up the right hand side of the nervous system, and vice versa.

3 *Neuron 3* synapses with neuron 2, the axon passing from the thalamus to the **sensory cortex** of the **cerebrum**.

Synapses are connections between neurons. Synapses use chemicals called **neurotransmitters** to bridge a gap that the synapse creates. This gap (called the **synaptic cleft**) and the neurotransmitters found there are important in the story of pain transmission. Beyond the nociceptor, therefore, three main parts of the nervous system are involved in impulse transmission that leads to pain. These are the spinal cord, the thalamus and the sensory cerebral cortex.

The spinal cord

Pain is *not* recognised as a conscious sensation at spinal cord level. All impulses pass through the cord and its synapses purely automatically at subconscious level. The posterior spinal cord is the site of the first synapse, between neurons 1 and 2. This connection permits the formation of a pain **reflex arc**; a mechanism that allows pain impulses to trigger another impulse in the corresponding **lower motor neuron (LMN)** in the cord which then causes muscles to contract and withdraw the affected part away from the source of pain. Here, also, is the location for a pain-blocking process called the '**gate-control theory**' (Figure 10.4). The gate control theory of pain works as follows.

In the centre of the spinal cord is an area of nerve cell bodies called **grey matter**. Part of this grey matter is a collection of neuronal cell bodies known as the **substantia gelatinosa** (or 'jelly substance'). This can be activated (switched on) by 'A' fibre stimulation, but de-activated (switched off) by 'C' fibre stimulation. Pain impulses arrive first via the 'A' fibres of neuron 1, and these impulses pass on up to the brain via neuron 2. At the same time, 'A' fibre impulses activate the substantia gelatinosa. The substantia gelatinosa then inhibits (= blocks) all further 'A' (and indeed 'C') fibre impulses, and the 'gate' is closed to pain (Figure 10.4). Slower pain impulses passing along 'C' fibres arrive later. They cannot pass through this 'gate', but 'C' fibre stimulation tends to switch off the substantia gelatinosa, thus opening the 'gate' to pain impulses again along both the 'A' and 'C' fibres. In reality, the so-called 'gate' will not be either fully

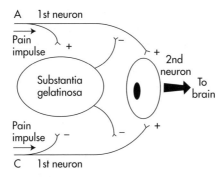

A   1st neuron

Pain impulse

Substantia gelatinosa

2nd neuron

To brain

Pain impulse

C   1st neuron

FIGURE 10.4 The gate control theory. The first neuron (from periphery to cord) is either an 'A' (fast) fibre or a 'C' (slow) fibre. Both carry pain impulses and both stimulate (+) the second neuron in the cord. The 'A' fibre also activates the substantia gelatinosa which then blocks impulses along both the 'A' and 'C' fibres using its own negative (−)(inhibitory) synapses. This closes the gate to pain impulses reaching the second neuron. 'C' stimulation shuts down the substantia gelatinosa using a negative (−)(inhibitory) synapse and therefore opens the gate to pain impulses reaching the second neuron. Generally the 'gate' is neither fully open nor fully closed but varies between these two states, and can be influenced by impulses from the brain.

opened or fully closed, but will fluctuate between the two states depending on which has the greater stimulus at any given moment, 'A' or 'C' fibres. Anything that promotes 'A' fibre stimulus will help to block pain at spinal cord level, and this may be how mechanisms like **TENS** (**transcutaneous electrical nerve stimulation**) or **acupuncture** may work (see pp. 272–273).

Also, what must not be overlooked is the fact that the 'gate control' mechanism is significantly influenced from above by the higher intellectual centres of the brain. Impulses descending from the **reticular formation** and other parts of the **brainstem**, also from the **hypothalamus** and from the cerebral cortex, modify the events at cord level. The brain does this because factors such as emotions, culture, personal beliefs and learning are all involved in the total pain experience. Descending neurons from the brain create synapses in the cord that use a variety of neurotransmitters such as **enkephalins**, **endorphins** and **dynorphins** (see p. 276) to block further pain transmission up the cord (Clancy and McVicar 1998).

At a local level, one important neurotransmitter at the synapse between neurons 1 and 2 is **substance P**. This neurotransmitter is a facilitator for pain transmission at cord level, and anything that inhibits or prevents substance P will decrease pain impulses from reaching the brain. The release of substance P is inhibited by another naturally produced chemical called **enkephalin** (see p. 276).

The thalamus

Pain impulses begin to become part of our consciousness as they pass through our brain. As impulses travel up neuron 2 and enter the brain they first pass through the **brainstem**. Here pain impulses are recognised as something different from other sensory impulses, but the true obnoxious nature of the stimulus is not known at this point. On arrival at the thalamus pain impulses are, for the first time, consciously recognised as unpleasant. As a sensory relay station, the thalamus is normally dealing with thousands of sensations every minute, all of which are still at subconscious level except pain. The thalamus must pass sensory impulses onto the conscious part of the brain, the *sensory cortex* of the cerebrum (in the *parietal lobe*), via neuron 3. With pain impulses this still happens, but the thalamus also communicates with the *motor cortex* of the cerebrum (in the *frontal lobe*) and thus influences movement in response to the pain (called a **thalamic response** to pain)(Figure 10.5). So, both synapses in the three-neuronal system, i.e. in the cord and in the thalamus, have motor connections facilitating responses to the pain impulses.

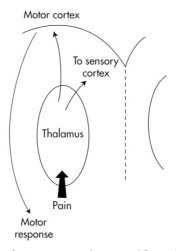

FIGURE 10.5 Pain impulses are not only passed from the thalamus to the sensory cortex, but also, by including the motor cortex, the thalamus can initiate a motor response to pain.

The cerebral cortex

Finally, the nociceptive impulses arrive at the sensory cortex of the cerebrum via neuron 3. This is the conscious brain, where the individual will become aware of the pain as a noxious and unpleasant sensation. The cells of the sensory cortex are laid out in a plan representative of the body (Figure 10.6), Having been 'relayed' from the thalamus, the pain impulses will arrive at that part of the cortex that represents that area of the body from where the pain has originated. Thus, pain impulses arising from the abdomen, for example, will arrive in that part of the cortex that specialises in the abdomen. Remember, there is also a crossover of the sensory neuron 2 in the cord, so pain impulses from the left of the body will arrive in the right cortex, and vice versa.

The conscious nature of the cortex allows for the individual to make decisions and to act on the pain, e.g. to rest, to take pain-killing drugs or to see a doctor. This is very different to the responses found at cord or thalamic levels that are less sophisticated, and are only there to save life and prevent further injury.

What is also interesting is that we are only conscious of the pain sensation when it reaches the cerebrum of the brain, but still we recognise the pain as arising from the body part affected. As an

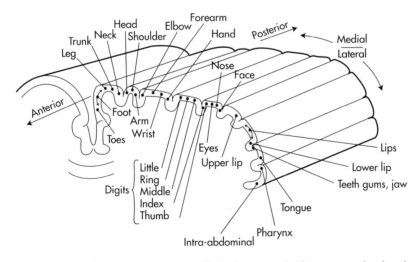

FIGURE 10.6 The sensory cortex of the brain is laid out as a body plan. Impulses from the body must be sent to the relevant part of the cortex, and directing these impulses to the appropriate part of the cortex is a function of the thalamus. (From Blows 2001, Figure 7.5.)

example, consider pain impulses arising from the bowel. These impulses are not conscious (and therefore not recognised as pain) until they reach the brain. Yet as soon as we are aware of them in the cortex we actually 'feel' the pain in the bowel, not the brain. This is because, as said before, the cerebral cortex receiving the impulses is laid out in a body plan. So, in our example, there is part of the cortex where the brain cells are representatives of the bowel. When these brain cells receive pain impulses they make the person aware of pain in the bowel, *not* in the brain.

And just to add a strange twist to this story, the brain *itself* does *not* feel pain! This has been demonstrated many times by surgeons who have operated on the brains of *conscious* patients. The scalp and other tissues require local anaesthesia, but the brain itself does not require any anaesthesia as it cannot 'feel' pain. When the surgeon stimulates the cortex, the patient feels sensations in that part of the body represented by the cerebral cortical cells stimulated. In our previous example, if the surgeon stimulated that part of the cortex representing the bowel, the patient feels sensation in the bowel. So, this means that the brain makes you aware of pain arising from all other parts of the body except itself. This should make sense because the cerebral cortex could not be both the *initiator* (i.e. the nociceptor) and the *receiver* of pain impulses at the same time.

This may raise questions about '*headaches*'. Suffice to say here that headaches are caused by many different problems related to the soft tissues of the head and neck (muscles, blood vessels, mucous membranes within bony sinuses, meninges and so on), but not the sensory cerebral cortex itself.

Endogenous opioids

These are chemicals produced naturally in the brain and cord which block pain impulses from entering the brain, thus providing some protection for the brain against noxious stimuli. They are produced at the time that pain is experienced. Further discussion of these substances is found in the section on analgesia (see p. 276).

Chronic pain in cancer

Chronic pain affects between 7 and 30% of the population. It is the most common complaint seen by **general practitioners** (**GP**s), mostly in the form of low back pain. Chronic pain changes the sufferer's lifestyle and personality, and causes dependence on others for help, insomnia, depression and fatigue. Chronic pain can be **nociceptive**, i.e. operates through nociceptors in the manner described (see p. 257), and can be severe. It may be from the main body structure (**somatic**) or from the internal organs (**visceral**). Alternatively, the pain may be **neuropathic**, i.e. caused by an abnormal process of sensory nerve conduction, such as occurs in a nerve pathology. It is often described as burning, dull, aching, tingling or shooting in character. The chronic pain suffered in cancer may have three causes:

1 Further advancement of the disease (the most common cause of the pain), where the cancer is growing into the surrounding tissues, or spreading as **metastases** (see p. 226). Such advancement puts pressure on surrounding structures, including pain nerve endings, it induces inflammation and predisposes to complications like obstruction.
2 The effects and side effects of cancer treatments.
3 The presence of any co-existing disease, i.e. some other disorder the patient is suffering from that is not related to their cancer.

Deafferentation pain is the term used to describe pain associated with loss of sensory input to the spinal cord and brain from one part of the body. As a result of this loss, the spinal cord or thalamus can become hyperactive and causes a burning or 'vice-like', or electric-shock-like pain, which is hard to manage with either drugs or adjuvant therapy.

Nursing skills: pain assessment and monitoring

The question arises 'how can you quantify and measure pain?' It is not difficult to identify when a person is in pain; they can usually tell you and they may show the signs of pain (Figure 10.7). But how *much* pain are they suffering (i.e. is it quantifiable?), and is it getting better or worse? How *much* pain is like asking 'how blue is the sky?' You can see it is blue, but measuring its 'blueness' accurately is very difficult. Pain is very much an individual (or subjective) concept: what is severe pain to one person would be mild to another. It raises questions like how much does conscious or subconscious exaggeration, or other factors, enter the equation?

Pain assessment requires judgement concerning the following factors:

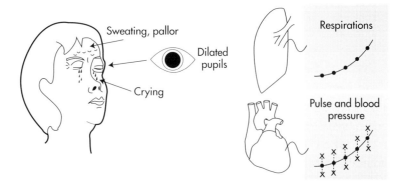

FIGURE 10.7 The signs of pain. The pulse, blood pressure and respiration rates rise. The pupils dilate, and the person may show sweating, pallor and may cry.

1 Pain site; i.e. where is the pain? Remember that not all pain occurs at the site of the pathology (or the cause of the pain). **Referred pain** occurs some distance away from the site of the cause (Figure 10.8). This is because pain impulses travel along

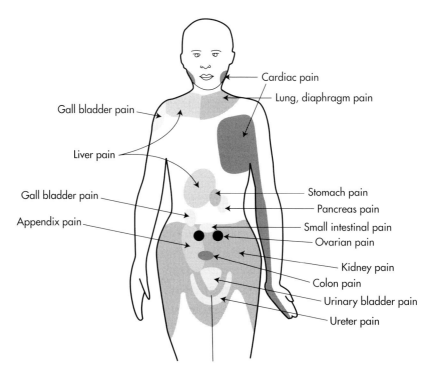

FIGURE 10.8 The areas where referred pain is experienced and the organs the pain is derived from. (Redrawn from LeMone and Burke 2004.)

nerve pathways and sometimes gives the brain a false impression of where the pain is originating from.

2 Pain intensity, which is very subjective and will vary between individuals and at different times in the same individual.

3 The nature of the pain; i.e. is it sharp like a knife, a dull ache or is it burning?

4 Is the pain associated with specific activities, like eating, vomiting or urinating, or with a specific movement or position?

5 Duration of the pain, i.e. is it sudden or acute, or is it chronic?

In an attempt to be as objective as possible about such a subjective phenomenon, **pain assessment tools** (**pain charts** or **pain scales**) have been devised. Pain assessment tools fall into three categories:

Verbal descriptor scales use words which may be appropriate to describe pain ranked in order of severity, e.g. *none (no pain)*; *slight pain*, *moderate pain*, *severe pain*, *agonising pain*. Patients indicate the word most applicable to their pain, and a numerical ranking alongside the words would aid in charting the response (Figure 10.9). The word list may provide rather limited choice when applied to some patients' pain, but it is easy to score and analyse.

Visual analogue scales consist of a line representing a pain continuum, with descriptive word 'anchors' at both ends. An example is the

Description	Score
No pain	0
Slight pain	1
Mild pain	2
	3
Moderate pain	4
	5
Severe pain	6
More severe pain	7
Very severe pain	8
	9
Worst possible pain	10

FIGURE 10.9 Verbal descriptor scale for pain.

continuum that stretches from 'no pain' at one end of the line to 'pain as bad as it could be' at the other end. Patients must indicate where along this line their pain ranks. Additional word descriptions may be added along the line to aid the patient in their choice (Figure 10.10). They are relatively easy to use and don't rely heavily on the choice of wording. However, they may not be suitable for all patients, particularly the elderly and confused, or those with educational disabilities.

Pain behaviour tools are based on the understanding that patients in pain demonstrate certain behaviour patterns. These behaviour patterns are most likely to consist of *verbal responses to pain* (e.g. crying or swearing); *pain-related body language* (e.g. holding affected area or rubbing); *specific facial expressions*; *certain behaviour changes* (e.g. seeking analgesia or medical attention); *changes in conscious level* and *pain-related physiological responses* (e.g. mild pain causes a rise in blood pressure; severe pain causes a drop in blood pressure). These scales can be used on patients with communication problems but they are more time consuming and complex than the previous tools, and they exclude the patient's own subjective assessment (Manchester Triage Group 1997).

Numerous variations of these tools will be seen in clinical practice where they have been combined or modified to suit specific patient needs.

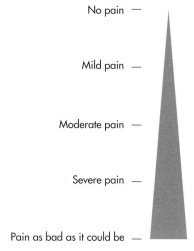

No pain —

Mild pain —

Moderate pain —

Severe pain —

Pain as bad as it could be —

FIGURE 10.10 Visual analogue scale for pain.

Pain in children

In **neonates** the first pain pathway to mature is the 'C' fibre, but slow myelination of motor pathways means that their responses to pain tend only to be generalised, e.g. crying rather than specific to the site of pain. **Infants** can localise pain better after about 3 months of age, and can produce more specific reactions. They still produce generalised reactions as well; crying and a change in facial expression being the most obvious. Some older children are better at discussing and describing pain. However, they often think in terms of extremes; i.e. it is either very bad or gone. They are also very good at pinpointing precise locations of pain, but because they do not understand the cause of pain, or often how to stop it, pain can cause confusion, fear and anger. Often the cause will be obvious, e.g. following a minor accident. But if the cause is less obvious, as in cancer for example, they do not understand why they are suffering from pain or what to do about it for themselves. They become entirely dependent on their parents or guardians at first, and later on nurses and other healthcare professionals to solve the problem of their pain. Nursing children in pain is a major challenge to all concerned, involving drugs, but also love, empathy, patience, tolerance and understanding.

Assessing pain in children is difficult, and to help to overcome the problems a number of pain charts have been developed specifically for children of any age, in some cases down to four years old. Some consist of a series of cartoon faces showing a range of expressions from happy (experiencing no pain) to very sad or crying (experiencing severe pain). Beneath each face are words describing the pain intensity in terms (verbal and written) that a child is likely to understand (e.g. the word 'hurt' instead of 'pain'). The most reliable indicator of pain in children is their verbal statements about the pain they are suffering, and what the child is saying should always be believed. A full assessment of child pain scales can be found in Wong *et al.* (1999). But scales are only part of the story. **QUESTT** is an overall pain assessment that incorporates scales where required (Baker and Wong 1987). **QUESTT** stands for:

Question the child.
Use pain rating scales.
Evaluate behaviour and physiological changes.
Secure parent's involvement.
Take the cause of the pain into account.
Take action and evaluate the results (Wong *et al.* 1999).

It is vital that children receive adequate treatment for their pain, including sufficient analgesia appropriate for their condition. Under-medication of children in pain is a major concern for the child and parents alike. Inadequate drug therapy may be due to inaccurate pain assessment, fear of the use of powerful drugs in children and worries about possible drug dependency. This last concern is unwarranted and should not be a factor when managing severe pain on a short-term basis. The Acute Pain Management Guideline Panel (1992) states: '*There is no known aspect of childhood development or physiology that indicates any increased risk of physiologic or psychologic dependence from the brief use of opioids for acute pain management*'.

In children with severe pain, as in the later stages of cancer, the **analgesic ladder** can be employed to ensure adequate pain therapy (see p. 271). Remember that pain generates fear in a child, and for this reason painful procedures must be reduced to the absolute minimum required. Full explanation is required from the parents and nurses for any procedures, especially if they are painful, including being honest about the possibility of pain. Children must not be left alone in pain.

Nursing skills: drug management of pain

Drugs have been the mainstay of pain control for a long time, and continue to be so. Two important sciences, **pharmacokinetics** and **pharmacodynamics**, describe the events inside the body once drugs have been administered. Pharmacokinetics involves the way drugs move through the body, from absorption through to distribution, metabolism and finally excretion. Pharmacodynamics describe how drugs actually work, i.e. how they achieve what they are given for.

Analgesia (an = without, algesia = increased sensitivity to pain) is the absence of pain *without* causing loss of consciousness (general anaesthesia) or loss of touch sensation (local anaesthesia). Two major groups of analgesic drugs exist: the **opioids** and the **non-steroidal anti-inflammatory drugs** (**NSAIDs**). Basically, they work very differently, not only in their mechanism of action but also in the location of action within the nervous system. NSAIDs act in the tissues where pain originates from, i.e. they work *peripherally*, while opioids work in the brainstem and spinal cord, i.e. they work *centrally*.

Analgesia can and should be given, so long as it is needed, in any setting from hospital to the patient's home or hospice care. In those patients where further treatment options are not possible the term

palliative care is used. Palliative care indicates the management of symptoms, like being pain or nausea free, so that the patient will live out their remaining life in comfort and will not suffer at the time of their death. Under these circumstances it is not necessary to be concerned about drug addiction risks, but care must be taken to prevent accidental drug overdose.

The analgesic ladder and adjuvant therapy

The **World Health Organization (WHO)**(1986) introduced the concept of a stepped approach to pain management known as the 'analgesic ladder' (Figure 10.11).

Step 1:   The baseline treatment to start with is a *non-opioid* drug, e.g. a **non-steroidal anti-inflammatory** agent, with or without **adjuvant therapy** (see below). Such non-opioids include aspirin (except in children), paracetamol, ibuprofen or indomethacin.

Step 2:   If pain persists or increases an **opioid drug** suitable for moderate pain is introduced, with or without the NSAID, and with or without the adjuvant therapy. Such an opioid drug is codeine, dihydrocodeine, pentazocine, dipipanone, oxycodone or dextropropoxyphene.

Step 3:   If pain continues to persist or increase a stronger opioid drug is introduced, one reserved for severe pain, such as morphine, diamorphine, pethidine, papaveretum,

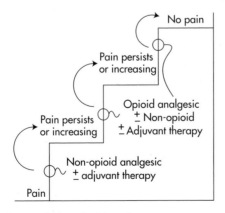

FIGURE 10.11 The analgesic ladder. If pain persists or increases the next level of analgesia must be attained. (Redrawn from Souhami and Tobias 2003.)

methadone, dextromoramide or fentanyl (see p. 276). The addition of the NSAID and adjuvant therapy remains an option as well. This is pursued until the patient is pain free.

In all cases, drugs must be given:

1 Enough to induce a pain-free state.
2 Regularly, not given on demand.
3 With a warning about potential side effects.
4 In conjunction with adjuvant therapy as required.

Adjuvant therapy is non-drug treatment for pain, and consists of a wide range of possibilities, from simple massage techniques to surgery. The following is a summary of adjuvant therapies available.

Local **radiotherapy** is very good for relief of symptoms including pain (see radiotherapy, p. 334).

Epidural infusion of local anaesthetic, perhaps given slowly via an infusion pump. Opiate drugs can be prescribed for delivery by this route when they cannot be tolerated by mouth. Infusions are into the **epidural space** (a space outside the **dura mater**; the outer of the three coverings of the central nervous system) within the spinal canal, and may be continuous or intermittent. Effectiveness is usually only for a few weeks after which tolerance becomes a problem, but it is very good for acute pain control without paralysis or disturbance of the autonomic nervous system.

Transcutaneous electrical nerve stimulation (**TENS**) is an electrical apparatus for delivery of a small charge across the skin surface, the purpose of which is relief of pain. It is effective, being used frequently in midwifery during labour, but its uses extend to other causes of pain. The analgesia comes on about 20 minutes or so after starting and continues for a significant period after use has stopped. There are no significant side effects. Limitations of use are few; i.e. it should not be used near the eye or over the heart if the patient has had a heart complication, not used on the head or neck in epileptic patients, and used with caution in pregnancy. It can interfere with the function of pacemakers and electrocardiographs (ECG) or electroencephalograms (EEG). How it works is not known but it may induce the closure of the spinal gate to pain (see gate theory of pain, p. 260);

Massage and **aromatherapy** can be used as adjuvant therapy.

Acupuncture; the Chinese art of inserting needles to relieve pain and other conditions. Like TENS, the way acupuncture works is unknown but it may prevent the flow of pain impulses through the gate control mechanism. The Chinese theory of *channels* and *collaterals* indicates the presence of 12 regular main trunks (*channels*) running horizontally and vertically across the body, connecting all the major parts of the body from inside out, from top to bottom. Thinner and smaller channels (*collaterals*) run as branches to all other areas of the body. These connections maintain the integrity and harmonious union of the entire body. It may be possible that these pathways coincide with the nervous system, as Western medicine recognises it. There are more than 300 standard acupoints along the channels and collaterals. Acupuncture prescription includes two or more points selected according to the symptoms and cause of the disease, and the functions of the points themselves. Applying needle stimulation to the prescribed points is said to regulate the body and restore any imbalance. It may release hormones from the endocrine system, stimulate the immune system and release antibodies and increase the body's resistance to inflammation (L. Zhang-Lheureux, personal communication).

Psychological support; i.e. staying with the patient, comforting, distracting their attention away from the pain (e.g. reading to them). Distraction, like television or favourite games, is particularly useful with children in pain.

Nerve block is carried out by injecting parts of the sensory nerves (e.g. the **dorsal root**) or sympathetic nerves with phenol or alcohol, thus blocking pain sensations. The destruction of the nerve by the chemical is irreversible, so the procedure is not carried out until other avenues have been tried.

Surgery is a last resort because it is also irreversible. The aim is to divide the pain pathways permanently and therefore stop the passage of pain impulses.

Non-steroidal anti-inflammatory drugs (NSAIDs)

To understand the **NSAIDs** we will begin with a visit to the margarine section of your favourite supermarket. Some margarines are rich in a substance called **linoleic acid**, a natural fat-based component of the diet. In the body linoleic acid is converted to another substance called **arachidonic acid**, and this becomes an important part of **phospholipids**, a large component of our cell membranes. But arachidonic acid is not only part of our membranes, it can be recovered from cell membranes if the need arises, since arachidonic acid is the basic substance (or substrate) from which other substances can be made (Figure 3.11, p. 86). One massive group of these other substances are **prostanoids**, a major class of chemicals that includes **prostacyclins**, **prostaglandins** and **thromboxanes**.

Prostacyclins, prostaglandins and thromboxanes act like hormones, mostly locally but sometimes systemically. Like hormones, they cause changes in the tissues, generally close to where they are produced. Prostacyclins, for example, cause several tissue changes, including local **vasodilation** (i.e. dilation of local blood vessels). Thromboxane A2 does the opposite by causing **vasoconstriction**. Prostaglandins are a large group of substances that have many effects, both locally and more widespread, including some like prostaglandin E (PGE) and prostaglandin F (PGF) groups, which cause pain. These prostaglandins are very important pain mediators which increase the sensitivity of nociceptors, making them respond more to other pain mediators, i.e. lowering the threshold to pain (see p. 257).

To produce all these chemicals from arachidonic acid requires the enzyme **cyclo-oxygenase** (**COX**), which occurs in two forms: COX-1 and COX-2. COX-1 is found in most cells most of the time (i.e. it is *constitutive*), whilst COX-2 is found in inflammatory cells when activated during inflammation (i.e. it is *induced*). NSAIDs work primarily by blocking (or inhibiting) COX-1 in peripheral tissues where the pain is generated. The best-known drug in this group is **aspirin** (a **salicylic acid**), which causes irreversible blockage of COX-1, thus preventing the formation of the prostaglandin pain mediators. **Indomethacin** (a derivative of **indole acetic acid**) also inhibits COX-1, **diclofenac** (derived from **phenyl acetic acid**) and **naproxen** (derived from **proprionic acid**) inhibit COX-1 and COX-2 equally, whilst **nabumetone** (derived from **naphthyl acetic acid**) blocks COX-2 specifically. Such selectivity for COX-2 means that nabumetone improves gastric tolerance when given by mouth, gastric intolerance being a problem noted for the COX-1 inhibitors.

Paracetamol, a well-known and popular analgesic drug is only a weak inhibitor of both COX-1 and COX-2, so its mode of analgesic action is still somewhat unknown. What is known is that some metabolites of arachidonic acid caused by the action of COX are **hydroperoxides**, and these in turn then further stimulate COX to produce more cytokines. Paracetamol blocks this feedback pathway, therefore inhibiting COX indirectly by stopping the activity of hydroperoxides. In this respect paracetamol is particularly active in the brain where it has an analgesic and an antipyretic effect, but no anti-inflammatory effect (Waller *et al.* 2001). As the group name NSAID suggests, most of these drugs are also **anti-inflammatory** (except for paracetamol as we have just seen), and reduction of inflammation may be of importance to some cancer patients, giving relief of some symptoms.

The NSAIDs are often marketed as tablets which have a combination of several drugs in one, and sometimes with **caffeine** added as this is said to enhance the analgesic property of the NSAIDs. Aspirin and other NSAIDs can be used in cancer pain control, especially in the very early stages and as a back-up measure when stronger drugs are in use (see analgesic ladder, p. 271). They are a very good means of controlling mild pain, but for severe pain there is often a need for an additional stronger analgesia: the opioid.

The opioid drugs

Opium, the natural product of the opium poppy plant, is a powerful analgesic and psychoactive drug. Its use in pain management, and also for sedation and even recreation, has been important for many years. It was used extensively in the last century as 'tincture of opium' (known then as **laudanum**), which contained **morphine**, an opium derivative. Laudanum is no longer used, but morphine is still used along with other opium derivatives, and these are a major means of solving the pain problem.

Unlike the NSAIDs, the opioid drugs work *centrally* within the central nervous system (CNS, i.e. the brain and spinal cord). They bind to special receptors within the brain and cord to provide a degree of analgesia at spinal cord level (called **spinous analgesia**) or brainstem level (called **supraspinous analgesia**). There are three main kinds of receptors on the surface of cells in the CNS that bind opioid drugs; the **mu** (μ), **kappa** (κ) and **delta** (δ) receptors. These receptors are referred to as **metabotrophic**, i.e. their activation changes the metabolism of the cell (see Blows 2003, pp. 41–3). The mu receptor is found mostly in the brainstem, and is the one mostly associated with supraspinous analgesia, respiratory depression, euphoria and dependence. This is the receptor that morphine and drugs like morphine mostly bind to. The kappa receptor is found in the upper spinal cord and provides spinous analgesia by blocking substance P (see p. 261). The relative importance of the delta receptor in pain control is not fully known.

But opiate receptors are not put on cell surfaces for the sole purpose of binding drugs; they bind naturally produced substances called **ligands**, i.e. ligands are products of the nervous system that bind to specific receptors. All nervous system receptors have their own particular ligand. In the case of the opioid receptors mu, kappa and delta, there are a number of *natural* ligands called **endorphins**, **enkephalins**, **dynorphins** and **endomorphines**. In addition, some less well-known small peptide ligands also exist, like **dermorphins** and **morphiceptins**.

Endorphins are the largest peptide molecules of the group. They come in various forms called **alpha (α)-endorphin**, **beta (β)-endorphin** and **gamma (γ)-endorphin**. They tend to be produced in the brain in response to severe pain and provide some degree of analgesia for around four hours or so.

Enkephalins are smaller peptide molecules. There are two types; **met-enkephalin** (where met = **methionine**) and **leu-enkephalin** (where leu = **leucine**). They are present in the ratio of about 4 met to 1 leu. They are produced in response to more mild pain and provide analgesia for around 2 minutes or so. Earlier, a neurotransmitter called **substance P** was identified as a facilitator for the passage of pain impulses across the synapse between neurons 1 and 2 of the pain pathways (see p. 261). Substance P is therefore a pain mediator at spinal cord level. By binding to kappa receptors in the spinal cord, enkephalin inhibits the release and therefore the function of substance P, thus reducing pain impulses at spinal cord level (see p. 262).

Dynorphins are of two known types, **dynorphin A** and **dynorphin B**, and are also small peptide molecules. Endomorphins are small peptide molecules that fall into two categories, **endomorphin-1** and **endomorphin-2**.

We take advantage of the receptors that naturally bind these ligands by delivering drugs that also bind to them; the **opiate drugs**. The principal members of this drug group include morphine, diamorphine, pethidine, codeine and fentanyl.

Morphine remains the major drug for pain relief in this group. It is the analgesic against which all others are compared. It is a potent analgesic for the management of severe pain, but it does cause respiratory depression (see p. 280), nausea, vomiting and constipation as side effects. It has found an important role in palliative care for the maintenance of a pain-free state, either given orally or by PCA (see

p. 278). Morphine also causes a state of euphoria (the reason for morphine addiction when taken in the absence of pain), and some degree of mental detachment (Blows 2003), which is useful in reducing the psychological response to pain.

Morphine has variable absorption when taken by mouth, and undergoes considerable **first-pass metabolism** in the liver, making injection more efficient as a route of administration. First-pass metabolism is the alteration of the drug in the liver after absorption from the bowel. These changes do not apply to the injected drug since only the drug delivered by the oral route is taken first to the liver by the hepatic portal vein. The metabolism of morphine in the liver results in a metabolite called **morphine-6 glucuronide**, which is a greater analgesic than morphine itself. **Morphine-3 glu-curonide** is also produced, but its pharmacological significance has not been fully evaluated. Morphine glucuronides are excreted through the urine, but also through the biliary system to the bowel where the morphine component is largely reabsorbed. Duration of activity is about 3 to 4 hours.

Diamorphine (**heroin**) is a powerful analgesic. It is more soluble than morphine and this is useful in palliative care to allow the injection of effective doses in smaller volumes. Diamorphine is converted to morphine in the body although diamorphine itself is more active as an analgesic than morphine. Diamorphine has greater powers than morphine in crossing the blood–brain barrier, and therefore enters the brain faster, especially when given intravenously (IV). This makes it attractive as a drug of illicit use. Diamorphine is active in the body for about 2 hours.

Pethidine provides rapid but short-lasting analgesia. It is less potent than morphine, even in higher doses, but it is less constipating. Severe pain on a long-term basis is better managed with drugs other than pethidine. Pethidine is metabolised in the liver to **norpethidine**, a metabolite with hallucinogenic and convulsant properties.

Codeine is made from morphine (codeine is **3-methylmorphine**), but is better absorbed when given by mouth than morphine, although it has only about 20% of the analgesic effect. Codeine is effective for treating mild to moderate pain but is not advisable for long-term use due to its side effect of causing constipation. It causes little or no euphoric effects and is therefore rarely addictive, and can be purchased without prescription.

Other opioid analgesia includes **fentanyl**, a drug with similar, but shorter-lasting actions to morphine, and is available in transdermal skin patches for the prevention of 'break-through' pain (i.e. transient periods of pain not prevented by other drugs). **Hydromorphone** and **nalbuphine** are others which have similar efficacy to morphine but with fewer side effects, especially nausea and vomiting.

Patient-controlled analgesia (PCA)

The ability for patients to take control of their own analgesia has become increasingly important and useful for patients and staff alike. Self-administration of even the more potent opioids in hospitals and hospices has provided the patients with greater and more consistent pain relief, and provided the staff with more time for other matters. The analgesia is delivered by means of a PCA pump (or *syringe driver*) attached to an intravenous (IV) or subcutaneous line (see Figure 10.12). This line consists of a cannula in a vein (IV) or under the skin (subcutaneous), usually in the arm, to which a delivery tube is attached. On the other end is the syringe driver, or PCA pump. The pump houses a syringe containing the analgesia, and by operating a switch, the pump pushes a controlled dose of a drug from the syringe, along the line into the patient. The line is usually separate from any other IV line, but could be combined with an IV fluid delivery system if this was desirable. Once operated by the patient, the pump usually provides a 'lock-out' period, perhaps about 5 minutes or so, during which the patient cannot operate it again. After the 'lock-out' period the pump is again ready for use. Patients can therefore keep pain under control according to their own needs. This saves the patient the need to alert staff whenever pain is a problem, and removes the difficulties for staff to try and assess the pain level that the patient is in (see p. 267). The drug and dose are prescribed by the doctor and prepared by the pharmacy, so the nurse has only to set up the pump and change the syringe when empty, according to the prescription chart.

A typical drug regime for PCA may consist of intravenous morphine, or subcutaneous diamorphine. Many units offering this treatment may prefer to use diamorphine as the drug of choice because its higher rate of solubility than morphine allows adequate dosages to be delivered in smaller fluid volumes.

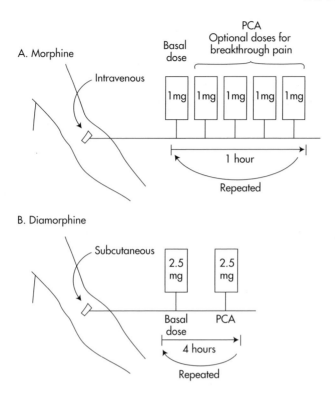

FIGURE 10.12 A diagrammatic representation of patient-controlled analgesia (PCA). Patients with severe chronic pain may be prescribed morphine or diamorphine. Morphine is usually given by continuous intravenous (IV) infusion, whilst diamorphine is the better drug to give by continuous subcutaneous infusion because larger doses of diamorphine can be concentrated in smaller volumes. Subcutaneous infusion is slower (0.1 to 0.3 ml per hour) than IV, and subcutaneous infusions are usually driven by a syringe pump. (A) *Morphine*: a basal rate of IV infusion of 1 mg per hour is a standard dose, with a bolus dose of 1 mg every 15 minutes that can be given by the patient themselves by pressing a button on the delivery apparatus if 'breakthrough' pain occurs. A total dose in 1 hour would be 5 mg. The delivery apparatus would be set to have a 'lock-out' period of 15 minutes, meaning the patient could not press the button twice in that time. (B) *Diamorphine*: a basal rate of subcutaneous infusion of 2.5 mg per 4 hours is a standard dose, with a 2.5 mg bolus dose available for the patient to self-administer to treat breakthrough pain (via pressing the button). The 'lock-out' time (and therefore the maximum 4-hourly dose) should be determined by the doctor. Irrespective of what drug or route is used, the patient should be reassessed for pain every 8 hours to determine if the basal infusion rate (and dose) needs adjustment (either up or down) to reduce the need for bolus doses.

The dosage of opioid analgesics has to be calculated accurately to combine a complete pain-free state without excessive drug administration, which would lead to unwanted side effects. Finding the right dosage level is called **titration** (see text for figure 10.12). Opioid drug titration is defined as *calculating the least amount of the drug required in circulation to achieve full analgesia.* A serious side effect that must be avoided is **respiratory depression**; i.e. the reduction in breathing caused by opioid drugs binding to receptors on the respiratory centre in the brainstem. Respiratory depression is particularly dangerous in the elderly (owing to reduced lung capacity) and in those with pre-existing respiratory disease, and both of these criteria apply to cancer. The elderly suffer cancers more commonly than the young, and if this is lung cancer it will already be seriously affecting the patient's breathing. Additional respiratory depression caused by the drugs could result in unnecessary complications. Opioid titration relies on feedback from the patient on their pain status, and this is where a pain assessment tool is of value. If they are still in pain then they require more analgesia. Each additional dose is less than the previous doses, and these 'top up doses' are given until a pain-free state is achieved (Figure 10.12). The other concern, that of drug addiction, does not apply to this situation. Giving opioids to treat pain does not cause addiction. Opioid addiction occurs only when the drugs are administered to individuals who are pain free from the start.

Key points

Pain

- Acute pain tends to be sudden and of short duration. Chronic pain has a longer duration of weeks, months or even years. Intractable pain is chronic pain unrelated to any detectable pathology.
- Localised pain is often caused by inflammation of the tissues involved.
- Pain mediators are released at the site; e.g. histamine, prostaglandins and bradykinins.

Pain pathway

- Nociceptors are pain nerve endings occurring in two types: mechanoreceptors and polymodal receptors.

- Two types of sensory nerve pathways carry pain impulses to the brain: fast 'A' fibres and slower 'C' fibres.
- The A and C fibres are the first neurons of a three-neuronal system from the periphery to the brain.
- The 'gate-control theory' describes a pain-blocking process in the spinal cord.
- The thalamic response to pain is to influence movement to help overcome the pain.

Pain assessment

- Pain assessment tools fall into three categories: verbal descriptor scales, visual analogue scales and pain behaviour tools.
- Child pain assessment tools often consist of a series of cartoon faces showing a range of expressions from happy (experiencing no pain) to very sad or crying (experiencing severe pain).
- Referred pain occurs some distance away from the site of the cause.
- The chronic pain suffered in cancer is caused by one or more of three effects: further advancement of the disease, the pain involved in treatment or pain from co-existing disease.
- Deafferentation pain is pain associated with loss of sensory input to the spinal cord and brain from one part of the body. It is a burning or 'vice-like', or electric-shock-like pain.

Analgesia

- The World Health Organization (WHO) introduced the concept of a stepped approach to pain management known as the 'analgesic ladder'.
- Adjuvant therapy is non-drug treatment for pain, and consists of a wide range of treatments from simple things like massage, TENS, acupuncture and aromatherapy, to nerve block and surgery.
- Analgesia is the absence of pain without causing loss of consciousness or loss of touch sensation.
- There are two major groups of analgesic drugs: the opioids and the non-steroidal anti-inflammatory drugs (NSAIDs).
- NSAIDs act in the peripheral tissues where pain originates, while opioids work centrally in the brainstem and spinal cord.
- Opioid drugs bind to the mu (μ), kappa (κ) and delta (δ) receptors within the brain and spinal cord.

- A drug acting on receptors at spinal cord level is called spinous analgesia, and at brainstem level is called supraspinous analgesia.
- The opioid receptors mu, kappa and delta are there to bind the naturally produced endogenous opioids called endorphins, enkephalins, dynorphins, endomorphins, dermorphins and morphiceptins.
- Palliative care is used for those patients where further treatment options are not possible. Palliative care indicates the management of symptoms, like pain, to allow comfort and improved quality of life.
- Morphine is the major opioid drug for pain relief, against which all others are compared. It is a potent analgesic for the management of severe pain, but it does cause respiratory depression, nausea, vomiting and constipation as side effects.
- Patient-controlled analgesia (PCA) is delivered by means of a PCA pump (or syringe driver) attached to an intravenous (IV) or subcutaneous line.
- Finding the right dosage level of analgesia is called titration.
- Opioid drug titration is defined as calculating the least amount of the drug required in circulation to achieve full analgesia.
- A serious side effect that must be avoided is respiratory depression.
- Respiratory depression is particularly dangerous in the elderly (owing to reduced lung capacity) and in those with pre-existing respiratory disease.
- Opioid titration relies on feedback from the patient on their pain status.

References

Acute Pain Management Guideline Panel (1992) *Acute Pain Management in Infants, Children and Adolescents.* AHCPR publication no. 92–0019, Rockville, Maryland.

Baker C. and Wong D. (1987) Q.U.E.S.T.T.: a process of pain assessment in children. *Orthopaedic Nursing*, 6 (1): 11–21.

Blows W. T. (2001) *The Biological Basis of Nursing: Clinical Observations*, Routledge, London.

Blows W. T. (2003) *The Biological Basis of Nursing: Mental Health*, Routledge, London

Clancy J. and McVicar A. (1998) Homeostasis – The key concept to physiological control (neurophysiology of pain), *British Journal of Theatre Nursing*, 7 (10): 19–27.

Jacques A. (1994) Physiology of pain, *British Journal of Nursing*, 13 (12): 607–10.

LeMone P. and Burke K. (2004) *Medical-Surgical Nursing, Critical Thinking in Client Care*, Pearson Education Inc., Prentice Hall, New Jersey.

Manchester Triage Group (1997) Pain assessment as part of the triage process, *in* Mackway-Jones K. (ed.) *Emergency Triage*, British Medical Journal Publishing Group, London.

Souhami R. and Tobias J. (2003) *Cancer and its Management* (4th edn), Blackwell Science, Oxford.

Waller D. G., Renwick A. G. and Hillier K. (2001) *Medical Pharmacology and Therapeutics*, W. B. Saunders, Edinburgh.

Wong D., Hockenberry-Eaton M., Wilson D., Winkelstein M. L., Ahmann E. and DiVito-Thomas P. A. (1999) *Whaley and Wong's Nursing Care of Infants and Children* (6th edn), Mosby, St Louis.

Wood S. (2002) Special focus: pain, *Nursing Times*, 98 (38): 41–4.

World Health Organisation (1986) Cancer pain relief. Geneva, Switzerland: Author.

Chapter 11

Nutrition and the cancer patient

- Introduction
- The elements of nutrition
- Nursing skills: nutritional considerations in cancer care
- Foods as a cause or prevention of cancer
- Key points

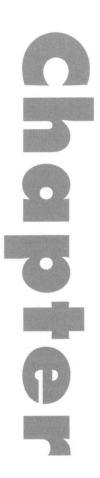

Introduction

Eating is fundamental to good physical, social and mental health, and is equally important in restoring good health during and after illness. This applies to cancer as much as the flu or any other illness. We need nutrition, not just for the provision of energy (although this is very important), but also for establishing resistance to infection, maintaining the healing process and ensuring that the metabolic processes of the cells continue to function normally. Without these functions the body would succumb to the disease process and die. And central to this need for nutrition is water. Without it the body becomes **dehydrated**, and all the cellular activities grind to a halt. Integral to nutrition, therefore, is **fluid balance** (Figure 11.1), the monitoring of water intake and output from the body. Patients with problems that affect the normal intake of food, e.g. vomiting, will have disturbance of fluid balance as well (Figure 11.2)

The elements of nutrition

The 'well-balanced diet' contains seven major categories of nutrients. They are **proteins**, **carbohydrates**, **fats**, **vitamins**, **minerals**, **fibre** and **water**. Of these, the proteins, carbohydrates and fats need some degree of digestion in order to render them available for absorption into the blood. Vitamins and minerals, however, need no digestion as they will be absorbed into the blood as they are. Fibre also needs no digestion simply because it is not absorbed; instead it remains in the gut and forms the bulk of faecal waste. This does not mean it is use-

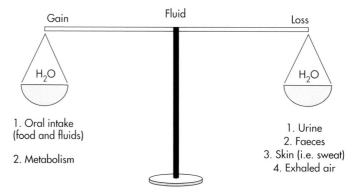

FIGURE 11.1 Normal fluid balance. Oral intake, and the much smaller amount of water produced by metabolism must match the output from urine, faeces and water lost through the skin and lungs.

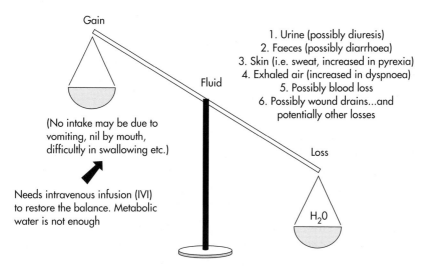

Gain

1. Urine (possibly diuresis)
2. Faeces (possibly diarrhoea)
3. Skin (i.e. sweat, increased in pyrexia)
4. Exhaled air (increased in dyspnoea)
5. Possibly blood loss
6. Possibly wound drains...and
potentially other losses

Fluid

(No intake may be due to
vomiting, nil by mouth,
difficultly in swallowing etc.)

Loss

Needs intravenous infusion (IVI)
to restore the balance. Metabolic
water is not enough

H_2O

FIGURE 11.2 Abnormal fluid balance. Oral intake is no longer available, and the loss of water may be increased (as shown), so intravenous infusion is required to correct the balance and prevent dehydration.

less and unnecessary to humans, as we shall see. Water, of course, also needs no digestion but is absorbed into blood directly.

Proteins

Proteins are our source of **nitrogen**, in the form of **amino acids**. Unfortunately we cannot avail ourselves of the free nitrogen in air (about 80% of air is nitrogen), instead we must eat it in the form of expensive protein.

Amino acids are the building blocks for proteins of all kinds. Amino acids consist of an **amino group** (**NH₂**), a **carboxyl group** (**COOH**) and a **radical** (**R**) or variable portion (Figure 11.3)(Blows 2003, pp. 39–40). The amino group contains the nitrogen, and changes in the radical produce the 22 different amino acids that we consume. Those that the body requires to be in the diet are called **essential amino acids** (tryptophan, lycine, methionine, phenylalanine, threonine, valine, leucine and isoleucine). They are essential because the liver cannot manufacture them, so dietary sources are critical. **Non-essential amino acids** (arginine, taurine, glycine, serine, glutamic acid, aspartic acid, tyrosine, cystine, histidine, proline and alanine) can be produced when required by the liver, by the conversion of the radical from one amino acid to another. However, their presence in the diet is desirable for day-to-day health.

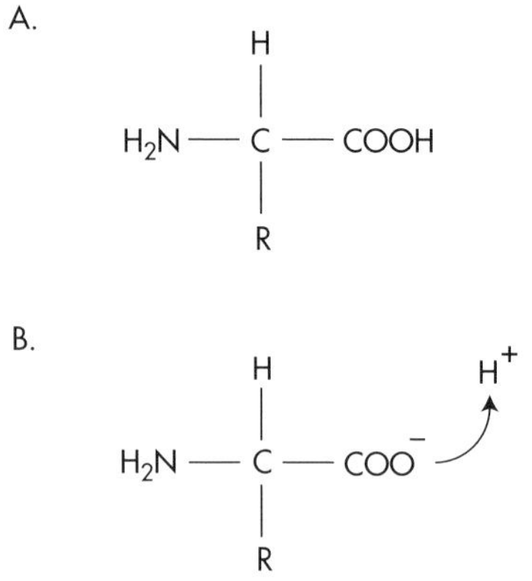

A.

$$H_2N \longrightarrow \underset{\underset{R}{|}}{\overset{\overset{H}{|}}{C}} \longrightarrow COOH$$

B.

$$H_2N \longrightarrow \underset{\underset{R}{|}}{\overset{\overset{H}{|}}{C}} \longrightarrow COO^- \quad \overset{H^+}{\curvearrowright}$$

FIGURE 11.3 (A) The basic structure of an amino acid (C=carbon; O=oxygen; H=hydrogen; N=nitrogen), where R is the variable radical. (B) Amino acids can liberate hydrogen ions (H⁺), and therefore are true acids.

The digestive process related to protein briefly works like this. Dietary *animal* proteins (like chicken, beef, lamb, fish and pork) and *plant* proteins are taken into the digestive system and reduced to their basic building blocks, i.e. amino acids, by protein-breaking enzymes. Most proteins are made from hundreds of amino acids. These amino acids are then collected from digestion by the blood and delivered to the body cells. Inside the cells the amino acids are rearranged and put back together as *human* proteins. So all the proteins in your body were originally from plants and animals, confirming the statement '*you are what you eat*'. Humans are mostly made of protein, and these include those needed to build the body (i.e. structural proteins, like muscle), enzymes, hormones, antibodies, and many others (Figure 11.4).

Carbohydrates

Carbohydrates are an abundant and diverse group of organic molecules. They are so called because they are made up of carbon, hydrogen and oxygen. A typical simple carbohydrate is **glucose**, chemically written as $C_6H_{12}O_6$, i.e. six carbons, twelve hydrogens and six oxygens. Glucose is the body's major energy source (see p. 305) and thus forms the end product of carbohydrate digestion and the basis of blood sugar.

Glucose is a sugar called a **monosaccharide**. Two such monosaccharides bonded together create a **disaccharide**, such as **sucrose**

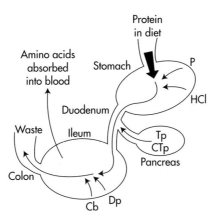

FIGURE 11.4 Summary of protein digestion. Proteins from the diet enter the stomach and are acted on by pepsin (P) in the presence of hydrochloric acid (HCl). Trypsin (Tp) and chymotrypsin (CTp) from the pancreas continue protein digestion in the duodenum, and carboxypeptidase (Cb) and dipeptidase (Dp) continue the process in the ileum.

(table sugar, which is a combination of the monosaccharides glucose and **fructose**). Fructose (fruit sugar) is not a typical blood sugar, so when it is absorbed from the digestive system it is quickly converted to glucose by the liver [note: the liver does a lot of converting of all sorts of things to glucose, as we will see later!]. So, glucose needs no digestion, it is absorbed just as it is; but disaccharides like sucrose must be digested to produce the two monosaccharides. Other carbohydrates are **polysaccharides** (i.e. the bonding of more than two monosaccharides to form a complex structure). Polysaccharides like **starch** (as found in flour) are capable of being broken down ultimately to monosaccharides. Other polysaccharides, however, are complex, and humans lack the enzymes to digest these, so they pass through the digestive system unchanged (see fibre, p. 298). Whilst polysaccharides, like starch, are bland to the taste, the more it breaks down into the simpler sugars the sweeter it becomes. Try this test: cut a 2 cm square of bread and hold it on your tongue absolutely still for a few minutes. An enzyme called **salivary amylase** in the mouth will break down the polysaccharide starch in the bread into disaccharide sugars, and the bread turns sweet in just a few minutes.

Dietary carbohydrates (mostly from fruits and vegetables) are taken into the digestive system and reduced to monosaccharides (mostly glucose). These enter the blood and are taken to the liver. Glucose may be converted to **glycogen** (a storage form of glucose created by a reversible chemical bonding of glucose molecules), or glucose may be delivered to body cells everywhere where it is used to form energy (see p. 302). Other monosaccharides are converted to glucose by the liver.

Fats (lipids)

Fat in the diet is in the form of **triglycerides**, which is a letter 'E'-shaped molecule, made from a **glycerol** backbone with three attached **fatty acids** (Figure 11.5). This is the form they arrive in the digestive system where they are split by the enzyme **lipase** into **monoglycerides** (the glycerol with one fatty acid attached) and two free fatty acids. In this form they are absorbed into the cells of the intestinal wall where they are reassembled as triglycerides again and combined with proteins. Protein aids fat transportation in a water medium since fats do not ordinarily blend with water. They are then further absorbed into the lymph at first, then on to the blood, in the form of **chylomicrons** (a collection of cholesterol, triglycerides and protein). The digestion of triglycerides is necessary only for absorption into the intestinal wall; the reassembled triglycerides are stored in the body as **adipose** tissue.

Fatty acids are essentially made from long chains of carbons. Each carbon atom has four possible bonds. In long chains the carbons bond to each other, but they still have vacant bonds to which other atoms could bond. Hydrogen has one bond, and will fill up carbon's vacant bonds very nicely. This results in two categories of fats, the **saturated** and the **unsaturated** fatty acids (Figure 11.6). Saturated fatty acids are so called because all the carbons are fully bonded to hydrogens.

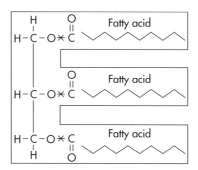

FIGURE 11.5 A schematic representation of the triglyceride molecule (the letter E shape, see text). It consists of a glycerol 'backbone' with three fatty acids attached (the bonds marked X are broken by the enzyme lipase).

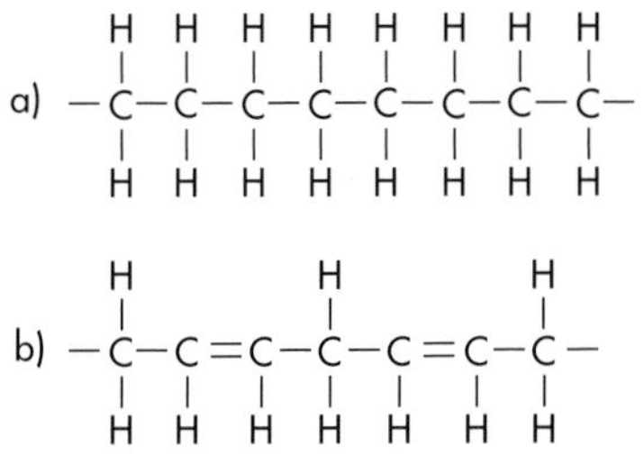

FIGURE 11.6 (a) Part of a saturated fatty acid, (b) part of an unsaturated fatty acid where some carbons (C) lack hydrogens (H) and are double bonded (=).

Saturated fatty acids are generally solid at room temperature, e.g. meat fats, and are not generally considered to be healthy in large quantities in the diet. Unsaturated fatty acids have vacant bonds along the carbon chains, so they are *not* fully saturated with hydrogens. These are generally liquid at room temperature, e.g. cooking oils, and are thought to be healthier than saturated fats as a dietary option. Everyone requires at least 10 to 15% (recommended to be 30%) of their daily calorie intake to be in the form of fats in order to obtain the minimum daily requirement of fat-soluble vitamins (see below). Fats are a rich and important energy source (see p. 303) and are the structural basis of cell membranes and some hormones, so their importance in the diet cannot be overstated. Also, some fatty acids are considered to be essential in the diet because they are unable to be formed by the body

Vitamins

The word **vitamin** comes from 'vital amine', and it classifies a group of elements that are essential in the diet for healthy tissue function. There are two main groups of vitamins, the **fat-soluble** forms (vitamins A, D, E, and K) and the **water-soluble** forms (the vitamin B group and vitamin C, plus others, see Table 11.1). Table 11.1 lists the major vitamins, their dietary sources and an overview of their functions. The table also indicates the diseases caused by a lack of the vitamin. You will notice that vitamins are given a letter of the alphabet, but some letters are not universally accepted and may not be found as such in many literature sources (e.g. vitamins F, H and P). Some vitamins are stored in the liver, notably vitamins A, K and B_{12}. There is about one month's worth supply of vitamin B_{12} in the liver.

TABLE 11.1 The major vitamins

Vitamin	Full name	Food source	a. Vitamin needed for b. Effects from lack of vitamin
A	Retinol	Liver, fish liver oils, butter, cream, cheese, whole milk, egg yolk	a. Growth, vision, healthy tissues, immunity b. Night blindness, dry and itching skin, reduced taste, bone growth failure
B_1	Thiamin	Yeast, cereals, legumes	a. Heart and circulation, growth, nervous system, energy b. Beriberi (fatigue, low appetite, weight loss, muscle wasting, diarrhoea, heart failure, oedema, paralysis), plus paraesthesia, depression
B_2	Riboflavin	Cereals, yeast, milk, eggs, green vegetable leaves, lean meat	a. Healthy skin, tissue healing, immunity, red blood cells b. Cheilosis (oral cracks and fissures, scaling of lips), sore tongue (glossitis), sensitivity to light (photophobia), and dermatitis
B_3	Niacin or niacinamide	Yeast, liver, kidney, meat, cereals, green vegetables, bran	a. Energy, skin, nervous system, cell metabolism b. Weakness, skin rash, memory loss, irritability, insomnia, pellagra (dermatitis, glossitis, diarrhoea, mental disturbance e.g. depression, confusion, hallucinations, delirium, leading to death)
B_5	Pantothenic acid	All plant and animal foods especially eggs, kidney, liver, salmon, yeast	a. Energy production, immunity, hormones b. Weakness, depression, low infection resistance

Vitamin	Full name	Food source	a. Vitamin needed for b. Effects from lack of vitamin
B$_6$	Pyridoxine	Pork, offal, fish, corn, legumes, seeds, grains, wheat, leafy vegetables, green beans, bananas	a. Protein metabolism, haemoglobin, nervous system b. Fatigue, nervous dysfunction, anaemia, irritability, skin lesions
B$_9$	Folic acid	Green leafy vegetables, liver, beef, fish, lentils, asparagus, broccoli	a. RBC maturation, growth, healthy tissues b. Anaemia, neural tube defects during very early pregnancy
B$_{12}$	Cyanocobalamine	Only from animal foods, liver, meat, milk, eggs, oysters	a. RBC (haemoglobin), growth, nervous system b. Pernicious anaemia: fatigue, glossitis, nerve degeneration
B$_{15}$	Pangamic acid	Sesame seeds, pumpkin seeds, whole brown rice, liver, offal	a. Unknown function b. No deficiency symptoms known
B factor	Choline	Yeast, milk, eggs, wheat germ, soya, offal	a. Nerve transmission, liver, cell membranes b. Growth problems, reduced liver and nerve function
B factor	Inositol	Milk, yeast, meat, fruit, nuts	a. Nerve transmission, fat metabolism b. Eye problems, constipation, hair loss
C	Abscorbic acid	Citrus fruits, strawberries, tomatoes, cabbage, potatoes, parsley, broccoli, sweet peppers	a. Collagen maturity, wound healing, maintains healthy gums, skin, immunity and blood b. Bruising, slow wound healing, anaemia, gingivitis, scurvy (fatigue and bleeding, later gum disorder)

TABLE 11.1 continued

Vitamin	Full name	Food source	a. Vitamin needed for / b. Effects from lack of vitamin
D	Calciferol	Milk, fish oil, liver, butter, egg yolk and ultraviolet light (UVL) in sunlight acting on skin	a. Absorption of calcium from the diet, good bones and teeth b. Rickets (children): soft, bent and fragile bones, deformity. Osteomalacia (adults): soft and painful bones, fractures
E	Tocopherol	Vegetable oil, whole grains, wheat germ, egg yolk	a. Antioxidant, maintenance of circulation and cell protection b. Poor muscle performance and circulation, RBC haemolysis
F	Unsaturated fatty acids	All sources of unsaturated fatty acids	a. Skin, blood and glandular products b. Acne, allergies, dry skin, brittle hair, eczema, brittle nails
H	Biotin	Liver, meat, eggs, nuts, milk, most vegetables, tomatoes, grapefruit, watermelon, strawberries	a. Skin, blood circulation, metabolism b. Depression, anorexia and non-specific skin rashes
K	Menadione	Lettuce, spinach, cauliflower, cabbage, egg yolk, soya bean oil, liver	a. Blood clotting mechanism b. Bleeding and diarrhoea
P	Bioflavonoids	Fruit, especially citrus	a. Healthy blood vessel walls b. Bleeding and bruising, colds, eczema

Other vitamins are not stored (e.g. vitamin C) and a daily intake from the diet is essential. Generally, fat-based vitamins are stored whilst water-based are not. Table 11.1 also indicates that 'vitamin B' is not a single entity but a range of numbered compounds (although not numbered strictly sequentially) that includes some B factors that are not numbered.

Minerals

Minerals are **non-organic elements** that are required by the body for maintenance of tissue function and health. The range of minerals in use in the body is large, but most are required in trace quantities, and thus are not often mentioned. Those that are well known, like calcium, are required in larger quantities, and will cause health problems if there is a lack in the diet. Table 11.2 shows the major minerals required in the diet.

Calcium is perhaps the mineral that is best known by most people. This is because mothers drum the importance of calcium into their children so that they drink their milk in the mornings. Calcium is well known to be important for bones and teeth, but it is also essential for blood clotting, muscle contraction and nerve conduction. However, mothers rarely say to their children '*drink your milk, you need it for good bones and teeth, blood clotting, muscle contraction and nerve impulse conduction*'. Perhaps they should, since the blood clotting mechanism, muscle contraction (especially cardiac muscle) and nerve conduction actually keep their children alive!

Minerals are capable of taking on an electrical charge, either positive or negative, to create **ions**. This happens when mineral compounds present in the diet, like **sodium chloride (NaCl)**, are dissolved in water, as in the human body. The mineral compound splits to form sodium (that takes on a positive charge $\rightarrow$ Na^+) and chlorine (that takes on a negative charge $\rightarrow$ Cl^-). The reason they take on these charges is because the sodium donates a negative electron to chlorine that accepts it readily. Having lost a negative electron, sodium's positive and negative balance is upset, and it becomes overall positive. Chlorine gains a negative electron, and that causes a greater overall negative charge than positive. Similar effects happen to **potassium chloride (KCl)** in the fluids of the body, to form K^+ and Cl^-. Positive ions are **cations**, whilst negative ions are **anions**. The word **electrolytes** is a term used for *ions in solution*, as in body fluids. It is important for electrolytes to balance in the body, i.e.

TABLE 11.2 The major minerals

Mineral (chemical symbol)	Mineral function	a. Food source, b. Deficiency causes . . .
Calcium (Ca)	Bones, teeth, muscle and nerve function, blood clotting mechanism	a. Milk and other milk products b. Weak bones and teeth, weak muscles, bleeding, poor nerve function. Severe loss of blood calcium causes tetany (a state of continuous muscle contraction)
Chromium (Cr)	Glucose metabolism, amino acid transportation, blood lipid and glucose levels	a. Full cream milk, seafood (e.g. oysters), whole grain, cheese, fresh fruit, nuts, vegetables, brewer's yeast and variable amounts in water b. Glucose imbalance, impaired growth, obesity, tiredness, increased cancer risk, heart disease and diabetes
Copper (Cu)	Haemoglobin in blood, collagen, heart function, energy production, iron absorption	a. Grains, nuts, liver, oysters and legumes b. Anaemia, muscle weakness, abnormal collagen synthesis, neurological defects
Iodine (I)	Thyroid hormones	a. Seafood b. Low thyroid hormone levels, goitre, cretinism, myxoedema
Iron (Fe)	Haemoglobin in blood, immunity, brain function	a. Liver, shellfish, oysters, lean meat, poultry, kidney, fish, beans and vegetables b. Anaemia, attention and learning difficulties, increased risk of infections
Magnesium (Mg)	Nerve and muscle function, bone formation	a. Leafy green vegetables, nuts, whole grain, peas, beans, dairy products, fish, cereals, legumes, meats b. Weakness, dizziness, abdominal distension, convulsions
Manganese (Mn)	Involved in calcium and phosphorus metabolism and bone formation	a. Legumes, nuts, whole grain cereal, tea, green leafy vegetables b. No specific deficiency syndrome identified
Phosphorus (P)	Bones and teeth, energy production, DNA formation, metabolism	a. Meat, poultry, fish, eggs, peanuts b. Serious problems with the nerve supply to muscles; skeletal, blood and kidney problems

Mineral (chemical symbol)	Mineral function	a. Food source, b. Deficiency causes ...
Potassium (K)	Intracellular electrolyte, factor in nerve conduction	a. Bananas, oranges, grapefruit juice, melons, nectarines, prunes, pears, avocados, cucumbers, potatoes, peas, beans, tomatoes, nuts, legumes, seeds, milk products, meats of all kinds b. Fatigue, depression, weakness, heart irregularities, dry skin, low blood pressure, oedema, muscle cramps
Selenium (Se)	Antioxidant, heart muscle, fat metabolism, tissue elasticity	a. Cereals, Brazil nuts, whole grains, seafood, meat, poultry, fish, dairy products b. Increased risk of cancer, myalgia (muscle pain) and muscle tenderness, heart disease (e.g. Keshan disease in China) and premature ageing
Sodium (Na)	Extracellular electrolyte, factor in fluid balance, blood pressure, muscle contraction, nerve conduction	a. Found widely in the diet, especially table salt, animal foods, processed foods b. Deficiency very rare
Zinc (Zn)	Gene expression in tissue growth/repair, cell reproduction, child growth, sperm and testosterone	a. Meat, poultry, fish, oysters, eggs, legumes, nuts, milk, yoghurt, wholegrain cereals b. Rare. Acrodermatitis enteropathica (rash over face, anus and distal parts), growth retardation in children, anorexia with diarrhoea, poor wound healing, depression, reduced reproductive ability

positives with negatives, for the normal function of body cells and tissues (Figure 11.7). Electrolyte imbalance causes serious changes in health. Our electrolytes are mostly derived from our diet, e.g. the sodium chloride (= table salt) put on fish and chips, and the calcium (Ca^{2+}) obtained from milk. Notice calcium, like some others, takes on a double positive charge (i.e. loses *two* electrons).

Sodium chloride (NaCl) is very important in the clinical area. A 0.9% strength solution is called **normal saline** and is used in a wide range of clinical functions, e.g. as a wound cleanser and for tissue and

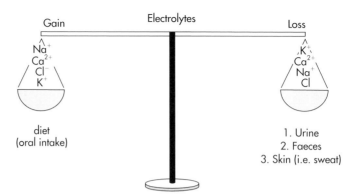

FIGURE 11.7 Electrolyte balance. Electrolytes (charged particles) in the diet (intake) must balance those lost in urine, faeces and through the skin.

eye irrigation. Sodium chloride 0.9% is **isotonic** (i.e. it has the same concentration as body fluids, notably blood plasma) and is therefore used as an intravenous infusion fluid. Sodium (Na^+) is the electrolyte found mostly in blood plasma and the extracellular (or tissue) fluid that surrounds the cells, whilst potassium (K^+) is the electrolyte found mostly *inside* the cells. Potassium in excess is potentially very dangerous and can cause fatal heart muscle irregularities. It is a sobering thought that we carry more than enough potassium inside our cells to kill us should it all ever get out into the blood! This would be a tragic example of electrolyte imbalance.

Selenium is interesting because, being a major **antioxidant**, it prevents the cell damage caused by **free radicals** (see p. 49). Patients with cancers have been found to have lower than average blood levels of selenium, and therefore selenium may protect against some cancers, especially those of the breast, lung, colon and prostate gland. It may even slow down that part of the process of ageing caused by free radical damage. Selenium levels in plant foods (see Table 11.2) are somewhat dependent on the selenium level in the soil. European wheat contains less selenium than American wheat for this reason, and therefore bread, a staple diet component, is apparently less selenium rich in Europe than it is in America (Rayman 1997). However, the UK imports more wheat from America than from Europe.

Fibre

Fibre (formerly called **roughage**) is the non-digested, non-absorbed component of foods. It remains in the digestive system and is eliminated from the bowel as a major component of faeces. At first, it may appear to be of no use to us and therefore is a complete waste as a dietary component. This is far from the truth. Fibre in the diet is as essential as anything else. Fibre is a collection of substances, notably **cellulose** and **hemicellulose** (both complex polysaccharides, see carbohydrates above), **pectins**, **gums** and **lignins**. Collectively these substances hold water by surface binding or by trapping it like a sponge. This helps to retain water in the bowel to make faeces soft and manageable. They also absorb and exchange **ions** (see electrolytes in the mineral section) and absorb **bile salts** (which are derived from the **bile**, a product of the liver). Bile salts are also irritants to the bowel and potentially toxic. Fibre therefore aids in the excretion of these substances. Fibre forms bulk in the stools, which is essential for the squeezing motions of the colon to act on. With low dietary fibre the colon struggles to push the faeces along, generating high internal pressures within the bowel and increasing the risk of bowel disease.

Whilst digestive enzymes do not affect fibre, small quantities of fibre can be digested by the natural bacteria that live in the colon. Known as the **intestinal flora**, these colon **commensals** (i.e. harmless bacteria that live in or on the body) are also essential for normal bowel function, and can synthesise some vitamins (e.g. niacin [vitamin B$_3$], thiamine [vitamin B$_1$] and menadione [vitamin K]) to our advantage.

The **caecum**, which is the first pouch of the colon near the appendix, is an important site for intestinal flora activity. Rabbits have a large extended caecum to be able to digest grass in significant quantities, since grass is full of fibre. Humans are unable to digest grass since our caecum is so small; most of our caecum appears to have been reduced to a structure we call the **appendix**.

Water

Water (**H$_2$O**) needs no digestion and is absorbed into the blood unchanged at most points along the digestive system, mostly from the colon. Water is absolutely essential for **metabolism** in the body, being the medium in which the majority of body chemical activities take place, and it is an important component of many chemical reactions.

Water is housed in three main compartments of the body: inside the cells (**intracellular fluid**), around the cells (**extracellular fluid**

[**ECF**], or just **tissue fluid**) and **blood plasma**. In a 75-kg adult the total amount of water in the body is about 45 litres. This is distributed as 30 litres intracellularly, 12 litres extracellularly and 3 litres in blood plasma (Figure 11.8). You may be wondering why there are only 3 litres of water in blood plasma when the total blood volume in circulation is about 5 litres. The answer is that the water constitutes the *plasma*, and therefore does not take into account the blood *cells* that make up the additional volume.

Water is constantly moving from one compartment to another, crossing semi-permeable membrane barriers, i.e. it crosses the capillary wall (between the blood compartment and ECF), and the cell membrane (between the ECF and intracellular compartment). In addition, water is both taken in and lost from the body. The average oral intake is about 2.5 litres per day, with an additional 500 millilitres (ml) of water added as a product of metabolism (= 3 litres per day). Urine water loss per day averages around 1.5 litres with additions from faeces (200 ml), through the skin (900 ml) and through respiration (400 ml) (= 3 litres per day). All these changes need constant regulation to prevent either too little water in the compartments (**dehydration**) or excessive water in the body. The matching and equalising of water intake with water loss is called **fluid balance** (Figure 11.1). Water is *gained* by the body mostly through oral intake; certainly drinking, but also the water present in food. Water is also

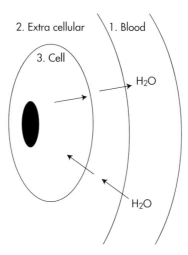

FIGURE 11.8 The three water compartments. Water in the blood (1) moves across the capillary membrane into the extracellular space (2) where it is called extracellular fluid (ECF, or tissue fluid). Water enters the cell (3) from the ECF. Water returns in the opposite direction.

gained from some forms of tissue metabolism, i.e. as a chemical by-product of certain chemical processes. This source of water is limited and would not be enough to sustain life, so oral intake is essential. Water is *lost* from the body by the process of elimination (mostly as urine, but also faeces), and through both the skin (evaporation of sweat) and the lungs (exhaled water vapour on breath) (Figure 11.1).

Because of the dangers of losing control of this balance in ill-health, it is vital to monitor both intake and output in those patients who are at risk of this problem; notably post-operative patients, the elderly, and the chronic and terminally ill. Also at risk are those who are prevented from taking oral fluids (i.e. due to nausea and vomiting, oral or oesophageal disease, or are deemed *nil by mouth*). Vomiting, a potential side effect of chemotherapy (see p. 323), would also increase fluid loss, as would diarrhoea, blood loss or excessive loss from post-operative drains (Figure 11.2). Oral or oesophageal disease may either prevent the normal mechanism of swallowing or block the passage of food to the stomach. Water lost through the skin, the faeces and the lungs is known as **insensible loss** because it cannot be measured on a day-to-day basis in the clinical area. It must, therefore, be *estimated* for the purposes of fluid balance each day, and it should be remembered that this route of loss would increase in **hyperventilation** (over breathing) or excessive **sweating** (due to high body temperature, as in some infections or fever).

Fluid replacement is best achieved orally whenever possible, not only to prevent dehydration, but also because drinking is a major means of keeping the mouth clean and preserving the mucosal membranes as barriers to infection. The alternative, for those who cannot drink, is an **intravenous infusion** (**IV**) of fluids (Nichol *et al.* 2000, pp. 43–58). This replaces fluids generally, but because the mouth is bypassed it becomes dry, sore and at risk of infection. Mouth infections can spread to the chest, ears and even the brain. If the patient is then allowed or becomes able to eat, but has a sore and dirty mouth, this alone may prevent them from eating. Special attention must be given to any patients on intravenous infusion to keep their mouth and teeth clean and healthy (Nichol *et al.* 2000, pp. 199–201).

Intravenous fluids must usually be **isotonic**, i.e. they must have the same concentrations of *solutes* (dissolved substances) as blood plasma. If this were not the case it would have serious, life-threatening consequences on the patient's blood cells. Isotonic fluids include **normal saline** (see p. 297) and **dextrose 5%**. The former provides water with minerals, whilst the latter provides water with sugar (and therefore energy). The choice of which fluid is used is usually based on the patient's hydrational needs. Full nutrition can also be given by the intravenous route (see p. 311).

Fluid balance monitoring is critical in all patients who are not drinking adequately, and especially if they are on IVI. The healthy adult should drink a minimum of about 2 litres of water per day although this is not always achieved. The ill person should try to achieve as much of this as possible, given their particular circumstances. Fluid balance monitoring will not only identify the potential for dehydration but also for circulatory overload; a particular problem if the patient is on IVI and has renal or cardiac complications (Nichol *et al.* 2000, pp. 131–2). The kidneys have a major role in fluid balance; excreting water when there is excess, and conserving water when there is little entering the body. The heart has the job of pumping blood (which is mostly water) around the body, and will suffer if the blood volume is too great.

Metabolism and energy

Metabolism is the collective noun for all the chemical processes taking place in the body. Of course, most of these processes occur inside the cells, but many also take place in body fluids (e.g. blood) and body cavities (e.g. the bowel). Metabolism falls mainly into two forms: the building up processes and the breaking down processes. Those that start with simple substances (e.g. amino acids) and build these into more complex structures (e.g. proteins) are called **anabolism**. Those that start with complex substances (e.g. polysaccharides) and break these down to form simple substances (e.g. monosaccharides) are called **catabolism**. Metabolism uses **enzymes** as agents of chemical change. These are proteins that promote change to take place without themselves becoming chemically involved in the change. Metabolism requires the raw material on which to act, and these raw materials are mostly the nutrients in our diet, delivered to our cells by the blood. Metabolism also generates wastes, like **carbon dioxide** (CO_2) and **urea**, which must be removed and excreted. Metabolism is ultimately responsible for all the cellular activities, including **energy** production.

Energy is produced in cells in the form of **adenosine triphosphate** (**ATP**), a high-energy molecule that can store the energy until required by the cell. Many foods are said to have an energy value because they contain carbohydrates, fats or protein, i.e. the nutrients that can fuel energy production in the cells. Carbohydrates have an energy value of 4 **kilocalories** (**kcal**) per gram (g), lipids have an energy value of 9 kcal/g, and proteins have an energy value of 4 kcal/g. One kilocalorie is 4.186 **kilojoules** (a standard international [SI] unit for energy), so the values for the three food types stated here in kilojoules are carbohydrates (4 × 4.186 = 16.744 kilojoules), lipids (9 × 4.186 = 37.674 kilojoules) and proteins (4 × 4.186 = 16.744 kilojoules). This final figure for protein is the same as for carbohydrates, and this is because when the time comes for protein to act as an energy source the amino acids are converted to glucose (see p. 234). Interestingly, **alcohol** also has some limited nutritional value because it provides energy, having an energy value of 7 kcal/g (7 × 4.186 = 29.302 kilojoules). However, alcohol does *not* provide any other nutrients.

Metabolism has its lower limits below which cellular chemistry must not fall. The **basal metabolic rate** (**BMR**) is described as the *minimum* rate of internal energy expenditure whilst *awake* but at *rest*. This means that if metabolism falls below this specific level it endangers health, and even life. This level is 1.25 kilocalories per minute for males of 65 kg weight and 0.9 kilocalories per minute for females of 55 kg weight. Sleep induces metabolic rates about 10% lower than the BMR, whilst physical exercise, as would be expected, drives metabolism higher than the BMR, although the BMR itself is raised in exercise.

Energy balance is a comparison between energy intake (in the form of food) and energy use by the cells. **Neutral energy balance** indicates that the energy intake and cellular expenditure match exactly. However, energy intake and expenditure often do not match. **Positive energy balance** is the consumption of more energy in food than is used by the cells. On a long-term basis this results in excess energy storage in the body, in the form of fats (**adipose tissue**), increasing the risk of becoming overweight (**obese**). The opposite is **negative energy balance**, where there is consumption of less energy in food than is used in the cells. The long-term effect is gradual loss of stored energy, with ensuing weight loss.

Energy, of course, is needed for the process of growth, both in height and weight. Measuring weight and height provides very good indicators of positive or negative energy balance. However, a third indicator is the **body mass index** (**BMI**), which compares weight with height. If you know the patient's weight (in kilograms) and their height (in metres) then you can calculate their BMI. The formula is:

$$BMI = Weight\ (kg) \div [Height\ (m)]^2$$

What this means is that the BMI is the weight divided by the height squared, i.e. the height is multiplied by itself. For example, if the weight was 55 kg, and the height was 1.5 m, the BMI would be 55 ÷ 1.5^2, or 55 ÷ (1.5 × 1.5), or 55 ÷ (2.25), which equals 24.4. Notice there are no *units*, it is just 24.4, hence it is an *index*. The ideal BMI falls between 20 and 25, whilst 30 or above is considered to be obese.

Whilst normal growth represents a healthy *anabolic state*, the cancer patient in the latter stages of the disease may be in a *catabolic state*, i.e. the forces of tissue breakdown are dominant over any tissue growth or repair (see p. 308). The BMI in cancer patients is at risk of falling seriously below the ideal levels, for the reasons we consider next.

Nursing skills: nutritional considerations in cancer care

Progressive cancer causes a loss of weight (both fat and muscle losses), plus it causes **anorexia** (loss of appetite) and eventually **cachexia** (see p. 305). All this is aggravated by the presence of nausea and vomiting associated with radiotherapy and chemotherapy treatments, and the emotional stress ill health causes. If the patient undergoes any surgery this further debilitates them, putting additional energy demands on their nutritional status (e.g. for wound healing) during the recovery period. The picture can easily become one of uncontrolled tumour growth whilst the patient wastes away.

Traditionally the patient has been encouraged to eat as well as possible to make good these losses. A high protein diet, for example, may help to replace wasting muscles, whilst additional carbohydrates replace the body's energy. However, some considerations may need to be made. For example, a fast growing tumour is likely to be accelerated in its growth by increased food intake. The tumour takes advantage of the supply of nutriments for its growth along with normal tissues. Slow growing tumours, on the other hand, may allow the patient to increase their food intake without adversely affecting the tumour growth pattern.

Patients should try to achieve optimum nutrition to ensure the maximum possible resistance to the effects of the malignancy and the debilitation caused by the treatment. This can become an uphill struggle for both the patient and their carer, particularly in patients who find the whole concept of eating tiresome and undesirable owing to their anorexia, nausea and general weakness. Generally, the tumour's growth increases demand for two major nutritional components: the nitrogenous amino acids derived from proteins, which causes depletion of the muscle stores of amino acids, and energy, derived from carbohydrate and fat stores in the body. Reinstating these stores to as near to normal as possible improves the patient's general condition so they feel better and can respond more favourably to treatment. Symptoms such as **ascites** (oedema in the abdomen, causing the abdomen to swell) may also improve under better nutritional conditions because low plasma proteins are one cause of oedema (Table 11.3). Plasma proteins are made in the liver from amino acids derived from dietary protein. Part of their role is to attract fluid from the tissues (called **extracellular fluid**, or **ECF**), back into the blood. Low plasma proteins will allow fluid to accumulate in the tissues (known as **oedema**). It is important to remember that this is only one of several causes of oedema (see Table 11.3), any of which may occur as a result of cancers.

Energy use and cachexia

Starvation is very much an undesirable state for anyone, but the cancer patient may be propelled into this condition if the disease is not controlled or halted and the patient's nutritional status falls into decline. As the body loses its oral intake of food it quickly uses up the carbohydrates in the blood (i.e. glucose) which are replaced from stored glucose in the liver, i.e. **glycogen**. Muscle also has stored glycogen which is available for the muscle's own use. These stores allow glucose levels to remain relatively steady for much of the patient's illness.

Carbohydrates are the first source of energy in the body, and a lack of glucose from the diet also increases a metabolic process called **gluconeogenesis**. This means the creation (= genesis) of new (= neo) glucose (= gluco); new in the sense that the glucose comes from *non-carbohydrate* sources, notably fats at first, and ultimately proteins. Fats (i.e. adipose tissue) are therefore broken down to release **glycerol** (see p. 290) which is taken to the liver via the blood and converted to glucose. Fats are the second source of energy in the body, coming into play when glucose is exhausted. Along with glycerol, adipose breakdown releases additional **fatty acids** (see p. 290) into

TABLE 11.3 Causes of oedema

Cause of oedema	Physical mechanism	In cancer
Low plasma protein level	Plasma proteins attract water out of the tissues back into blood. Low levels will have the effect of leaving the tissue fluid to accumulate in the tissues	This can be the result of poor diet, notably low protein, due to prolonged anorexia, weakness or vomiting
Low plasma sodium level	Plasma sodium similarly attracts water out of tissues back into the blood, and low levels fail to do this	This can be the result of prolonged vomiting or diarrhoea coupled with poor dietary sodium intake
Lymphatic obstruction	A major route for the return of tissue fluid to the blood is via the lymphatic system. Obstruction of this system allows tissue fluid accumulation (called lymphoedema)	Due to lymphatic node obstruction by the cancer cells (i.e. nodal secondaries), or caused by surgical removal of lymph nodes
Venous blood obstruction or congestion	Tissue fluid normally returns to venous blood plasma. Venous obstruction or congestion prevents the plasma from taking further tissue fluid and it accumulates in the tissues	Obstruction of the veins by a tumour pressing on them from outside, or by infiltrating and blocking the veins
Increased capillary permeability	The capillaries in the tissues are semi-permeable membranes that allow fluid through from the blood at a specific rate. Increasing that permeability causes a rise in the rate of fluid passing through the wall, and this excess fluid can accumulate in the tissues	This occurs in inflammation and is the cause of the swelling associated with inflamed areas. Some cancers cause inflammation in the tissues surrounding them

circulation, some of which can be used to drive energy production, but much of which will be converted to **ketones** by the liver. Under normal nutrition, ketones are produced in small quantities, and these are taken up by the muscles as an energy source, hence none are found in normal urine. But in starvation, when fatty acid levels in the blood are raised and muscle itself is likely to be deteriorating, excess ketones are produced. These cannot be used by the muscle and they are therefore filtered into the urine through the kidneys, creating a **ketonuria**. Ketones are acids, and this means that significantly raised amounts in the blood reduce the blood **pH** (the measure of the **acid–base balance**) from the normal pH 7.4 (which is just slightly alkaline). This pH change due to ketones causes serious complications called **keto-acidosis**. Once all the fat stores in the tissues are exhausted the body is in crisis. There is little option but to turn to protein as an energy source.

In the long term, therefore, proteins (especially muscle) will suffer a similar fate to fat, i.e. they will be broken down to form glucose, if the glucose shortage continues. Protein is the third and final source of energy, and when it is depleted the body has no further energy stores. Amino acids from muscle proteins are also broken down in the liver, and later by the kidneys (a breakdown process called **deamination**) to produce glucose and **urea** (the waste product containing the nitrogen; see p. 234). **Lactic acid** is also a potential source of glucose energy made available by the liver once it is delivered to the liver by the blood from muscles. Lactic acid is a byproduct of **anaerobic metabolism** in muscles, i.e. cellular chemical processes taking place without adequate oxygen. Muscles cannot themselves convert lactic acid to glucose (only the liver can do this), thus large quantities of lactic acid can seriously affect muscle activity unless the blood removes it quickly. Lactic acid, like ketones, is acidic (i.e. it has a low **pH**) and is therefore going to seriously reduce the pH of the muscles if it is allowed to accumulate there, or may contribute to a lower blood pH in circulation, leading to acidosis. The deamination of amino acids causes difficulties with fluid balance due to the elimination of increased levels of nitrogenous urea and acidic wastes, both of which require ample water to dissolve in; water which is lost along with the wastes. The picture becomes one of profound weight loss, dehydration and acidosis, all of which seriously affect tissue function, leading to organ malfunction. Ultimately the patient is likely to die from cardiac, renal or other organ failure, combined with a keto-acidosis, a profound hypoglycaemia and protein deficiency. The time taken to reach this end varies with the amount of stored adipose tissue the starved patient started with; but typically around eight weeks unless nutritional support can be maintained.

Cachexia is a *syndrome* (i.e. a collection of symptoms) that marks a particularly bad stage of a disease, which may occur during the end stage of the disease (i.e. during the final weeks and days of the patient's life) or be demonstrated by a slow decline throughout. It marks the onset of specific biochemical changes that begin the process of cellular and tissue breakdown. The syndrome is identified by significant **muscle wasting** (loss of muscle tissue leading to reduced muscle bulk and strength), **adipose atrophy** (i.e. a **lipolysis**, or fat breakdown) causing a loss of fat tissue (adipose) and leading to a profound loss of weight and profound **weakness** (energy loss). Muscle wasting and adipose atrophy together indicate that the patient is in a serious *catabolic state* (**catabolism** being a metabolism characterised by tissue breakdown). The effect of these changes causes the patient to become extremely thin, with little flesh over the bones. They are so weak they become immobile, and therefore at risk of skin breakdown and multiple infections.

The patient suffers a severe loss of appetite (**anorexia**) and starts the metabolic process of survival based on their body reserves of fat and muscle. As these dwindle (see p. 307) the patient sinks to a physical low point from which recovery is difficult or impossible. Add to this a sense in the patient that the *end is near*, i.e. they take on a mental attitude that death is inevitable, and they are basically giving up on life; then the risk of death for this patient becomes obvious. They move from a state of anxiety, through depression, then to the point of being resigned to their fate. The process is gradual, perhaps taking weeks rather than days for most patients, depending on the rate of growth of their tumour. And neither is cachexia confined to cancer patients, but sometimes can also be found in other terminal conditions such as **AIDS** and **tuberculosis**.

What happens in cachexia is complex and not fully understood. What appears to be happening is that a substance called **tumour necrosis factor-α** (**TNF-α**, also called **cachetin**) is produced by activated **macrophages**. TNF-α, in conjunction with another chemical called **interleukin-1** (**Il-1**), has some *valuable* functions. It activates immune cells (called **lymphocytes**, **eosinophils** and **natural killer** [**NK**] cells) to attack the tumour, and it may damage the tumour directly by harming its blood supply. However, it also has some *harmful* effects on the body, especially in the long term. These unwanted effects include:

1 An increase in the adhesion of **granulocytes** (white blood cells that have granules containing chemicals) to **endothelium** (the inner surface cells of blood vessels), where these granulocytes then **degranulate** (i.e. discharge their granules). Chemicals from the granulocytes form **free radicals** (see p. 49) which then attack healthy tissues around the body and can induce circulatory collapse.

2 Endothelial cells losing their usual anti-coagulant properties, thus allowing increased deposits of fibrin on blood vessel walls. This leads to **diffuse intravascular coagulation** (i.e. many small blood clots forming throughout the circulatory system). Blood clotting factors may become low and this leads to bleeding.

3 In the short term combined TNF-α and Il-1 re-route nutrients away from the periphery to the liver, promoting an acute response to tumour formation; but in the long term they cause abnormal carbohydrate, protein and fat metabolism.

4 Anorexia is a consequence of long term TNF-α and Il-1 activity, and may be increased by a dietary zinc deficiency, lost or abnormal taste of food or the presence of liver metastases (see p. 240).

Two other chemicals are also implicated in cachexia, **interleukin-6** and **interferon-γ [gamma-interferon]**. *Interleukin-6* normally initiates a non-specific inflammatory response to infection, including NK cell activation, and thus helps to mediate natural immunity, and *interferon-γ* is a growth inhibitor (in normal and malignant cells) and activates inflammatory cells (including NK cells and macrophages) against viral-infected and tumour cells. In cachexia, however, these substances have been identified as playing an important role in abnormal fat breakdown (interferon-γ) and protein breakdown (i.e. muscle wasting) (interleukin-6). The picture is complicated by a cascade effect involving other cytokines which make it difficult to assess which cytokine is responsible for the clinical state. In addition, some products released by the tumour itself contribute to the overall effects, e.g. some **lipolytic hormones**, which break down fats and cause anorexia and a negative **nitrogen balance**. Proteins are the source of nitrogen in the diet, thus anorexia combined with muscle (human protein) breakdown and wastage causes more nitrogen to be lost from the body than taken in (i.e. a negative nitrogen balance).

The metabolic changes seen in cancer patients are:
Increases in all of the following:

1 Gluconeogenesis.
2 Glucose usage.
3 Insulin resistance.
4 Blood levels of lactic acid.
5 Adipose breakdown.
6 Glycerol turnover.
7 Blood fatty acid levels (a **hyperlipidaemia**).
8 Whole body protein turnover.
9 Skeletal muscle breakdown.
10 BMR.

Decreases in the following:

1 Building of skeletal muscle.
2 Appetite (an **anorexia**).
3 Glucose tolerance.
4 **Lipoprotein lipase** activity, an enzyme that breaks down fats (i.e. triglycerides) that are combined with protein (a combination called **chylomicrons**, see p. 290) in circulation. Failure to break down these fats results in further hyperlipidaemia (high blood fat level).

The management of cachexia is particularly difficult and provides the caring professions with a major challenge. The problem is how to supply adequate nutrition when:

1 The body has serious adverse chemical processes going on.
2 The patient does not want to eat, and may have lost the will to live.

Some mechanisms for feeding the patient are required to give nutritional support even if the outcome is not expected to be good. No patients should die from starvation if they are terminally ill, since starvation will only add to their suffering. To die in comfort means more that just being pain free and psychologically at peace, they must also be as free as possible from nutritional inadequacies, including dehydration. The problem, however, is that in cachexia the nutrients provided are not being metabolised and used correctly by the body, making nutrition difficult to achieve. Feeding may not always help, and certain feeding regimes, like **total parenteral feeding (TPN)** (see below) may sometimes exacerbate the problem. Each case must be assessed individually to determine the way forward.

Feeding the patient

The normal mechanism of oral feeding is by far the preferred method of feeding for all patients because it is the easiest to achieve, the most natural method and is the least invasive. Oral feeding may require considerable patience and some skill to achieve in some cases. Careful monitoring of the amounts consumed is important in order to identify at what point inadequate nutrition may be a possibility. Maintaining a fluid balance record will help to identify the potential for dehydration.

As has been mentioned, oral feeding is not always possible, and other means of feeding are then required. These alternatives may be via the **enteral** and **parenteral** routes. **Enteral feeding** means the delivery of nutrition directly into the digestive tract, using a tube that bypasses the oral route and therefore avoids the swallowing of food. Tubes may be inserted through the nose into the stomach (a **nasogastric tube**) or into the intestines (a **nasointestinal tube**), or inserted through the abdominal wall into the stomach (a **gastrostomy tube**, or **percutaneous endoscopic gastrostomy [PEG]** tube) or into the jejunum (a **jejunostomy tube**). Note that '-stomy' means *opening into*, in this case either the stomach (gastrostomy) or the jejunum (jejunostomy). By avoiding the mouth, oesophagus and swallowing mechanism they can be used when disease prevents the normal function of these structures. Enteral feeds may be given as *intermittent* (300 to 500 ml of enteral formula given several times per day, a total of about 1500 ml per day), or given as *continuous* (enteral formula delivered over 24 hours by an electric enteric infusion pump). Enteral formula deliver about 1 calorie per ml, and they contain the required mix of proteins, fats, carbohydrates, vitamins, minerals and water, and may be purchased commercially or prepared individually for the patient following assessment by the dietician. Being in liquid form, it is difficult (but not impossible) for enteral formulas to contain fibre, but the fibre content is likely to be significantly reduced below what might be consumed normally.

Parenteral feeding (or **total parenteral nutrition; TPN**) is the delivery of nutrition directly into the bloodstream by the intravenous route. This is done to avoid the entire digestive system when normal or enteral feeding is not possible. Delivery of nutrition directly to the blood means that digestion will not happen, so the nutrients themselves must already be in the form of the end products of digestion. Thus, the fluids used must already have proteins reduced to amino acids, carbohydrates reduced to glucose, and so on, with no fibre (since fibre never reaches the blood normally). Intravenous TPN is mostly delivered via a **central venous catheter**, i.e. an intravenous line established into a central vein rather than a peripheral vein, and often maintained by an electric infusion pump. It is demanding on both the patient and the carer and still carries a risk of complications. The procedures and care of enteral and parenteral feeding can be found in detail in Nichol *et al.* (2000, pp. 86–94).

Foods as a cause or prevention of cancer

Some foods are said to be a potential cause of cancer, mainly because they contain substances claimed to be **carcinogenic** (see p. 45). On the other hand, other foods are claimed to be protective, i.e. they prevent cancer, again because they have certain ingredients. This is always a complex, large and controversial subject because there are constant uncertainties, such as:

1 If a food substance causes cancers in rats, does it cause cancer in humans?
2 If a food ingredient is thought to be carcinogenic to humans what, if any, is a dangerous dose?
3 Are there any other unknown substances, good or bad, in our food? Research is suggesting that there are plenty of both.
4 Does organic production or the genetic manipulation of food change its health status, for good or bad?
5 Does cooking, prolonged storage or going beyond the 'sell by' date change the health status of our food?

And there are many other questions like these that need to be answered before we know the whole story about the food that we eat. It boils down to inadequate research, but science is catching up with the problem. Here are some of the claims made so far, often with significant scientific support. First, some of the reports that indicate *bad* findings.

Acrylamide, a known cancer-causing chemical, has been found in significant quantities in starch-based foods cooked at high temperatures (i.e. frying and baking, *not* boiling) such as chips, crisps and breakfast cereals (Starck 2003).

An excess of 250 calories per day above that normally required in the diet during childhood increases the risk of cancer later in life by 20% (Frankel *et al.* 1998).

Now, some of the reports that indicate *good* findings.

Flavonoids (or **bioflavonoids**) are a large group of agents, some of which are antioxidants, and as such they may have anti-cancer properties. Examples under examination are **naringenin** (found in grapefruit), **isoflavones** (found in soya), **hesperetin** (found in oranges) and **quercetin** (found in onions). People who eat foods rich in flavonoids are said to have an overall lower risk of cancers (Anon. 2003a).

Other flavonoids are found in tea, and these also have antioxidant activity. These flavonoids are **catechins** (simple flavonoids found mostly in green tea), and **theaflavins** and **thearubigins** (more complex flavonoids found in black tea). Green tea is protective against many cancers, especially lung, stomach and early breast cancer. This may be due to their ability to prevent the growth of new blood vessels, and of course tumours need new blood vessels to develop further.

The phenols in tea include **phenolic acids**, and these have more powerful antioxidant activity than vitamin C, E or A. Black (Indian) tea, the type mostly drunk in the UK, is a fully oxidised form of the same leaves as green (Chinese) tea, and contains similar quantities of phenols as green tea. These phenols appear to repair the mutagenic damage to DNA (see p. 38), which is responsible for some cancers, especially colon cancer (Anon. 2003b). This effect on DNA damage includes some protection against ultraviolet (UV) light damage from sunshine (see p. 57).

Another green tea component is **EGCG**, a **urokinase** (**uPA**) inhibitor, which blocks the uPA enzyme. This enzyme helps cancers to invade tissues and form metastases. EGCG in Chinese green tea may help to protect against breast and prostate cancers, if drunk in large enough quantities. Black tea lacks EGCG (Jankun *et al.* 1997).

Eating five or more portions of fruit and vegetables per day cuts our cancer risk by 20% (Anon. 1998a), and this has become government policy. A 'portion' is recognised as 80 grams (or 2.8 ounces). Spinach and beans of all kinds are especially healthy and protective against cancer. Between 66 and 75% of all gastric cancers are preventable by appropriate diet (Anon. 1998b). Green vegetables are particularly valuable in the diet for many reasons, including as a protection against cancers. A chemical called **allyl-isothiocyanate**

(**AITC**), which is a breakdown product of a compound called **sinigrin**, is released when green vegetables are chopped, chewed or cooked. AITC gives green vegetables a bitter taste, and is probably why children particularly do not like eating greens. The **brassica** family of vegetables, such as cabbage, broccoli, cauliflower, sprouts and swede, appears to be an important source for AITC. Two or three portions of the brassica family per week in the diet are now recommended, with the best cancer protection occurring if they are cooked in a little water and for the shortest time as possible.

AITC blocks reproduction of colon cancer cells and can trigger **apoptosis** (cell death, see p. 13) in malignant cells. The chemical also has a protective role against lung cancer, and possibly prostate cancer.

Those persons who eat very few green vegetables have double the risk of cancer compared with those who eat them regularly, indicating the anti-cancer protective role for green vegetables is significant. The emphasis is on prevention, not as a cure, so a life-long habit of eating green vegetables regularly is a healthy lifestyle that should be established early in childhood.

Grapes contain a natural product called **resveratrol** which appears to inhibit all the stages of cancer development, namely **initiation**, **promotion** and **progression** (see p. 45) (Jang *et al.* 1997).

Omega-3 fatty acids found in fish, but especially salmon, inhibit various cancers, particularly bowel and breast cancers (as well as being protective against a range of other diseases). Walnuts are also a good source of omega-3 and antioxidants, and are also protective against many diseases including cancer.

Citrus fruit *peel* has another compound called **limonene** which reduces the risks of skin cancers.

Anthrocyanin in blueberries protects the skin against the harmful effects of sunlight and boosts brain function. Blueberries are a fruit that contains five different types of anthrocyanins.

Lycopene from tomatoes (particularly cooked tomatoes as in tomato ketchup) is protective against cancers, especially gastrointestinal cancers and prostate cancer in men.

Yoghurt protects against cancers by reducing the chemical activity that otherwise would lead to the formation of carcinogens (see p. 45).

Soya beans when digested produce a substance called **equol**, and this blocks the production of the male hormone **dihydrotestosterone** (**DHT**). DHT causes growth of the male reproductive tract, including the prostate gland, and so may be involved in the cause of prostate cancers. By blocking DHT, equol may have a protective role against prostate cancer, as suggested by the lower rates in Japan where soya beans are eaten widely.

Soya beans also contain **genistein**, a component that helps in breast development and appears to be protective against breast cancers. Eating soya products during adolescence reduces the risk of breast cancers later in life, and those women having a soya-rich diet appear to have a 60% less risk of developing large amounts of dense breast tissue which could lead to cancer.

The Chinese mushrooms called **shiitake** and **reishi** contain the chemical **lentinan** which boosts the immune system to destroy tumour cells (see p. 66).

The above claims are based largely on scientific research which indicates a trend, and more research is constantly underway to confirm these trends. The trends do suggest that a healthy diet provides far more beneficial chemicals for our health than harmful ones, and diet should be given much greater consideration in sickness and in health. Clearly we have not heard the last about diets and cancer yet, not by a long way.

Key points

Diet

- The 'well-balanced diet' contains proteins, carbohydrates, fats, vitamins, minerals, fibre and water.
- Negative energy balance is the consumption of less energy in food than is used in the cells. The long-term effect is gradual loss of stored energy, with ensuing weight loss.
- Proteins are a source of nitrogen, in the form of amino acids.
- Glucose may be stored as glycogen, or delivered to body cells everywhere where it is used to form energy.
- Fats, in the form of triglycerides are stored in the body as adipose tissue.
- The two main groups of vitamins are the fat-soluble forms (vitamins A, D, E and K) and the water-soluble forms (e.g. the B group and C).
- Minerals are non-organic elements that are required by the body for maintenance of tissue function and health.
- Water and fibre are also essential components of the diet.

Intravenous infusion and BMR

- Special attention must be given to any patient on intravenous infusion to keep the mouth and teeth clean and healthy.
- Fluid balance monitoring is critical in all patients who are not drinking adequately, and especially if they are on IVI.
- Intravenous fluids must usually be isotonic, i.e. they must have the same concentrations of solutes as blood plasma.
- Isotonic fluids include normal saline and dextrose 5%.
- The basal metabolic rate (BMR) is described as the minimum rate of internal energy expenditure whilst awake but at rest.

Cancer

- Progressive cancer causes a loss of weight, anorexia (loss of appetite) and eventually cachexia, a syndrome identified by muscle wasting, adipose atrophy, weakness and a sense of hopelessness.
- Some mechanisms for feeding the patient are required to give nutritional support even if the outcome is not expected to be good.
- Oral feeding is by far the preferred method for all patients. However, patients may be fed via enteral means (tube feeding into the digestive tract) or parenteral means (intravenous feeding).

References

Anonymous (1998a) Health, the 5+ a day way, *World Cancer Research Fund, Newsletter (on diet, nutrition and cancer)*, issue 33: 3.

Anonymous (1998b) Stomach Cancer . . . facts in focus. *World Cancer Research Fund, Newsletter (on diet, nutrition and cancer)*, issue 30: 3.

Anonymous (2003a) Flavonoids, **http://www.hollandandbarrett.com/healthnotes/Supp/Flavonoids.htm**

Anonymous (2003b) Understanding complex phenols and tannins. **http://www.flair-flow.com/consumer-docs/ffe44701.html**

Blows W. T. (2003) *The Biological Basis of Nursing: Mental Health*, Routledge, London.

Frankel S., Gunnell D., Peters T., Maynard M. and Smith G. (1998) Childhood energy intake and adult mortality: the Boyd Orr cohort study, *British Medical Journal*, 316: 499–504.

Jang M., Cai L., Udeani G. *et al.* (1997) Cancer chemo-preventive activity of resveratrol, a natural product derived from grapes, *Science*, 275: 218–20.

Jankun J., Selman S., Swierca R. *et al.* (1997) Why drinking green tea could prevent cancer, *Nature*, 387: 561.

Nichol M., Bavin C., Bedford-Turner S., Cronin P. and Rawlings-Anderson K. (2000) *Essential Nursing Skills*, Mosby, Edinburgh.

Rayman M. (1997) Dietary selenium: time to act, *British Medical Journal*, 314: 387–8.

Starck P. (2003) Cancer risk in chips, french fries, bread – study, **http://www.icnr.secure sites.com/acrylamide.htm**

Chapter 12

The treatment of cancer

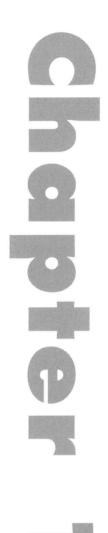

- Introduction
- Surgery
- Chemotherapy
- Nursing skills: the administration of cytotoxic drugs
- Radiotherapy
- Hormonal treatment and immunotherapy
- Adjunct therapy
- Prevention of cancer
- Key points

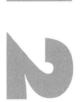

Introduction

The treatment of cancer is multifaceted, meaning that a number of different ways of tackling the problem are employed, often at the same time, to give the maximum possible benefit to the patient. These treatment methods include not only the mainstream therapies of surgery, radiotherapy and chemotherapy, but other important and developing scientific approaches such as immunotherapy and hormonal treatments. Other additional treatments are also available where required (like stem-cell therapy, see p. 108), and supportive treatments (such as blood transfusions) are vital in many cases to maintain the normal state of the body. Some patients also believe in other adjunct treatments such as herbal medicines and aromatherapy, and these can give the patient comfort and hope. Mixed in with this cocktail of treatments is the need for pain control (the subject of Chapter 10) and management of the stress and anxiety that the diagnosis of cancer will bring. This chapter looks at the biology behind the main treatments of surgery, chemotherapy, radiotherapy, immunotherapy and hormonal therapy.

Surgery

The reasons for surgery in cancer treatment are obvious. If the patient has a new growth it makes sense for this new growth to be removed. **Excision** (cutting out) of new growths wherever possible is important for several reasons. First, surgery removes as much of the malignancy as possible to prevent further growth and spread. Second, it reduces the bulk of a tumour which otherwise is a burden to the body, i.e. the tumour will consume energy and nutrients, it may produce unwanted amounts of hormones or other harmful substances and it may obstruct, squeeze or infiltrate surrounding tissues. Third, surgery can interfere with tumour growth in circumstances where it cannot be removed, e.g. it may be possible to reduce the blood supply to a tumour and this will cause it to regress. Fourth, surgery often corrects the defects that are caused by the tumour, e.g. creating a bypass around the obstruction can often relieve obstructions that cannot be cleared. Fifth it can be a major component in pain relief. Many of the procedures listed above will make the patient more comfortable and improve their quality of life and reduce the need for large doses of analgesic drugs. Finally, surgery may offer the patient some hope towards a future cure. It is not usually a cure in itself; in the vast majority of cases surgery needs follow-up treatment to answer the problem of secondary growths. But surgery will often make the postoperative treatment period shorter and with a much greater chance of success.

Surgery sounds like a vital first step in cancer management, and so it is in many cases. But surgery has its own set of problems, and whether or not to go ahead with an operation is often a matter of weighing the facts in favour of surgery against the facts that would prohibit it. Some of the important problems are the following.

First, since cancer is more frequently a disease of the older aged population than any other age group, surgeons find themselves deciding whether or not to operate on the elderly, i.e. those who are least well equipped physically to withstand surgery. Cancer surgery is often extensive, putting an enormous burden on the older person during the days immediately after the operation. Many of the elderly may not have the optimum respiratory fitness in order to tolerate an anaesthetic, quite often due to a lifetime of smoking. Alongside this is the fact that this older person is already ill, and may have been for quite a while, and is therefore not at their peak physical condition. Surgery, and the accompanying anaesthetics, put yet another burden on the patient's health, and it may be, in many cases, a burden too far. In these cases, surgery is no longer an option, and the benefits of surgery are therefore lost to that patient.

Second, surgery is not, even today, entirely safe, at any age. Whilst every effort is made to reduce the risks, complications can and do arise, and this will add a further burden on the patient's health and quality of life. Complications are numerous and varied, including problems such as haemorrhage and infections, and these may be enough to cause the patient to deteriorate, again, especially if they are elderly.

Third, surgery may cause disfigurement. Here too great efforts are made to prevent any such disfigurement, but sometimes it is unavoidable. Facial disfigurement (e.g. following surgery for facial, mouth or jaw cancers) is one of the hardest for patients to come to terms with, and the follow-up reconstructive surgery only adds to their physical and psychological burden. Other forms of disfigurement, such as loss of a limb, are also major traumas for the patient to live with. It involves a rapid reassessment of one's own body image by the patient, after many decades of being used to the way they look and feel. The burden is increased when the patient has to re-learn a basic function, such as feeding, walking or elimination, e.g. following a **colostomy** (see p. 142), or the patient faces the rest of their life in a wheelchair. It is easy to see that, in the elderly particularly, surgery can tip the balance in favour of the patient wanting to end it all, leading to a rapid decline in the patient's health as they lose interest in life.

Postoperative care following cancer surgery is always a major challenge for health-care professionals of all kinds, particularly nurses. This means not only for the physical care needed (e.g. the pain relief), but also for the psychological support these patients will need. This is particularly important when the surgery is **palliative** (i.e. it only relieves the symptoms or improves the quality of life, but the tumour remains), or when further postoperative treatment is required, or complications occur. Some surgery may be required simply to confirm a formal diagnosis, and if the cancer proves to be at an inoperable stage the patient will have to be told the bad news when they awake. This requires a very sensitive approach with support for the patient from the family as well as the nurses.

Surgery is a life-saving vital first step in many cancer treatment regimes, and the success of other subsequent treatments will often depend on it. Like all therapies, it needs to be considered carefully in all cases, on an individual basis, looking at all the known facts about the patient's diagnosis, prognosis, current health status, the risks involved and, not least of all, the patient's own desires and concerns. A joint consultation is usually planned between the patient, the family and the surgeon, where every aspect of the patient's illness and the surgery can be discussed, and this meeting will usually point the way towards the decision on how to take the treatment forward.

Chemotherapy

Chemotherapy (drug treatment) is the main approach to anti-cancer treatment, either on its own or after the initial surgery. The drugs used in the treatment of cancer are of the type that prevents the reproduction of cells, i.e. cell division. The faster the rates of cell division, the more the cells are affected by the drugs. Since tumour cells divide quickly they are susceptible to drug treatment. Cells that divide quickly are those that are constantly passing around the cell cycle in quick succession (see cell cycle, p. 8 and Figure 1.5). In normal tissues the cells of the bone marrow, the gonads (sperm in males and ova in females), mucous membrane and those of stratified epithelium (e.g. the outer layer of the skin, see p. 16) have the fastest cell division, and are therefore the cells most affected by these drugs. Complications of cytotoxic drug therapy include, particularly, the risk of damage to these tissues and, although normally they heal or recover quickly, this may not be the case during the course of chemotherapy because the drugs may interfere with the healing process.

A good account of cytotoxic therapy can be found in Waller *et al.* (2001). The main groups of chemotherapy drugs are:

1 Alkylating agents.
2 Platinum compounds.
3 Topoisomerase I and II inhibitors.
4 Cytotoxic antibiotics.
5 Antimetabolites.
6 Drugs disrupting microtubule function.
7 Others.

The side effects of cytotoxic therapy are very unpleasant, making this one of the treatments feared the most by patients with cancer. These unwanted effects are:

1 Distressing nausea and vomiting will be accompanied by **anorexia** (loss of appetite) and intolerance to oral fluids makes the patient reluctant to drink.
2 Bone marrow suppression, where bone marrow produces too few cells leading to low numbers of red blood cells (causing an **anaemia**) and white blood cells in circulation.
3 **Alopecia** (hair loss, which will slowly grow back in most cases after treatment is stopped).
4 **Teratogenesis** (the ability of the drug to cross the placenta during pregnancy and affect the developing foetus).
5 **Hyperuricaemia** (high levels of uric acid in the blood which is filtrated into the kidneys where it forms crystals and can inhibit kidney function) (see also p. 333).

The alkylating agents

These include four groups of drugs: (1) the **nitrogen mustards** (e.g. **cyclophosphamide, melphalan** and **chlorambucil**); (2) the **sulphonate esters** (e.g. **busulphan** and **treosulphan**); (3) the **cyclic** nitrogen derivatives (e.g. thiotepa); and (4) the nitrosoureas (e.g. carmustine and lomustine).

The original drug (chlormethine, also called mustine) was developed from sulphur mustard gases used as a weapon in First World War trenches. The nitrogen mustards, sulphonate esters and cyclic nitrogen derivatives kill cells during cell division by binding to DNA (deoxyribonucleic acid, see p. 4) during G_0 and G_1 of the cell cycle (see p. 11) (Figure 12.1) and in so doing block DNA and RNA synthesis. This may cause the formation of cross-links between opposing guanine bases on opposite strands of the DNA, i.e. a bridge link between the strands, a process called intercalation, that prevents the DNA from unwinding (Figure 12.2). Alternatively the binding of these drugs may cause misreading of the DNA code, and therefore disrupt RNA synthesis. The nitrosoureas bind to proteins and therefore block DNA repair. In either case the affected cell will die.

The alkylating agents have two main complications associated with their prolonged use. First, they may interfere with gametogenesis, the formation of sperm or ova, and this can lead to infertility.

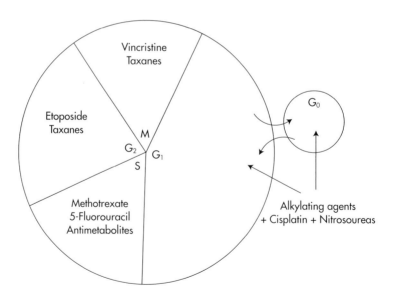

FIGURE 12.1 The cell cycle and the points where the major anti-cancer drugs act. Those that interfere with cell division act during mitosis (i.e. cell-cycle dependent), and since cancer cells pass through mitosis often they are more vulnerable to these drugs. M = mitosis, G_0 = 'resting phase' (leaving the cell cycle), G_1 and G_2 = growth phases, S = synthesis phase (see also Figure 1.5).

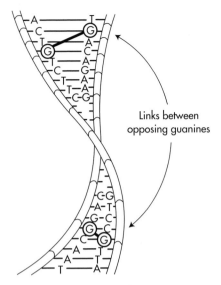

Links between
opposing guanines

FIGURE 12.2 Intercalation. The action of some anti-cancer drugs is to bind opposing guanines (G) with links that prevent the DNA strands from separating. This blocks any further attempt at RNA or DNA synthesis and the cancer cell will die.

Second, again on a long-term basis, they have been linked to **acute non-lymphocytic leukaemia**, especially if used in combination with radiotherapy. However, this does not appear to be a problem with short-term use of these agents. The side effects, however, can be very unpleasant (see p. 323).

Platinum compounds

The drugs in this group include **cisplatin, carboplatin** and **oxali-platin**. They are a good choice of drug in the treatment of ovarian and testicular cancers. Like most of the alkylating agents, these drugs also cause cross-linking of guanine bases on the DNA during G_0 and G_1 of the cell cycle (see p. 11), making DNA unavailable for RNA and DNA synthesis, and the cell will die (Figure 12.2). They are given by the intravenous route rather than by mouth because they have such poor absorption from the digestive tract. They are excreted by the kidneys but can be a cause of renal toxicity, and the patient should drink well to aid in the drug's safe elimination. This may be easier said than done as the side effects (see p. 323) include nausea and vomiting, and drinking may not be tolerated by the patient. They can also cause **ototoxicity** (damage to the ears) causing hearing losses and **tinnitus** (i.e. continual noises, buzzing or whistle sounds heard in the ears). **Peripheral neuropathy** (the term means damage to the nerve tissues in the extremities) is another complication of these drugs, where tingling or burning sensations are felt in the feet or hands.

Topoisomerase I and II inhibitors

The enzymes **topoisomerase I** and **II** between them cut one or both strands of DNA (**cleavage**) in order to allow these two DNA strands to unwind and separate, a necessary process for DNA and RNA synthesis. They also allow the reverse to occur (where the two strands reform the usual double helix formation), and rejoin the original cut ends. By blocking the function of topoisomerase I, the drugs **ironotecan** and **topotecan** prevent the separation of the DNA strands and therefore both DNA and RNA synthesis cannot take place, killing the cell. They are large molecules and are delivered by intravenous infusion (IVI), with most of the metabolism and excretion occurring via the liver. Side effects of these drugs are as noted for all cytotoxic drugs (see p. 323), but also include **myelosuppression** (reduction in the production of cells in the myeloid bone marrow cell line, see p. 97), and gastrointestinal effects like **diarrhoea** (loose or watery stools).

Etoposide is a drug with a slightly different means of action. It binds to the complex formed by the joining of DNA and the enzyme **topoisomerase II**. This enzyme is involved in the cleavage, uncoiling and recoiling of the DNA double helix during DNA replication, and works along with topoisomerase I. The drug causes DNA strands to break and blocks DNA replication mostly whilst the cell is in G_2 of the cell cycle. The cell will therefore die. Etoposide can be given by mouth but absorption is not easily predictable and it is therefore often given by the intravenous route. It may cause the usual side effects (see p. 323). Etoposide is protein-bound in circulation and excretion is via the kidneys (Souhami and Tobias 2003).

Cytotoxic antibiotics

Antibiotics are thought of generally as drugs that act in killing foreign cells like bacteria, but some will kill malignant cells. These include **doxorubicin, epirubicin, mitoxantrone, bleomycin** and **mitomycin**. They act partly like other drugs in that they prevent DNA synthesis by causing intercalation (see p. 324) between the two

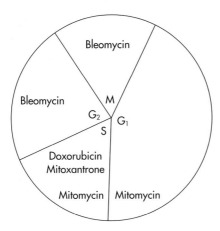

FIGURE 12.3 The points on the cell cycle where the anti-cancer antibiotics work (see also Figures 1.5 and 12.1).

DNA strands (Figure 12.2), but they also have other ways of damaging and destroying cells. They create **metabolites** (i.e. products of metabolism) which are called **free radicals.** These free radicals are highly reactive molecules which interact with the structures inside the cells, including DNA, and damage them. They also interfere with membrane function, including free radical membrane damage. The cells cannot survive this degree of intracellular destruction and loss of function, and will die. Most of these antibiotics work in all parts of the cell cycle, but others are particularly active in the S phase (doxorubicin and mitoxantrone), in the G_1 and early S phase (mitomycin) and G_2 and mitosis (bleomycin) (Figure 12.3). Poor digestive absorption means these drugs are given by intravenous infusion. They have the general side effects of all cytotoxic drugs (see p. 323) but may also cause cardiac complications (known as **cardiomyopathy**), especially doxorubicin. This drug will also cause extensive tissue damage if the delivery cannula becomes extravasated (see p. 332).

Antimetabolites

These drugs work by becoming incorporated as a component of the DNA at the time it is produced by the cell and blocking the function of normal enzymes that act on it. Other antimetabolites become an irreversible attachment to cell enzymes, thus causing these to fail. The cell is no longer able to survive. Antimetabolites fall into two main groups: folate antagonists and purine or pyrimidine base analogues.

Folate antagonists are drugs where the component is a **folate** (or **folic acid**) **analogue**, i.e. analogue means the drug very closely resembles the structure of a vital component of metabolism but, being slightly altered, it does not act as such. In this case the structure of the drug is very close to that of folate, and these drugs include **methotrexate**. When incorporated into the folic acid metabolic pathway, methotrexate inhibits the enzyme **dihydrofolate reductase**. Folic acid is essential for the formation of DNA, and when the metabolism of folic acid fails the cell dies (Figure 12.4).

Purine or **pyrimidine base analogues** (they closely resemble the purine bases, i.e. **adenine** and **guanine**, or the pyrimidine bases, i.e. **cytosine** and **thymine**, all major components of DNA, see p. 6) include **cytarabine** (also called **cytosine arabinoside**, a pyrimidine analogue), **5-fluorouracil** (or **5-FU**, a pyrimidine analogue) and **6-mercaptopurine** (a purine analogue).

Methotrexate is well absorbed from the digestive tract and is also given by intravenous infusion and via the **intrathecal** route, i.e. directly into the **cerebrospinal fluid** via a **lumbar puncture**, a needle placed between the lumbar vertebrae. Antimetabolites cause

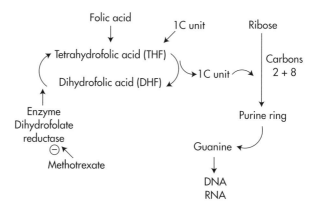

FIGURE 12.4 Folic acid is converted to THF which receives units containing one carbon (1C). THF then donates these units to the sugar ribose as part of the formation of the purine ring. THF contributes two such 1C units to the ring, these become the carbons at positions 2 and 8 of the ring. By donating a 1C unit it becomes DHF, and to receive further 1C units it must be converted back to THF by the enzyme DHF reductase. Methotrexate inhibits the function of DHF reductase and this prevents THF conversion, and thus blocks the purine ring synthesis. The purine ring forms the basis of guanine, a vital component of both DNA and RNA, and without the ring guanine and DNA/RNA synthesis stops.

similar side effects to those seen generally for cytotoxic drugs (see p. 323).

Drugs disrupting microtubule function

The **vinca alkaloids** (e.g. **vincristine, vinblastine** and **vindesine**) are drugs that bind to a protein inside the cell called **tubulin**. This protein forms the building blocks for **microtubules**, essential components of the cell's protein **cytoskeleton** (the internal framework of the cell). Like our *bony* skeleton, the cell's *protein* 'skeleton' provides shape and support to the cell. But it is also the framework that forms the **mitotic spindle**, to which chromosomes attach during **metaphase** of **mitosis** (see p. 10). When drugs of this group bind to tubulin they disrupt the mitotic spindle, causing failure of cell division, and the cell will die. The drug is active, therefore, only during mitosis.

The vinca alkaloids are especially useful drugs in the treatment of lymphomas (see p. 107) and leukaemias (see p. 98). They are given by the IV route only, and can induce the general side effects of cytotoxic drugs (see p. 323) as well neurotoxicity symptoms, like peripheral neuropathy (see p. 265).

Taxanes (i.e. the drugs **paclitaxel** and **docetaxel**) bind to microtubules and promote their assembly (and conversely inhibit their breakdown). The resultant stabilised microtubules cannot be removed by the cell, including the mitotic spindle which should normally disappear after mitosis. This means the cell cannot complete mitosis and will die. The main action occurs during G_2 and mitosis (Figure 12.1). Poor oral absorption means that delivery is by intravenous infusion. They can cause the general side effects of most cytotoxic drugs (see p. 323), but also **neutropenia** (low blood levels of **neutrophils**, see p. 95), **arthralgia** (joint aches) and **myalgia** (muscle aches). Paclitaxel can also induce neuropathy (disorder of the nerves), depending on the dose.

Other cytotoxic drugs

An assortment of other drugs are available for anti-cancer therapy. **Razoxane** (which is not commonly used) binds metal ions, making them unavailable for cancer cell use. **Amsacrine** has a similar action to that of doxorubicin, i.e. it causes intercalation (see p. 324) between base pairs on DNA. **Crisantaspase** is an enzyme called **asparaginase**, and this removes the amino acid **asparagine** from all protein synthesis. Without this amino acid many proteins will fail to assemble or function. **Pentostatin** inhibits the enzyme **adenosine deaminase**, and this in turn inhibits the formation of **deoxyribonucleotides** (the building blocks of DNA). **Procarbazine** prevents the incorporation of both adenine and thymine into DNA (see p. 6).

Hydroxyurea inhibits the formation of deoxyribonucleotides (see also pentostatin above). **Altretamine** binds to large molecules (called **macromolecules**) and this includes DNA. The cell dies but the killing mechanism is not fully known. **Dacarbazine** and the structurally related **temozolomide** have an alkylating function (see p. 323) and block DNA repair. **Tretinoin** is the acid form of **vitamin A** (**retinol**) known as **retinoic acid**, and this binds to intracellular receptors triggering gene transcription involved in regulation of epithelial growth and differentiation (it is used also in the treatment of acne and skin damage by excessive light, i.e. sunburn).

Nursing skills: the administration of cytotoxic drugs

Chemotherapy agents are potentially dangerous if they are not handled properly. To give some idea of this, the original drugs used in cancer were derivatives of a nerve gas agent used as a weapon in the First World War (see p. 324). Because of this, these drugs must be used with great care, and cautions are put in place to prevent chemical injuries to staff and patients alike. The biggest dangers come from drugs getting onto skin, or splashed into the eyes. Guidelines, policies or protocols are usually in place in oncology units to protect nurses and doctors against the harmful effects of these drugs during preparation and administration, and with good reason, so these local policies must be followed. It is the responsibility of all nurses before handling these drugs that these safety instructions are known, understood and carried out. Generally, nurses should:

1 Preferably be fully trained in the preparation and administration of these drugs.
2 Restrict drug preparation to one designated area of the ward or unit only, to prevent dispersal of the drugs around the unit.
3 Wear gloves, as any drug getting on the skin will act on the epidermis and cause open sores which may be difficult to heal.
4 Wear eye and face protection, usually in the form of a transparent face mask. Drug sprayed or splashed into the eyes may cause

irreparable damage to the cornea with potential permanent loss or disturbance of vision. Again, the skin of the face is also at risk and drug damage may cause facial scarring.

5 Wear protective clothing, like a gown. This prevents drug contamination of uniforms or other clothes, and therefore prevents the potential spreading of these drugs to other patients or staff (LeMone and Burke 2004).

6 Special attention should be given to the safe disposal of wastes, such as syringes, which will have drug traces remaining in them.

7 Pregnant staff should avoid all contact with these drugs.

Nurses should also be aware that excreta, urine and faeces, from patients undergoing treatment with these drugs should again be managed with caution as the excreta is likely to contain waste products derived from the drugs.

Like any drug being administered, chemotherapy agents must be checked for accuracy of drug chosen, dosage, route and time of administration, and the patient's identity. Remember the golden rule of drug administration, the five *rights*:

1 Check the **right dose** (the dose prepared is checked against the prescription).

2 Check the **right drug** (the drug is checked against the prescription).

3 Check the **right patient** (the patient name is checked by asking them if possible and also by checking the name on the wrist band against the name on the prescription, being very aware of any two patients with the same name on the ward. Also check the patient number on the wrist band against the patient number on the prescription).

4 Check the **right time** (check the current time against the time of administration, as prescribed).

5 Check the **right route** (check the route chosen against the prescribed route).

Failure to apply the appropriate checks each time drugs are delivered to the patient could easily result in drug errors. Mistakes in any drug administration are often disastrous for all concerned, and in chemotherapy such errors can be fatal, mainly because they are powerful tissue-destroying agents and because they are often delivered intravenously, the fastest possible route. In addition, because these drugs damage tissues, it is necessary to prevent any extravasation during administration by the **intravenous (IV)** route. **Extravasation** means *outside the vein*, where fluid containing the drug is injected or leaks into the tissues surrounding the vein, instead of going into the blood. This can happen when the **intravenous infusion (IVI)** that is delivering the drug goes *subcut* (short for *subcutaneous*, which means 'under the skin'), i.e. the cannula that was in the vein has become displaced and is now out of the vein, delivering fluid to the tissues. Movement of the patient's arm can cause this, or it may sometimes be due to inappropriate positioning of the cannula during original siting of the IVI. Extravasation of fluids containing cytotoxic drugs will cause enormous damage to the tissues around the vein, including death of many cells (dead tissue is known as **necrosis**) and this damage will be difficult and lengthy to heal. It will cause further distress to the patient, not least because it is quite often preventable.

Oncogenic emergency

This is a rapid deterioration in the patient's condition due a catalogue of metabolic changes which happen as a result of aggressive treatment of large, rapidly growing cancers. Many chemical substances are released from dying tissues, and these result in a massive metabolic disturbance from which the body may not recover (Figure 12.5). The effects are dependent on the size of the tumour (the larger

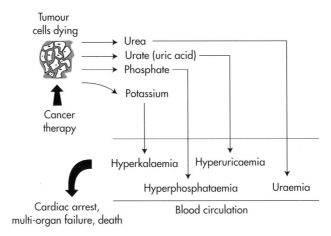

FIGURE 12.5 Oncogenic emergency (sometimes called cell lysis syndrome), is caused by the massive destruction of tumour cells by cancer treatment. The cells release a cocktail of chemicals that in circulation can be life threatening.

the tumour the greater the effect), the rate of cancer cell growth and turnover within the tumour (the faster the growth rate the greater the effect) and the response of the tumour to treatment. The consequences of oncogenic emergency can be life-threatening as the chemical changes may cause, amongst other things, acute renal failure. The effects of the metabolic changes typically occur about 24 to 48 hours after starting the treatment and comprise hyperuricaemia, hyperkalaemia and hypherphosphataemia.

Hyperuricaemia (high levels of blood **uric acid**) is caused by cell death and breakdown which releases the nucleic acids **DNA** (**deoxyribonucleic acid**) and **RNA** (**ribonucleic acid**). These are converted first to **hypoxanthine** and **xanthine**, then converted to uric acid. Normally, uric acid is excreted in the urine, and in hyperuricaemia the excess uric acid filtered from the blood may crystallise in the urinary tract and obstruct urine flow; a step towards renal failure.

Hyperkalaemia (excessive **potassium** $[K^+]$ levels in the blood) is caused by potassium coming from the dying and dead cells. About 98% of the K^+ in the body is stored inside cells, and will be liberated if the cell dies. Potassium is excreted via the kidneys, but this removal mechanism may be impaired if the kidneys are damaged or begin to fail (see hyperuricaemia above), allowing the blood level to rise. Excess potassium in the blood and extracellular fluid reduces cardiac function, slowing the heart rate (called **bradycardia**) and causing **heart block** (inability of the impulse within the heart to travel from the atria to the ventricles properly). The ultimate result could be **cardiac arrest**, when the heart stops beating.

Hyperphosphataemia (excessive phosphates in the blood) is caused by phosphates being released from dying cells. More than 99% of the body phosphates are inside the cells, and some malignant cells have higher than average phosphate levels. Large quantities are released from tumour cells when the drugs act to kill these cells. Increase in blood serum phosphates causes a corresponding loss of blood serum calcium, since the two substances have interrelated balances, and **calcium phosphate** molecules form. The resulting **hypocalcaemia** (low blood calcium) causes increased excitability of nerve tissue, **tetany** (severe muscle contractions linked to reduced calcium levels) and low conduction of impulses through the ventricles of the heart. The accumulation of calcium phosphate in the tissues precipitates the onset of organ failure, including the kidneys (Figure 12.5).

Radiotherapy

Radiotherapy is the use of radiation to kill cancer cells. Radiation was reviewed in Chapter 2 (see p. 53) as a potential cause of cancer, and this was because radiation damaged DNA causing mutations. But it is because of this DNA damaging quality that it can also be used to treat cancers. The damage is dose related, the higher the dose the more damage incurred, and therefore the less chance of the cell surviving. Short exposures to higher dosage can therefore be used to kill cancer cells, while the prolonged exposure to lower dosage can cause cancers.

Radiotherapy comes in several forms. The usual method is to deliver high-voltage X-rays (see p. 57), delivered by a machine known as a **linear accelerator** (Figure 12.6). As a guide to the dose to use consider a standard diagnostic X-ray procedure, say for a broken arm. This would use a power of around **50 kV** (**kV** is **kilovolts**) to generate, but therapeutic X-rays used in radiotherapy require voltages up to **30 MV** (**MV** is **megavolts**), that is perhaps 600 times greater power. The standard 50 kV X-ray has a relatively long wavelength (see p. 57), but an increase in the voltage causes shorter wavelengths which penetrate the body better. The very high voltages used in radiotherapy have great penetrating and cell killing power in order to reach and destroy the deep-seated solid tumours that standard X-rays could not even pass through.

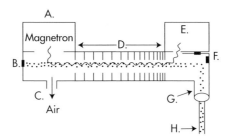

FIGURE 12.6 A diagrammatic view of a linear accelerator. Microwaves are produced by a magnetron (A) and these microwaves pick up electrons (B) at one end of a vacuum tube (air is pumped out, C). Baffles positioned along the tube (D) at decreasing intervals shorten the wavelength and therefore increase the energy. This energy is transferred to the electrons which reach very high speeds. At the other end of the tube the microwaves are removed (E) and the high-speed (high-energy) electrons are directed (F) onto a target (G) which then generates a high-energy beam of X-rays (H). The longer the tube (D) the higher the energy.

X-ray radiation is measured in the **rad** or the **gray** (**Gy**). The gray is the **Système International unit**, or **SI unit** for radiation, and the relationship between the gray and the rad is 1 Gy = 100 rad. This is a measure of the total absorbed dose by the tissues. The **centigray** (one hundreth of a gray) is often used since this is an equal term to the rad (1 centigray = 1 rad). A linear accelerator (Figure 12.6) works first by using a **magnetron** to produce microwaves. These microwaves are fed past a source of electrons and on into a vacuum tube called a **wave guide**. The microwaves now carry the electrons along, speeding them up to a point, in some cases, close to the speed of light. The tube is long, and this length is important to the power of the radiation beam produced, i.e. the longer the tube the greater the electron speeds and therefore the greater the power produced. As the electron-laden microwaves speed down the tube they encounter baffles with ever shorter distances between them. This has the effect of shortening the wavelength (remember: shorter wavelength = greater tissue penetrating power). At the end of the tube the microwaves are removed leaving a beam of extremely fast, high-energy electrons which hits a tungsten target, causing a very powerful X-ray beam emission. In modern machines this X-ray beam is very precise and can be aimed accurately at a tumour; it also produces very little harmful X-ray scatter, thus reducing the risk to the patients and staff. The ability to create a narrow accurate beam means that the lower-dose (and therefore potentially carcinogenic) outer rim of the beam (the **penumbra**) is reduced to a minimum.

Radiotherapy affects cells during their most vulnerable point of the cell cycle, mitosis, when DNA is exposed and being manipulated. Consequently, like chemotherapy, those cells passing round the cell cycle rapidly, and dividing at a fast rate, are most susceptible to this treatment (i.e. they are more often going through mitosis). Therefore, as in chemotherapy, cancer cells are particularly affected by this treatment, but also the normal cells noted earlier (see p. 322) that divide quickly: the skin, bone marrow and mucous membrane. Of these the skin, or more accurately the **epidermis** (see p. 16) is particularly vulnerable to the effects of radiation therapy. A linear accelerator source of radiation is external to the body, and any beam must first penetrate the epidermis in order to enter the tissues. The epidermis, therefore, is in a position to receive the full dose of the beam, with the dose falling off as the beam penetrates deeper (Figure 12.7). It is unfortunate that a rapidly dividing tissue (the epidermis) is going to receive the highest dose. Clearly this problem had to be addressed. One way was to spread the beam over a wide area of skin so each patch of skin received only a fraction of the total dose, whilst the tumour remained in target throughout treatment, and so received the maximum dose (Figure 12.7). Also, it became regular practice to break-up the total dose into separate daily doses, known as **fractionation**, spread over a period of about 10 or more days, maybe up to 25 days, per episode. Sometimes several episodes like this are planned, with breaks in between to allow normal tissue to recover.

If the skin does suffer the effects of the radiation this will become evident by the following early changes in the epidermis:

1 The skin becomes red (known as **erythema**).
2 Dry or moist **desquamation** (loss of epidermis by scaling) occurs.
3 Increased pigmentation.
4 Loss of sweat gland function.
5 **Epilation** (loss or removal of hairs by their roots).
6 Formation of tissue **oedema** (fluid collection in the tissues causing swelling).
7 The area affected will become very painful.

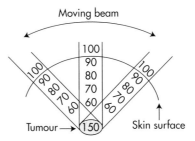

FIGURE 12.7 A diagrammatic representation of the principle behind radiation dosage. If this tumour needed a dose of 150, a single beam aimed at the tumour would deliver a dose much higher than 150 because the beam strength drops as it penetrates the tissues. The skin at the point where the beam enters would suffer from a very high radiation dose. To spread this dose, several beams are used at different angles (three are illustrated here), or a moving beam is focused on the tumour from above. Each single beam delivers a lower dosage so the skin suffers less, but the beams intersect at the tumour so their combined strength is focused on the tumour. In the illustration shown here, the three beams are each delivering a dose of 50 to the tumour, so the tumour gets 3 × 50 = 150, but the skin only gets 100 (the figures are arbitrary).

On a long-term basis the irradiated skin may also show the following developments:

8 Formation of fibrous tissue (called **fibrosis**).
9 Pigmentation loss (i.e. opposite to that seen in the early stages).
10 **Telangiectasis**, which are localised red spots made from dilated capillaries.
11 Loss of connective tissue from the dermis, with hair loss and even nail loss.

Nurses need to be very aware of the skin problems associated with radiotherapy, and manage their patients carefully. Instructions on skin management may be issued for patients individually and these must be observed. Generally the care of the affected skin area should include:

1 Washing without using soaps, creams, talc, deodorants or any similar substances.
2 Protection against injury, including rubbing, scratching or scrubbing, and protection against exposure to sunlight (which is additional radiation, see p. 57).
3 Keep the skin area at a moderate temperature (do not apply heat or cold).
4 Wear loose soft clothing over the area.
5 Eating a well balanced diet, for the nutrition needed for skin re-growth (see Chapter 11).

In addition to the skin, nurses must also be aware of the acute sensitivity of the **gonads** (the ovaries or testes) to radiation and ensure precautions are taken to protect the gonads on behalf of the patient. And of course, nurses themselves should also never be exposed to sources of radiation. Of the two, the testes are more sensitive because the rate of sperm replication far exceeds that of the ova. Exposure of the gonads to radiation causes the sperm count to drop significantly, inducing male infertility, and can cause artificial **menopause** in women.

Radiotherapy damages cells, in particular the DNA, to the point of cell death. Figure 12.8 shows the way radiotherapy separates the cancer from normal tissue. Before treatment there is a mix of normal with cancer tissue. Daily treatments of radiotherapy cause the cancer cells to decline in numbers quicker than the normal cells, because

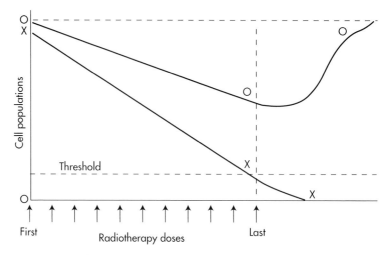

FIGURE 12.8 A diagrammatic representation of the separation of normal cells from cancer cells by radiotherapy. The arrows along the base line are the individual daily doses of radiation over the selected treatment period. At the start of treatment the cancer cells (X) and the normal cells (O) are mixed in the tissue. As a result of radiotherapy both populations of cells decline, but the cancer cells decline faster than the normal cells. The cancer cells reach threshold first, i.e. the point where the number and quality of the cells is so poor that survival is no longer possible. From here they go on to extinction. Because the normal cells have not reached threshold at this point

they reproduce faster and are therefore more vulnerable. Eventually the cancer cells reach a point where they are either all dead or damaged enough to die, and the tumour can no longer survive. But enough normal cells remain to regenerate and restore the tissue.

Hormonal treatment and immunotherapy

The sex hormones

The sex hormones are the **oestrogens** (female) and **androgens** (male). A full discussion of these hormones is given in Chapters 7 and 8 (see page 174) and in Silverthorn (2001). **Oestrodiol** is the most potent of the female hormones, and the most potent male hormone is **testosterone**. As seen in Chapters 7 and 8, these hormones often increase the rate of tumour development if the cancer cells have receptors that bind the hormone. Tumour cells with oestrogen receptors are said to be ER+ (i.e. oestrogen receptor positive), and they may also be positive for the female hormone **progesterone**

(**PgR+**) as well. Male cancer cells may be testosterone receptor positive (**TR+**), particularly those cancers associated with the reproductive tract. Treatment with hormone receptor antagonist drugs, or those drugs that reduce the amount of hormone produced, may cause some regression of the tumour. The mechanisms and drugs involved are discussed in Chapter 7 (see p. 189).

Immunotherapy

Immunotherapy (i.e. the concept of using the immune system to fight the cancer) has been under intense investigation for some time. However, progress is slow as the results of many experiments have not been encouraging. Immunotherapy involves using monoclonal antibodies, modified immune cells and cytokines, and the prospect of anti-cancer vaccines for the future.

Monoclonal antibodies

Monoclonal antibodies have been developed specifically against certain tumour cells. Work has been done with antibodies that: (1) activate NK cells after binding to the cancer cell; (2) have a toxin attached to them, and once the antibody has bound to the cancer cell surface the toxin kills the cell; or (3) have a radioactive substance attached to them, and once the antibody has bound to the cancer cell this substance kills the cell and others nearby.

The drugs currently available that contain monoclonal antibodies work by causing lysis of B-cell lymphocytes. These are **rituximab** and **alemtuzumab**. Rituximab causes lysis of B-cell lymphocytes and is used in chemotherapy-resistant advanced **lymphoma** (see p. 107). It is given by intravenous infusion. Careful monitoring of the patient's condition should be maintained during treatment with this drug, and full resuscitation facilities must be available.

Alemtuzumab also causes B-cell lymphocyte lysis and is used to treat **chronic lymphocytic leukaemia** (see p. 101). Both drugs can cause **cytokine release syndrome**, which appears as fever, flushing, chills, nausea, vomiting, pain in the area of the tumour and allergic reactions such as **bronchospasm** (a narrowing of the bronchus, part of the airway), **pruritis** (itching), **dyspnoea** (breathlessness) and **angioedema** (swelling of the lips, tongue and eyes, and may threaten to close the airway).

Modified immune cells

Attempts have been made to make the cancer cells more **immunogenic**, i.e. the cells would stimulate a greater immune response. This has been attempted by inserting genes that increase T-cell activation into tumour cells, or by making vaccines (see also p. 341) from modified versions of the patient's own cancer cells. In this case modified means the cell is rendered harmless and at the same time rendered more immunogenic. It is early days with this work and more will be heard of this approach in the future.

The cytokines

Various chemical agents called cytokines (see p. 84) have been employed to help reduce the tumour. **Interferons** (**IFN**) were discussed in Chapter 3. IFN can be given as anti-cancer treatment, particularly in **chronic myeloid leukaemia**, **melanoma** (16% of patients respond to IFN), **multiple myeloma** (20% of patients respond to IFN), and it has been shown to prolong life in **non-Hodgkin's lymphoma**. In **hairy cell leukaemia** (a CLL variant, see p. 101) up to 90% of patients have shown good responses to IFNα, giving long-term benefits for the patients. The interferons IFNβ and IFNγ have proved to be less useful in malignant disease than IFNα (IFNβ is licensed for use in the treatment of **multiple sclerosis**), and all the IFNs have little value in the treatment of solid tumours. IFNα, in combination with other anti-cancer drugs, has shown better responses to treatment and improved prognosis. IFNα has been given by various routes. The intravenous (IV) route gives a peak serum level in 30 minutes with rapid renal clearance within 6 hours. The intramuscular (IM) route gives a peak serum level in 2 to 6 hours and is eliminated within 36 hours. Antibodies can be formed against the interferon anything from 8 weeks to 7 months after administration, and this reduces its effects. Toxic symptoms can occur, notably **fatigue** and a **flu-like syndrome**, e.g. fever, then chills, **tachycardia** (fast pulse rate), **malaise**, **myalgia** (muscle ache) and headaches. IFN can also cause **ocular** (visual) effects and depression. All these problems are dose related. The drugs containing IFNα are **Intron A**, **Referon-A** and **Viraferon**.

Interleukins (**Il**) are also cell-signalling agents between lymphocytes (see also Chapter 3, p. 84). They bind to their own specific receptors and stimulate activity in TC, NK and LAK cells (see p. 78). Table 3.2 (Chapter 3, p. 85) gives the functions of the main interleukins. **Aldesleukin** is Il-2 produced artificially in the *E. coli* organism. Its use is primarily in the treatment of **renal cell carcinoma (RCC)** (see p. 165). About 14% of patients respond to the treatment, 5% completely and 9% partially. It is given by subcutaneous injection, and side effects at low dose include fever, chills, nausea, skin desquamation (see p. 336) and inflammation at the injection site. In high doses the side effects also include **dyspnoea** (breathlessness), **malaise**, diarrhoea, **hypotension** (low blood pressure), **oliguria** (poor urine output), weight gain and **cardiac arrhythmias** (abnormal heart rhythms). The combination of Il-2 with IFNα has shown great promise as a treatment in cancer since both have anti-cancer properties and they work well together. Il-2 combined with cytotoxic therapy, and also combined with artificially produced NK cells are also treatments being explored, so far with mixed results.

Interleukin-1 RA (Il-1 RA) is a substance that binds to the same receptors as Il-1α and Il-1β. It has biological activity on this receptor and serves as a receptor antagonist, keeping Il-1α and Il-1β off the receptor. Since naturally produced Il-1α and Il-1β can cause side effects such as fever, rigors, hypotension, nausea, headaches and inflammation, it may prove useful to give Il-1 RA as a means of blocking these unwanted effects.

Cancer vaccines

The principle behind all vaccines is the ability to introduce a small quantity of an antigen into the body in order to stimulate the immune system, the defence mechanism of the body (see p. 66). This boost to the immune system provides additional cells and antibodies to attack the antigen. Vaccines have been highly successful against foreign organisms, viruses particularly but also bacteria, and now research is well underway to extend this to cancer cells. Vaccines that protect against infections are **prophylactic** (or preventative) in nature, whilst most cancer vaccines act as another arm to treatment in people who already have cancer.

Some cancer vaccines are currently passing into phase III trials, where they can be tested on patients with early stages of cancer. The phase II trials were very successful, with late-stage cancer patients living for years after a course of vaccinations, and this suggests that vaccines will become a useful means of cancer treatment for the future (Anon. 2004). There are three main types of cancer vaccines on trial.

Dendritic cell vaccines, where dendritic cells are immune cells, i.e. white blood cells (WBCs, see p. 94), that warn other immune cells to attack antigens. In the vaccine these cells carry tumour antigens, thus prompting other cells to attack similar antigens on malignant cells.

Heat shock protein vaccines use certain tumour antigens called **heat shock proteins** (**HSP**) to produce a vaccine which is injected after removal of the tumour, in order to boost immunity against any remaining malignant cells. HSP are also known as **stress proteins** and are found within all cells if subjected to stress. But in tumour cells they appear as cell surface antigens, and exposed on the membrane surface they can trigger an immune response. The vaccine boosts this immune response in a similar way.

Viral vector vaccines involve a virus that is normally harmless to humans, and this virus is processed to carry a cancer antigen into the body and thus boost immunity. Hiding a cancer protein in a virus is the reason these vaccines are known as '**Trojan horse**' vaccines, after the wooden horse trick said to be played on the city of Troy during the Trojan wars.

Examples of current vaccines in trial are those for colon cancer (a viral vector type); prostate cancer and melanoma (both are dendritic cell vaccines), and pancreatic and kidney cancers (both HSP vaccines). The search is on for a generic vaccine, i.e. one that will work for all cancers. Such a vaccine is likely to target the enzyme **telomerase**, a component of cancer cells, since it is generic to virtually all cancer cells. Telomerase lengthens the end portion of a chromosome known as the **telomere**, which in normal cells progressively shortens with each cell cycle, until it is so short that it triggers cell death (apoptosis) in that cell. Cancer cells can prolong the cell life by using telomerase to lengthen the telomere, and therefore significantly delay apoptosis. Research is moving fast and vaccines will be in regular use clinically in a few years.

Adjunct therapy

Apart from the main treatments of surgery, drugs and radiation, patients may choose to follow various other courses of additional (**adjunct**) therapies. These are mostly introduced into the treatment regime by the patient themselves according to their own wishes and desires. In choosing a total treatment package the wishes and desires of the patient must never be overlooked. Such special adjunct therapies such as herbal medication, acupuncture and aromatherapy may not be a cure for cancer, but can provide some symptom relief, help to overcome stress and to ease pain. They give psychological comfort to the patient. If such therapies are considered by a patient, they should first be discussed with the medical staff to check to see if anything the patient wants to use contradicts their regular treatment (e.g. some herbs may interact with the drug treatment). If the proposed additional therapy is approved then the nurse can assist the patient with this. Massage is a simple therapy that provides comfort and perhaps pain relief, and is unlikely to interfere with the patient's main treatment regime.

Prevention of cancer

The treatment of cancer has made great advances over the last fifty years or so, backed up by a strenuous research campaign which is destined to continue. New developments like cancer vaccines give us hope that one day this particular collection of diseases can be overcome. But there is a catch. Progress will always be slow until the root causes of cancer are tackled in a meaningful way. Prevention is better than cure? Yes, but not in the case of cancer it seems. The human race is struggling to find the cure, but not doing anywhere near enough towards prevention. So cancer will continue until there is both the political and individual will to stop the menace of smoking (which is increasing in women and young people), to stop introducing technologies like mobile phones that expose users to more radiation, and to tackle the problem of air pollution (from car exhausts especially), particularly in the cities where most people live and work. Improvements that would help in the prevention of cancer would be to:

1 Ban smoking from all indoor public places like restaurants, pubs, terminal train stations, and so on, and consider ways to make smoking much harder for young people to start.
2 Ban all advertising of any tobacco product anywhere and give greater resources to anti-smoking measures.
3 Make all major shopping areas in the city centres, like Oxford Street in London, for pedestrians only.
4 Double the effort and resources needed to make electric cars a reality, and introduce them gradually to replace the internal combustion engine.
5 Convert all bus routes back to electric tram routes.

6 Give serious consideration to finding a solution to the growing menace of pollution by the aviation industry.

7 Introduce legislation that stops the expansion of new technology before the consequences to health have been fully explored.

The real answer to cancer rests in society itself, not in the laboratory or the hospital. The fight against cancer must be with a double-edged sword, one edge is research and the other is prevention. It is this second edge to our sword, prevention, which is seriously lacking at the moment.

Key points

Palliative care and surgery

- Palliative treatment is where the emphasis is on relief of the symptoms to improve the quality of the patient's life, but the tumour remains.
- Surgery is a life-saving vital first step in many cancer treatment regimes, and the success of other subsequent treatments will often depend on it.

Chemotherapy

- The drugs used in the treatment of cancer (i.e. chemotherapy) prevent cell division. The cells mostly affected by the drugs are those with faster rates of cell division.
- The main groups of chemotherapy drugs are the alkylating agents, the platinum compounds, the topoisomerase I and II inhibitors, the cytotoxic antibiotics, the antimetabolites and the drugs that disrupt microtubule function.
- The side effects of cytotoxic therapy are very unpleasant. They are distressing nausea and vomiting with anorexia (loss of appetite) and fluid intolerance, bone marrow suppression causing anaemia and low white blood cells in circulation, alopecia (hair loss), teratogenesis (the drugs cross the placenta during pregnancy and affect the foetus) and hyperuricaemia (high levels of uric acid in the blood).
- It is the responsibility of all nurses before handling cytotoxic drugs that the safety instructions are known, understood and carried out.

- Like all drugs being administered, chemotherapy agents must be checked for accuracy of drug chosen, dosage, route and time of administration, and the patient's identity.
- Oncogenic emergency is a rapid deterioration in the patient's condition due to a massive release of metabolic substances from dying cells as a result of aggressive treatment of large, rapidly growing cancers.

Radiotherapy

- Radiotherapy comes in several forms. The usual method is to deliver high-voltage X-rays from a linear accelerator.
- The skin suffers the effects of the radiotherapy because the epidermis has rapidly dividing cells. Such effects will become evident by the skin becoming red (erythema), dry or moist desquamation (loss of epidermis), increased pigmentation, loss of sweat gland function, epilation (loss or removal of hairs by their roots), formation of tissue oedema (fluid in the tissues causing swelling) and the area affected will become very painful.

Hormones

- Oestrodiol is the most potent of the female hormones, and the most potent male hormone is testosterone. These hormones often increase the rate of tumour development if the cancer cells have receptors that bind the hormone.

Other treatments

- Monoclonial antibodies in drug form are rituximab and alemtuzumab. They causes lysis of B-cell lymphocytes.
- Interferons (IFN) can be given as anti-cancer treatment, particularly in chronic myeloid leukaemia, melanoma, multiple myeloma, non-Hodgkin's lymphoma and hairy cell leukaemia.
- Aldesleukin is Il-2 and is used in the treatment of renal cell carcinoma.
- There are three main types of cancer vaccines: dendritic cell vaccines, heat shock protein vaccines and viral vector vaccines (also known as 'Trojan horse' vaccines).

References

Anonymous (2004) Cancer vaccines – on the verge of victory, *in* Bredenburg J. (ed.) *Medical Breakthroughs 2004*, The Reader's Digest Association, London.

LeMone P. and Burke K. (2004) *Medical-Surgical Nursing, Critical Thinking in Client Care*, Pearson Education International, Prentice Hall, New Jersey.

Silverthorn D. U. (2001) *Human Physiology, an Integrated Approach* (2nd edn), Prentice Hall, New Jersey.

Souhami R. and Tobias J. (2003) *Cancer and its Management*, (4th edn), Blackwell Science, Oxford.

Waller D. G., Renwick A. G. and Hillier K. (2001) *Medical Pharmacology and Therapeutics*, W. B. Saunders, Edinburgh.

Index